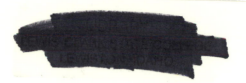

More praise for *Global Health Watch 5*

'*Global Health Watch* again meets our expectations for a critical analysis of the two great challenges of our time: the ecological crisis, and continuing economic disparities. It holds us accountable, and moves us toward an alternate vision.' **Vic Neufeld, Special Advisor, Canadian Coalition for Global Health Research**

'This encyclopaedic work offers a thorough discussion of the state of human health worldwide, a deep analysis of the social causes of persistent health deficits, and constructive ideas for reform. An indispensable second opinion to government propaganda.' **Thomas Pogge, Yale University**

Praise for the *Global Health Watch* series

'Provides us with compelling evidence about all that is wrong with the governance of health care systems across the world. At the same time it also provides us with hope, in the many stories about what can be done and what is being done.' **Halfdan Mahler, former Director-General of the World Health Organization**

'An incisive socio-political critique of contemporary global health issues.' **K. Srinath Reddy, President, Public Health Foundation of India**

'Reading *Global Health Watch* is a necessary step in understanding how challenging and urgent change is, but that it is increasingly necessary for the survival of our planet Earth.' **Eduardo Espinoza, Vice Minister for Health of El Salvador**

'*Global Health Watch* confirms the failure of the UN, capitalism and liberal democracy. It also convinces us that we shall need a radically new manner of thinking if mankind is to survive.' **Suwit Wibulpolprasert, former Senior Adviser on Disease Control, Ministry of Public Health, Thailand**

'Challenges us to look at health and health care from a critical perspective. Essential reading for the movers and shakers in health policy the world over.' **Gill Walt, London School of Hygiene and Tropical Medicine**

The Global Health Watch is a broad collaboration of public health experts, non-governmental organizations, civil society activists, community groups, health workers and academics. It was initiated by the People's Health Movement, Global Equity Gauge Alliance and Medact as a platform of resistance to neoliberal dominance in health.

GLOBAL HEALTH WATCH 5

AN ALTERNATIVE WORLD HEALTH REPORT

People's Health Movement

Medact

Third World Network

Health Poverty Action

Medico International

ALAMES

ZED

Global Health Watch 5: An Alternative World Health Report was first published in 2017 by Zed Books Ltd, The Foundry, 17 Oval Way, London SE11 5RR, UK.

www.zedbooks.net

Typeset in Plantin by seagulls.net
Index by John Barker
Cover design by Emma J. Hardy
Cover photo © Brian Sokol/Panos

A catalogue record for this book is available from the British Library

ISBN 978-1-78699-224-6 hb
ISBN 978-1-78699-223-9 pb
ISBN 978-1-78699-225-3 pdf
ISBN 978-1-78699-226-0 epub
ISBN 978-1-78699-227-7 mobi

MIX
Paper from responsible sources
FSC® C020471

Printed and bound in Great Britain by CPI Group (UK) Ltd, Croydon CR0 4YY

CONTENTS

LIST OF ABBREVIATIONS

ACCHOs	Aboriginal Community Controlled Health Organizations
ACT UP	AIDS Coalition to Unleash Power
AMR	antimicrobial resistance
ANC	African National Congress
APLHWA	All Pakistan Lady Health Workers Association
ARV	antiretroviral
ASHAs	Accredited Social Health Activists
AU	African Union
BCG	Boston Consulting Group
BMGF	Bill & Melinda Gates Foundation
BoD	Burden of Disease
CBD	Convention on Biological Diversity
CCWs	community care workers
CDC	Centre for Disease Control
CEPI	Coalition for Epidemic Preparedness Innovation
CFCs	chlorofluorocarbons
CHWs	community health workers
CMS	Centers for Medicare and Medicaid Services
COSATU	Congress of South African Trade Unions
CSR	corporate social responsibility
DAH	development assistance for health
DfiD	Department for International Development
DoH	Department of Health
DUHS	Duke University Health System
ECOWAS	Community of West African States
EIAs	environmental impact assessments
EIs	extractive industries
EITI	Extractive Industries Transparency Initiative
EPA	(US) Environmental Protection Agency
ERLs	Essential Regulatory Laboratories
ESA	East and Southern Africa
ESCR	(International Covenant on) Economic, Social and Cultural Rights
ESPs/SAPs	Economic Stabilization Programmes and Structural Adjustment Programmes
EU	European Union

FCHV	Female Community Health Volunteer
FENSA	Framework for Engagement with Non-State Actors
FIND	Foundation for Innovative New Diagnostics
FMLN	FrenteFarabundo Marti para la Liberacion Nacional
FNIH	Foundation for the National Institute for Health
FNS	Foro National para la Salud
FTAs	free trade agreements
FTT	financial transaction tax
GATT	General Agreement on Tariffs and Trade
GAVI	Global Alliance for Vaccines and Immunization
GDP	Gross Domestic Product
GEAR	Growth, Employment and Redistribution
GFATM	Global Fund to Fight Aids, Tuberculosis and Malaria
GHIs	global health initiatives
GISN	Global Influenza Surveillance Network
GISRS	Global Influenza Surveillance and Response System
GNI	gross national income
GOBI	growth monitoring, oral rehydration, breast feeding and immunization
GSD	genetic sequence data
H5RL	H5 Reference Laboratories
HDI	Human Development Index
HiAP	Health in All Policies
HICs	high-income countries
HRH	human resources for health
HSS	health systems strengthening
IADB	Inter-American Development Bank
ICESR	International Covenant on Economic, Social and Cultural Rights
ICPD	International Conference on Population and Development
ICSID	International Centre for Settlement of Investment Disputes
IDs	identity documents
IFC	International Finance Corporation
IHR	International Health Regulations
ILO	International labour Organization
IMF	International Monetary Fund
INCB	International Narcotic Control Board
IPCC	Intergovernmental Panel on Climate Change
ISDS	investor-state dispute settlement
ISSS	InstitutoSalvadoreno de Seguridad Social
IVPP	influenza viruses of pandemic potential
IVTM	Influenza Virus Tracking Mechanism
KEI	Knowledge Ecology International

LDCs	least developed countries
LFAs	local fund agents
LMICs	low- and middle-income countries
MDGs	Millennium Development Goals
MERS	Middle East respiratory syndrome
MIC	medical–industrial complex
MINSAL	Ministry of Health of El Salvador
MNEs	multinational enterprises
MoH	Ministry of Health
MoHFW	Ministry of Health and Family Welfare
MSH	Management Sciences for Health
NACLA	North American Congress on Latin America
NAFTA	North American Free Trade Agreement
NCDs	non-communicable diseases
NDPS	Narcotic Drugs and Psychotropic Substances
NGOs	non-governmental organizations
NHI	National Health Insurance
NHS	National Health System
NHSC	National Health Services Commission
NIH	National Institutes of Health
NPM	new public management
NRHM	National Rural Health Mission
NSAs	non-state actors
ODI	Overseas Development Institute
OECD	Organization for Economic Cooperation and Development
OHS	occupational health and safety
PAC	Policy Advisory Center
PEPFAR	President's Emergency Plan for AIDS Relief
PHEIC	Public Health Emergency of International Concern
PIP	Pandemic Influenza Preparedness
PMA	Pharmaceutical Manufacturers Association
PMTCT	prevention of mother-to-child transmission
PPPs	public–private partnerships
R&D	research and development
RCT	randomized controlled trial
RDP	Reconstruction and Development Programme
REACH	Registration, Evaluation, Authorization and Restriction of Chemicals
RPHC	Re-engineering of Primary Health Care
SADC	Southern African Development Community
SAPs	Structural Adjustment Programmes
SDGs	Sustainable Development Goals
SDH	social determinants of health

SDT	special and differential treatment
SGP	Stability and Growth Pact
SMEs	Small and Medium Enterprises
SMTAs	Standard Material Transfer Agreements
STIs	sexually transmitted infections
SUN	Scaling up Nutrition
TAC	Treatment Action Campaign
TNCs	transnational corporations
TPP	Trans–Pacific Partnership
TRIPS	Trade-Related Aspects of Intellectual Property Rights
UHC	universal health coverage
UNCTAD	United Nations Conference on Trade and Development
UNDP	United Nations Development Programme
UNECA	UN Economic Commission for Africa
UNFPA	United Nations Population Fund (formerly the United Nations Fund for Population Activities)
UNICEF	United Nations International Children's Emergency Fund
UNMEER	UN Mission for Ebola Emergency Response
USAID	United States Agency for International Development
VA	Veterans' Administration
VCS	voluntary specified contributions
WHA	World Health Assembly
WHO	World Health Organization
WHO CC	WHO Collaborating Centres
WTO	World Trade Organization

BOXES, TABLES AND FIGURES

Boxes

ACKNOWLEDGEMENTS

A unique feature of all volumes of the *Global Health Watch* is the wide canvas of analysis and proposals that are featured in its contents. This has been possible through contributions received from a number of academics, scholars and activists. The contents of *Global Health Watch 5*, as for the previous volumes, have been collectively developed. While all those who have contributed to the contents are listed at the end of the volume, it gives us great pleasure to acknowledge all contributors and to express our special gratitude to all of them for having worked on their contributions without any honorarium, a spirit of volunteerism that we value immensely. Individual contributors have been involved in writing specific sections of the *Watch* and the overall views expressed in the volume are the collective responsibility of the editorial group.

We wish to thank our funding partners – Open Society Foundations and Medico International – for the generous support provided. The views in the *Watch* are not necessarily those of our funding partners.

The production of the *Watch* is supported by a coordinating group of six civil society organizations – People's Health Movement, Asociación Latinoamericana de Medicina Social (ALAMES), Third World Network, Medact, Health Poverty Action and Medico International. We would like to thank those involved, from all these organizations, in producing the *Watch*. Specifically, we would like to acknowledge the contributions of Rafael Gonzalez Guzman (ALAMES), K. M. Gopakumar (Third World Network), Natalie Sharples (Health Poverty Action), Andreas Wulf (Medico International), David McCoy (Medact) and Gargeya Telakapalli, Anneleen de Keukelaere, Bridget Lloyd and Hani Serag (People's Health Movement). We also wish to acknowledge Mala Ramamoorthy for her painstaking efforts in copy editing the first drafts of the contributions and Rodrigo Millán for his translation of the Spanish contributions.

It has been a pleasure to work with the team at Zed Books associated with the production of the *Watch*. Specifically, we would like to thank Kim Walker, Amy Jordan, Dominic Fagan and Ruben Mootoosamy for their patience, understanding and support.

Amit Sengupta

On behalf of the *Global Health Watch 5* editorial group: Anne-Emanuelle Birn, Chiara Bodini, David Legge, David McCoy, David Sanders, N. B. Sarojini, Pol de Vos and Amit Sengupta

INTRODUCTION

The fifth edition of the *Global Health Watch*, similar to the previous editions, provides an alternate discourse on health. The Global Health Watch was conceived in 2003 as a collaborative effort of activists and academics from across the world. *Global Health Watch 5* has been coordinated by six civil society organizations – the People's Health Movement, Asociación Latinoamericana de Medicina Social (ALAMES), Health Poverty Action, Medico International, Third World Network and Medact. *Global Health Watch 5*, like the preceding volumes published in 2005, 2008, 2011 and 2014, provides policy analysis, debates technical issues and provides perspectives on current global processes that shape people's health in different parts of the world.

The Watch provides information and analysis embedded in a vision of the world and of human society that is more just, more equal and more humane. As in the case of the previous editions, the contents of *Global Health Watch 5* are divided into five interlinked sections. The section on the 'The global political and economic architecture' draws causal links between decisions and choices that impact on health and the current structure of global power relations and global governance. The section 'Health systems: current issues and debates' looks at contemporary debates on health systems in different parts of the world, to draw appropriate lessons and propose concrete actions. The third section, 'Beyond healthcare', examines multiple social and structural determinants of health. The section on 'Watching' critically analyses global processes and institutions which have a significant impact on global health. The final section foregrounds stories of action and resistance, from different regions of the world.

While the book covers a very large canvas, this edition has a particular focus on two areas: the recently announced Sustainable Development Goals; and the rapid transition in global governance for health from a nation-driven process to one that promotes the influence of private foundations, consultancy firms and corporations.

The global political and economic architecture

The section on political and economic architecture speaks to the urgent need for a new global economic and social policy platform. It asks the question: Can the new Sustainable Development Goals (SDGs) offer help in creating such a platform?

The broad struggle surrounding the SDGs is about constraining the predatory nature of capitalism. The headline intent of the SDGs appears to oppose the premises of global capitalism. However critics argue that the SDGs represent a fundamental contradiction. They propose growth strategies that seek to perpetuate the current neoliberal model – ever-increasing levels of extraction, production and consumption. It is precisely this model of growth that has perpetuated poverty, destroyed the planet and is threatening the basis of our existence. It is clear that a change in this paradigm will not occur by itself, and definitely not by a mechanical application of the SDGs. Real change can only result from the clash of opposing forces, in which the Watch clearly positions itself on the side of 'well-being for all' and a healthy planet, and against profit for a few.

Latin America's experience of the past decade in pushing for change that represented a departure from the neoliberal discourse on politics and economics in general, and on healthcare services in particular, is critically examined in this section. While impressive progress was made in expansion of public services to provide universal access, progressive movements and governments that emerged in the region were unable to complete the task of dismantling the power of the previous neoliberal regimes. An ideological counter-offensive is underway in the region that promotes the idea that the public health system is 'poor healthcare for the poor'. The recent changes in Latin American countries are not isolated examples. In many European countries public health systems are being dismantled while resistance mounts from peoples' and workers' organizations. It is imperative that just as the neoliberal project seeks to globalize its policies, progressive forces must find a way to globalize their struggles and demands.

The final chapter in the section focuses on migration, especially in the context of the acute humanitarian crisis associated with flows of forced migration. Over the past four decades, globalization and neoliberal economic policies have become one of the most significant forces fuelling migration. Migrants face a triple burden of victimization. First, they suffer the consequences of a model of development that dislocates them and drastically reduces their options, while resulting in ecological mayhem that further disrupts their connection to the land. Second, they face isolation and detention imposed on them by those who benefit, at least in the short term, from that same model of development. And finally, they are victimized due to misconceptions, biases and hypocrisy that distort the largely technocratic and bureaucratized debate on global human displacement.

Health systems: current issues and debates

The struggle for health is closely linked to demands for functioning health systems. The first chapter in the section on health systems notes that universal health coverage (UHC) is the *slogan de jour* in global health systems policy but its meaning is highly contested. At one pole are those who use the term simply to refer to financial protection. The other view recognizes the need to advance tax-based funding, single payer systems, capped programme funding and effective clinical governance. The differences in emphasis between the primary healthcare (PHC) and UHC approaches are significant. The former involves a focus on building and supporting the primary healthcare sector and envisages a prominent role for community health workers and community involvement in planning, accountability and prevention. By contrast, the UHC discourse starts with a focus on financial protection and essentially argues for care that is 'purchased' from a range of private and public providers. This has legitimized the dismantling of public services in many parts of the world and the increased participation of private providers in the delivery of healthcare.

While efforts to promote UHC are largely concerned with ensuring the acceptability of health services, community control has the more ambitious goal of providing space for community power to control healthcare, to increase the community's control over its own health and to improve the responsiveness of the health service to the local community. A number of health services in Australia have been transferred from state government management to community control, providing an opportunity to examine what benefits community control may bring. Experiences related to these indicate that involving citizens in the management of health services is likely to make them strong advocates for non-commercialized healthcare and provide a counter voice to the powerful corporate voices baying for more chances for profit. For indigenous peoples, it also provides greater self-determination and control over health and healthcare, and more culturally respectful services that take into account holistic, indigenous conceptions of health and healing.

The concept of a 'Medical-Industrial Complex' (MIC) was proposed more than four decades back in the United States to depict the functioning of its health system. The chapter 'Healthcare in the USA: Understanding the Medical-Industrial Complex' analyses how, in the USA, the essential problem with the health system is the commodification of health and the idea that health is an economic good. The US experience shows that, despite all claims to the contrary, healthcare does not make a good commodity and 'marketplace solutions' have been a failure

The chapter on South Africa follows the development of civil society activism in South Africa on one hand and, on the other, the trail of broken promises that underpin the story of healthcare services in the country. The AIDS 'denialism' of the Mbeki era sparked the re-awakening of social movements in health with the launch of the Treatment Action Campaign (TAC). The central role that the TAC played in mobilising people and influencing policy showed how citizen action can bring about change from below. The rise and success of the TAC campaign occurred in a period when influential external donors started funding HIV/AIDS activities undertaken by non-governmental organizations (NGOs), which have come to dominate the health civil society. This NGO-ization of health civil society is not confined to South Africa and reflects the changed nature of donor funding under neoliberalism, characterized by the directing of substantial funding through private and non-government recipients in a climate of cuts in public spending by the state under austerity.

Conservative economists often berate low and middle-income countries (LMICs) for their failure to pursue neoliberal reforms while restructuring healthcare services. The failures are sought to be explained as being caused by inefficient and corrupt financial and administrative systems in these countries. However evidence indicates that neoliberal reforms in restructuring healthcare services, such as through Public Private Partnerships (PPPs), are inherently flawed and represent a transfer of public resources to the private sector and do not lead to any increased efficiencies. This is illustrated in the chapter on the 'new' Karolinska hospital in Stockholm.

Over the last decades, issues related to migration have emerged as a fundamental and defining factor in European societies. The chapter on migrants' health in the EU discusses how there has been an increase in the number of countries in the EU who deny basic healthcare to migrants. Undocumented migrants are often blamed to divert attention from unpopular social sector cutbacks. Even in countries where the law allows access to healthcare for undocumented migrants, actual implementation is flawed and migrants continue to face exclusion from the healthcare system.

There is a perceptible trend towards use of non-standard forms of employment in public services in general and in the health sector in particular. The chapter on 'informalization of employment' presents evidence that the remuneration of health workers has decreased in relation to total health expenditure globally. Women are among the worst impacted -- while the global health workforce is predominantly female in many countries, women are concentrated in lower skilled jobs, with less pay and stay at the bottom of professional hierarchies. Of particular concern is the plight of community health workers, who make a major contribution to health outcomes of rural and poor communities in South Asia. Recently, CHWs have successfully organized themselves and are finding avenues to improve their conditions of work.

Beyond healthcare

Despite a broad consensus and a shared understanding that climate change requires concerted global action, the global response has been timid and late in coming. The chapter on climate change reviews the underlying forces within the broader crisis of environmental degradation, and the consequent effects on human health and health inequities. Although manifesting distinctly in different locales, environmental degradation and its health consequences are interrelated across the world, transcending place and ultimately affecting everyone. Addressing the myriad environmental challenges and their interconnected health effects is complex and difficult, and will require broad cooperation, creative ideas and intense political struggle. Unfortunately, the present reality is one of substantial political recalcitrance to transformative change by some of the largest polluters.

Historically, women's ability to make choices and exercise autonomy in matters of sexuality and reproduction have been conditioned and constrained by economic and political structures, based on a model that prescribes 'normative' behaviour and abhors 'deviant' behaviour. The chapter titled 'Gendered Approach to Reproductive and Sexual Health and Rights' through a discussion on the struggles of sex workers and transgender communities, and of women demanding abortion rights, argues for an alternate public health discourse that advances a more nuanced approach to sexual and reproductive health rights. A separate chapter on sexual and reproductive health rights in Chile depicts how, even in relatively high income countries, women's sexual and reproductive health rights are frequently ignored. Governments must not only commit to promoting women's health concerns but must simultaneously address the deeply embedded gendered norms within society and in healthcare systems.

Trade agreements have seldom been analysed in terms of their impact on the health of workers. The chapter 'Trade Agreements and Health of Workers ' looks at the possible risks that free trade agreements (FTAs) pose to the health of workers. Changing power relations have shaped the global trade framework in the last few decades, and trade agreements impact on various aspects of health, such as government revenue (for funding social services), nutrition, and access to medicines and healthcare services. Importantly, trade agreements impact employment and working conditions, and the health of workers.

Countries rich in mineral resources also experience high levels of inequality and poverty—a situation often referred to as 'the resource curse'. The chapter on the extractive sector argues that while extraction and export of unprocessed raw materials may lead to rapid growth, this is often unsustainable and not accompanied by higher value-added processing activities in African countries. Of particular concern is the impact of the extractive sector on the health of workers in the sector and of communities living in the vicinity of extractive activities.

A growing recognition of the failure of the war on drugs and a move towards adopting a public health approach are gathering pace around the world. The chapter on this issue argues that the debate is often polarized between two extremes – prohibition on the one hand and free market legalization on the other – and neither of these simplistic positions provides a viable solution to what is a complex public health problem.

Watching

Underpinning the deficiencies in the World Health Organization (WHO) is its deep funding crisis, which constrains its ability to carry out its normative activities. The chapter on the WHO's funding crisis discusses how the WHO, similar to many UN agencies today, faces challenges to its norm-setting activities, given its growing dependence on private donors and funding that is tied to specific programmes. This has implications for WHO's account-ability to member states, and represents a serious erosion of the principles of democratic governance of the organization. With the shift to operational and implementation control by donors and their various 'stakeholder' partners, rights-based approaches and the governing role of member states in the public interest are being undermined, often intentionally.

In recent years, substantial attention has been focused on the growing influence of philanthropic foundations in global development and the risks and side-effects of this trend. The chapter on private philanthropic founda-tions argues that actions of philanthropic foundations are aimed at preserving rather than redistributing wealth, and are a way for elites to pursue and legitimate their actions. International organizations, individual governments and civil society organizations need to weigh the cost of engagement with such foundations against the role they play in undermining the accountability of public institutions.

While many global health actors have been critically examined, the role of management consulting firms, which can be linked to all significant global health institutions over the past decade and to critical junctures in countries in crises, has remained by and large hidden from the public eye. The activi-ties of these firms are examined in a chapter that concludes that there is no evidence that the ascent of consulting firms in the health sector has led to approaches and solutions to radically improve health outcomes for the poor and most marginalized. The framing of health as a technical exercise and the related focus on 'value for money', 'efficiency gains' and rapid results has led to the exclusion of those most in need, the sidelining of systemic long-term solutions and the downgrading of community voices.

Global public private partnerships (PPPs) have emerged as the new medium of global governance, replacing over time the nation-state driven governance system which was embodied in the UN system. The examination of arguably the two largest PPPs in the health sector, the Global Alliance for Vaccines and Immunization (GAVI) and the Global Fund to Fight AIDS, Tuberculosis and Malaria (GFATM) suggests that the unfettered power of both PPPs represent a threat to the hitherto nation-state driven system of global governance for health. They clearly represent instances of private sector influence on activi-ties which are public funded and essentially take place in the public sphere.

Nearly all developing countries have signed bilateral investment treaties (BITs) with developed countries. Increasingly, free trade agreements (FTAs) also feature investment protection chapters. The discussion on investments treaties shows how they affect social, environmental and health policies of sovereign governments. National polices that promote public interest are now being challenged by foreign investors on the plea that they put their invest-ments at risk. These challenges involve the Investor-State Dispute Settlement

(ISDS) mechanisms that are embedded in trade and investment treaties. ISDS mechanisms often place an onerous burden on countries as they are conducted outside the nation's own legal systems, in international courts of arbitration.

In the last couple of decades, political actors' perceptions of what constitutes a threat to international security has broadened – the subject of a chapter titled 'Framing of Health as a Security Issue'. The 'health security' discourse was extensively articulated in the aftermath of the Ebola epidemic in West Africa. This is symptomatic of how health issues, particularly those related to infectious diseases, have increasingly been presented as security threats. The 'securitization' of health encourages feelings of selfishness and fear rather than compassion. It can result in the misallocation of scarce resources in a manner that undermines efforts to secure access to healthcare and improve the social determinants of health.

Data, information and knowledge are core resources for policy, practice and activism in relation to healthcare and population health. However, as a chapter on this issue proposes, they are not simple representations of an objective reality but are produced in social practice and bear the imprint of power. This chapter calls for the need to develop a more nuanced understanding regarding the politics of data, information and knowledge.

In 2011 the members of the WHO adopted a Pandemic Influenza Preparedness Framework (PIP Framework), linking access to pathogens to fair and equitable sharing of benefits arising from their use. The chapter, analysing the framework, argues for extending similar mechanisms to other areas that involve the sharing of biological materials by countries with manufacturers of medicines and vaccines.

Campaigns on Community Led Total Sanitation (CLTS) are being extensively promoted in a range of resource poor settings. An integral part of these campaigns is the 'naming and shaming' of errant individuals and households. Practitioners of CLTS claim that the 'shame' comes from self-critique and not from externally imposed humiliation. The chapter on this subject, drawing on case studies from India, however, suggest that in practice CLTS programmes in many countries appear to thrive on coercive practices that often lead to gross violation of the rights of poor people.

Struggles, action and change

Low and middle-income countries face challenges to adequately resource their health systems. In many countries, the challenge for people's movements is the lack of a political will to opt for a model that is truly fair and that effectively avoids wastages created by private interests and private sector participation in healthcare delivery. The chapter on advances made in El Salvador describes how the country's current government has exhibited the political will to propose and advance progressive reforms. Yet, this is not sufficient, as even a well-structured system needs to be adequately financed.

The case study on the situation in El Salvador shows that a transformation of economic and fiscal structures is required in order to achieve adequate financing for healthcare services. Further, as the case study highlights, private interests and local elites can take democratic institutions hostage and sabotage reforms that benefit the majority. In such a situation, strong and independent people's movements and organizations have a key role to play to protect and further progressive reforms. The dilemma faced by the progressive government in El Salvador is typical of what other progressive governments face. In a globalized world where the global economy is integrated through myriad mechanisms, countries find it extremely difficult to create the fiscal space for welfare. This calls for international mobilization designed to break the power of the international financial institutions, the international trade regime and multinational corporations.

India is among the 20 countries worst affected by hunger in the world. The alarming situation of malnutrition in India demands a comprehensive approach that addresses the needs of children who are malnourished and require treatment. Unfortunately, the approach followed has been informed by a biomedical rather than public health perspective, where malnutrition is often treated without considering its broader social determinants. The chapter on this issue provides evidence from community led initiatives which point to the efficacy and sustainability of comprehensive community-based nutrition programmes that incorporate the use of locally devised solutions.

A story of consistent struggles waged by People living with HIV (PLHIV) in India, supported by national and international solidarity, lies behind the successes achieved as regards HIV treatment in India. This is the story of the struggle conducted by People living with HIV in India. The Indian experience shows the benefits of using the legal system for making full use of the flexibilities under the TRIPS agreement. The story also illustrates how the struggles of community groups lie at the heart of successful struggles that are challenging unfair trade rules.

The neoliberal order affects people's lives in myriad ways and it is thus contingent that the struggle for health be conceived and constructed as a very broad struggle. It incorporates different strands, different objectives of an immediate nature and diverse strategies, while upholding the vision of a globe that is free of the ills of neoliberal globalization. The final chapter depicts two struggles from Italy of communities, defending and reclaiming their rights, in the face of the neoliberal onslaught. It tells the story of *Genuino Clandestino,* an Italian network of collectives, associations and individuals who advocate and practice the re-appropriation and collectivization of land for autonomous, self-managed small scale farming. The chapter also relates the story of citizens' resistance in Casale Monferrato against asbestos-related health and environmental hazards.

Towards a shared narrative for change

A single volume cannot claim to cover the complex terrain of health and healthcare. The analysis, proposed actions and stories of struggles and change are presented with the view that it is necessary to propose an alternate vision and alternate strategies. We hope that *Global Health Watch 5* will stimulate readers to reflect more concretely about what needs to change, how things can be done differently, and how people can be at the centre of bringing about desired change. This volume is essentially an effort to build a community of believers who believe that change is necessary and urgent. It hopes to contribute to the construction of a shared narrative, located in a vision of equity and justice, and imbued with the urgency that the present global health crisis demands.

SECTION A

THE GLOBAL POLITICAL AND ECONOMIC ARCHITECTURE

A1 | SUSTAINABLE DEVELOPMENT GOALS IN THE AGE OF NEOLIBERALISM

Introduction

In the previous edition of *Global Health Watch* (GHW4), the opening chapter A1 was on "The Health Crises of Neoliberal Globalization". Neoliberalism 3.0 (the austerity agenda) was in full force. Massive US-led regional trade and investment deals were in negotiation or near finalization (the Trans-Pacific Partnership and the Transatlantic Trade and Investment Partnership). There was little movement on climate change, wealth inequalities were worsening and the UN world was still trying to come up with a set of new global plans to replace the waning Millennium Development Goals (MDGs). Much has changed in just three years.

The Sustainable Development Goals (SDGs) were adopted by more than 150 nations at a special UN General Summit in September 2015. A new climate change agenda was signed by 197 nations in December 2015 in Paris, and reached ratification and 'entry into force' in October 2016. The International Monetary Fund (IMF) in May 2016 featured a cover story in its flagship *Finance & Development*, "Neoliberalism: Oversold?" (Ostry, Loungani, Furceri, 2016), a belated response to (but no apology for) the extent to which the neoliberal policies they had helped to diffuse globally had exacerbated inequalities while failing to stimulate much growth. Globalization itself, at least as it was generally considered by the popular media, appeared to be tottering on

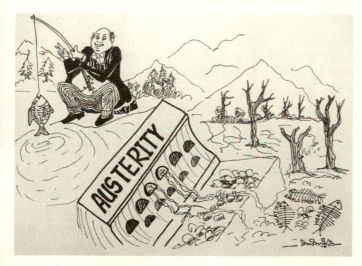

Image A1.1 The austerity agenda was in full force (Indranil Mukhopadhyay)

its last legs. Was the world taking a slow U-turn towards a more just, locally grounded and environmentally sustainable future?

Not so much. The world continues to grow hotter, each of the last three years being the warmest on record. Wealth inequalities persist in getting worse. Oxfam in its "Even it Up" campaign calculated in 2010 that it took the wealth of 388 billionaires to equal that of the world's poorest 3.6 billion people (the bottom half of humanity). In 2014 the number had dropped to just 85, and then to 67, and then further to 62. By the end of 2016 it was a mere 8. The top 1 per cent of the 'uber-elites' (the ones who gather annually at the World Economic Forum in Davos, Switzerland) now control more wealth, and the privilege and power that brings, than the 99 per cent rest-of-us. (Oxfam, 2017).

2016 also saw the UK choose to 'Brexit' by the slimmest of voting margins, after a campaign filled with false statements that marked the start of the 'post-truth' era and the possible break-up of the European Union (EU). This surprise outcome has since become fodder for the rise of the 'alt-right' (alternative right) in much of Europe, a previously slumbering movement built on xenophobic, nationalistic and racist motives with unhealthy doses of misogyny. But the year's biggest shock came with the November election of Donald Trump as US President, after a vitriol-laced campaign in which the elite billionaire presented himself as the anti-elite champion of the disenfranchised blue-collar worker. Trump subsequently stocked his new administration with even more billionaires, mostly white, mostly men. This kleptocratic group will somehow re-create the mythical America of the 1950s when the USA was the world's industrial juggernaut, Mexicans stayed on their side of the border, a woman's place was in the home and the uber-rich were growing increasingly ill-content with their declining share of national wealth. As the recently passed and ever insightful sociologist, Zygmunt Bauman, characterized Trump (and Russia's Putin, China's Xi, India's Modi, Turkey's Erdogan, the Philippines' Duterte, the resurrecting Latin American oligarchs and the suite of European alt-right wannabes): They are 'decisionists', autocratic individuals who fill a void of citizens' existential uncertainty as economies falter, environments grow more fragile, migrations strain nations and borders, the rich world's middle-class hollows out, and the hegemonic assuredness of neoliberalism's old order begins to fray (Bauman, 2016).

Trump's election has thrown a large political spanner into globalization's economic machinery. His threatened protectionism and prompt withdrawal from the mega-trade and investment treaties could begin to unravel the world's economy as we have come to know it these past forty years. Whether this means that the USA will abandon neoliberalism's underlying tenets remains to be seen, although there are reasons to doubt. Powerful swathes of American transnational corporations have built their wealth upon neoliberalism's market openness, including Trump's own global businesses. It is more probable that the global trade tilt will be less away from neoliberalism (or from globalization, for that matter) than towards new rules, agreements or simply unilateral actions that give even greater favour to American ("America first!") interests. More immediately troubling is the Trump administration's climate-change denialism, Islamophobia, militaristic intentions, antagonism to Mexico, and abandonment of women's reproductive rights.

Not all who voted for Trump, or who support the world's other 'decisionists', necessarily agree with all of their economic or social policies. One also wonders what might have transpired in the US election had Bernie Sanders and his centre-left populism become the Democrat candidate unlike Hillary Clinton who, setting aside the sexist hatred levelled at her by the Trump campaign, was widely perceived as continuing policies that had been disappointing many working class Americans for decades. Like Trump, Sanders spoke to this same disaffection but did so from a more inclusive, non-divisive and self-described 'socialist' platform (more accurately a somewhat social democratic politics, hardly radical).

We can only guess at what such a different US electoral outcome might have signalled to the rest of the world. The huge protests that met Trump's inauguration in January 2017 and that continue with each new outrageous Presidential executive order are necessary and encouraging. But what is needed now is a left-populism to counter that violence of the ascending right-populism, a new global economic and social policy platform that speaks both rationally and emotively to the human need for caring and sharing, and to the ecological urgency of sustainability.

Can the new Sustainable Development Goals (SDGs) offer help in creating such a platform?

The SDGs: Plus ça change, plus c'est la même chose?[1]

Many development activists were quick to embrace the hopefulness of the SDGs, with one lauding them as "a gigantic global version of Franklin Roosevelt's New Deal, a plunge into public investment in order to stave off not just recession but also climate change, famine, and a few other horsemen of the apocalypse" (Van der Zee B, 2016). The breadth of the SDGs, the extent of public consultations that went into their finalization, and their normative binding on *all* of the world's countries decidedly set them apart from their predecessor MDGs. As one of the lead negotiators that led to their eventual creation described them, they "signalled the need to redesign the global and national development landscape." (Farrukah Khan, 2016). This redesign, originally meant to set targets for a green economy and to address the most pressing environmental problems, merged with developing countries' deep concerns with poverty reduction and inequalities in global power and decision-making. As such the twin crises of our era were given political voice "in an international process going right." (Farrukah Khan, 2016)

Other views, from both the right and the left, were not so generous. *The Economist*, standard bearer for the status quo, described them as "stupid"

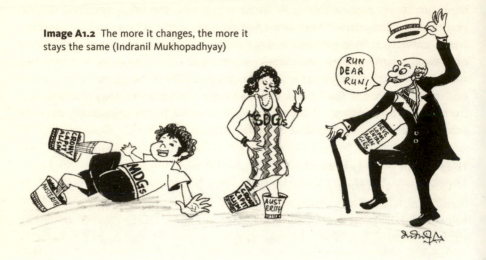

Image A1.2 The more it changes, the more it stays the same (Indranil Mukhopadhyay)

development goals, "so sprawling and misconceived…that the entire enterprise is set up to fail." (The Economist, 2015). This was a common refrain from mainstream economists who preferred the narrow, precise and non-threatening style of the MDGs, non-threatening because these did not question the underlying logic of either neoliberal globalization or global capitalism. The new set of 17 goals with 169 targets (and 230 indicators) unquestionably comprises a sprawling agenda for change (see Table A1.1), but such an agenda is "misconceived" only if one holds to a simplifying market fundamentalism that views human development as a matter of a few inexpensive interventions

TABLE A1.1: Sustainable Development Goals

1	NO POVERTY
2	ZERO HUNGER
3	GOOD HEALTH AND WELL-BEING
4	QUALITY EDUCATION
5	GENDER EQUALITY
6	CLEAN WATER AND SANITATION
7	AFFORDABLE AND CLEAN ENERGY
8	DECENT WORK AND ECONOMIC GROWTH
9	INDUSTRY, INNOVATION AND INFRASTRUCTURE
10	REDUCED INEQUALITIES
11	SUSTAINABLE COMMUNITIES
12	RESPONSIBLE CONSUMPTION AND PRODUCTION
13	CLIMATE ACTION
14	LIFE BELOW WATER
15	LIFE ON LAND
16	PEACE, JUSTICE AND STRONG INSTITUTIONS
17	PARTNERSHIPS FOR THE GOALS

Source: https://sustainabledevelopment.un.org/sdgs

here and there. Patrick Bond, an incisive critic on the left, expressed similar skepticism, calling them "Seriously Distracting Gimmicks" that risked diverting social movement and political activist attention away from the depredations of a twenty-first century capitalism on disequalizing environment-destroying steroids. (Patrick Bond, 2015). There is good reason to be cautious of an uncritical acceptance of the SDGs, which in their present form remain abstracted from an understanding of why the world now faces the entwined crises of ecological collapse and gross economic inequities.

The myth of poverty reduction

Consider, first, the new poverty SDG, *End poverty in all its forms everywhere*. Significantly, and likely at the insistence of the G77 + China (the negotiating voice for developing countries), this sits prominently as the first in the list of 17. Superficially, it is a much more ambitious poverty goal than the MDG's

---

Box A1.1: The SDGs: universally binding or selectively cherry-picked?

In most international resolutions, declarations or agreements, there are 'preambular' paragraphs that set the interpretative context for what countries have agreed to. Paragraph 55 of *The 2030 Agenda for Sustainable Development* (United Nations, 2015), which finalized the SDGs and their targets, is revealing for how it illustrates the governance dilemma between universal obligation (even if only a non-enforceable one) and national or sovereign choice.

> The SDGs and targets are integrated and indivisible, global in nature and universally applicable, taking into account different national realities, capacities and levels of development and respecting national policies and priorities. Targets are defined as aspirational and global, with each government setting its own national targets guided by the global level of ambition but taking into account national circumstances. Each government will also decide how these aspirational and global targets should be incorporated in national planning processes, policies and strategies. (¶ 55)

While the goals themselves are seen as universal and indivisible, the targets give nations considerable latitude in defining their own "level of ambition". On the one hand this can be interpreted as recognizing differences in the resource capacities and circumstances of differing countries. On the other, it can be a 'get out of jail free' card (a reference to the board game, *Monopoly*), allowing countries at whatever level of development or wealth to choose their own particular targets.

call for a halving in the proportion of people living below the 'absolute' poverty line between 1990 and 2015, set initially at $1/day but later adjusted by the World Bank to $1.25/day to reflect higher price levels in developing countries (Millennium Development Goals and Beyond, 2013). With great fanfare this MDG poverty goal was announced as "mission accomplished" five years ahead of schedule (The World Bank, 2016). Much of this success is attributed to China and a handful of other developing countries which benefited from the outsourcing by American and European transnational firms of industrial production (think manufactured goods and electronics) and services provision (think call-centres). Globalization's opening of borders to the freer flow of capital, goods and services has created new pockets of the not-absolutely-poor, although huge increases in income inequalities within those countries benefiting from this (now declining) growth has been the socially disrupting price paid for it. Remove China from the global headcount, however, and the number of those living in absolute poverty today is about the same as the number back in 1981, trickle-down neoliberal globalization not keeping pace with population growth. (Hickel, 2016). A sixth of the world's population still struggles below the absolute poverty level, which has since been re-adjusted to $1.90/day.

The SDG now commits governments to eliminate absolute poverty by 2030. *The Economist* likes this target, because it is simple and just possibly achievable (although since 2015 there's been backsliding rather than forward progressing). There is another poverty target that calls on countries to reduce by "at least half" the proportion of people living in poverty "in all its dimensions according to national definitions." Less ambitious than "eliminate" this target partially addresses the need to improve income growth for the 2 billion people who now live at the not-quite-absolutely-poor level averaging globally at around $2.90/day (Shaohua Chen and Martin Ravallion, 2012), a level characterized by insecure or informal employment that is highly vulnerable to small economic or environmental shocks. Targets in the SDGs, it is important to note, are "aspirational", with each country able to set its own level of ambition (see Box A1.1). Given the ubiquity of the World Bank's absolute poverty measure it is likely that, without powerful and persistent civil society prodding, this will become the default metric for SDG 1, with little attention given to the income distributional needs of those who have been 'lifted' a dollar-a-day higher. The absolute poverty target is also not well-liked by most development activists, for the simple reason that it is so low that achieving it would still leave people with insufficient resources for a reasonable life expectancy, generally pegged at around 70 years. Estimates of the income required for this still modest outcome (since many in high-income countries can expect to live well past 80 years) range between $5/day and $7.40/day (Hickel, 2016). Using the $5/day level (the minimum the United Nations Conference on Trade and Development considers to qualify as a poverty line, and below which over

4.3 billion people presently live) (Hickel, 2016) and based on current poverty reduction trends, when 2030 dawns:

- 15% in Latin America and the Caribbean would still be poor, rising to
- 30% in East Asia and the Pacific, and
- 50% in Middle East and North Africa, but an astounding
- 90% in South Asia and sub-Saharan (United Nations Conference on Trade and Development, 2013)

At the current rate by which the global economy has been reducing poverty, it would take 200 years to eliminate poverty at the $5/day level, and over 300 years at the $7.40/day (Woodward, 2015). Even if these more appropriate poverty targets were eventually achieved, what would be the cost to all of the environmental SDGs if our prevailing economic growth model continues? This question cuts to the contradiction at the heart of the SDGs: The belief that the same global economic rules and power relations that have created an increasingly unequal and unsustainable world can somehow engineer the reverse.

The contradictory hearts of the SDGs

The strongest expression of this contradiction is found in SDG 8, that calls on all the world's countries to *Promote sustained, inclusive and sustainable economic growth, full and productive employment and decent work for all*. Its first target emphasizes "sustained per capita economic growth" exceeding "at least 7 per cent...in the least developed countries." This is the clarion call of conventional economists, which has grown louder since the financial crisis of 2008. Although countries going through prolonged recessions or depressions generally do not do well health-wise (Karanikolos et al., n.d.; Arne Ruckert & Labonte, 2017), and economic growth itself is not necessarily or at least not always a bad thing, the problem once again is with the metric, and secondarily with where the emphasis is placed. Regarding the metric, the GDP has long been critiqued for measuring only economic transactions regardless of whether they are good for poverty reduction, the environment or human health, with the oft-cited cliché that wars, pollution and disasters increase GDP hence, at least in theory, also reduce poverty. (Wars do have a way of reducing competition for well-paying jobs by killing workers-as-soldiers.) With respect to the misplaced emphasis, assuming that "sustainable economic growth" means growth that is environmentally sustainable (a questionable assumption given it could equally mean growth that goes on and on and on), the noun in the phrase (economic growth) dominates the modifying adjective (sustainable). This phrasing is reminiscent of the 1980s when "sustainable development" was the policy rage. Some countries established multi-stakeholder Roundtables (government, business, civil society) to debate the way forward, much the way multi-stakeholder governance for the SDGs is still imagined (on which

Box A1.2: Decent work

The tripartite ILO (with representatives from government, industry and labour) defines decent work with the same idealistic flair found in the best of the SDGs:

> Decent work sums up the aspirations of people in their working lives. It involves opportunities for work that is productive and delivers a fair income, security in the workplace and social protection for families, better prospects for personal development and social integration, freedom for people to express their concerns, organize and participate in the decisions that affect their lives and equality of opportunity and treatment for all women and men. (International Labor Organization, 2017)

Few reading this passage (at least few workers) would disagree with these aspirations, which are buttressed by the ILO's responsibility to oversee ratification of and compliance with core labour rights. These rights are also referenced in SDG 8 (target 8.8). Leaders in the G20 and G7 country groups, the European Union and the African Union have signed on to this agenda although, as with all normative commitments, the agenda flounders on a lack of enforcement measures. Nonetheless, labour rights and the Decent Work agenda can be useful rhetorical tools for health activists who approach the SDGs through the lens of employment rights or alongside movements advocating for a living wage (there are several operating in different countries).

more later). When one environmentalist emerged from yet another fruitless meeting, frustrated by the lack of any ecosystem understanding on the part of the business representatives, a friend explained, "It's simple. You see. They (business) got the noun (development) while you (environmentalists) got the adjective (sustainable)." Nouns as subjects of the sentence control the action. Adjectives only modify from their secondary status.

The way in which the employment targets are stated deepens the contradictions. The reference to *decent work for all* is useful, as it gives traction for the Decent Work agenda of the International Labour Organization (ILO) (see Box A1.2). The call for full employment (elaborated under target 8.5) is also nice to see, albeit one that is frequently promised by governments but rarely delivered. Yet it is almost immediately contradicted by another of SDG 8's targets (8.2), which calls for "higher levels of economic productivity", the indicator for which is "annual growth rate of real GDP per employed person." Increased productivity is another axiom of conventional economics, since as the amount of output per labour input rises, so does the time-value of labour, with productivity gains leading to lower prices for what is produced. Or so the theory goes, often with historic narratives such as how, 250 years ago, over 90 per cent of Americans worked in agriculture. Today it is less than 2 per cent who, with technology, now produce far more per farmer than in the eighteenth century. (Ross, 2015). This theory, however, assumes that the labour displaced by increased productivity will simply be re-employed in new forms of better-paying work. Figure A1.1 begins to question this theory, at least for developed economies, by illustrating a widening gap between workers' productivity and workers' wages. This gap is shown even more starkly in Figure A1.2, which shows changes in manufacturing output and employment since 1980 in the USA. It is this particular gap that came to dominate the Trump campaign and arguably led to his electoral victory. Blame was placed on China, and outsourcing to China (and elsewhere) is estimated to have destroyed between 700 thousand and 2.4 million US manufacturing jobs. But other studies suggest that over 5 million jobs were lost due to automation, with a recent US business school study attributing as many as 87 per cent of American manufacturing jobs since 1987 lost due to technology-enabled increased productivity. (Hicks and Devaraj, 2015).

Globalization's inclusion of hundreds of millions of new workers in global production and service supply chains (allowing transnational companies to take advantage of 'labour market arbitrage') has led to a world of too many workers competing for too few jobs to produce too many goods or services for too few consumers with too little income to afford them without increasing their already high levels of personal debt.[2] (Debt in the form of risky mortgages, real estate bubbles and corrupt banking practices, as the last GHW4 pointed out, is what precipitated the 2008 financial crisis.) This statement may seem an oversimplification, but consider that since the 2008 financial crisis and recession global unemployment is at its highest-ever recorded level and is expected to rise again in 2017. (International Labour Organization, 2017). Much of this burden will be borne by low and middle income countries, with unemployment falling slightly in developed economies. Most of the employment gains in high income countries, however, are a result of increases in part-time, insecure and low wage jobs, creating what the labour economist, Guy Standing, has called the 'precariat'. (Caldbick, Labonte, Mohindra, & Ruckert, 2014). Even Germany (the economic 'powerhouse' of Europe) is affected, reporting the highest instance across Europe of workers earning below 60 per cent of the median wage, indicative of the loss of mid-level occupations (Mezger, 2017).[3] Similarly insecure and often hazardous informal employment continues to dominate the labour markets in many low income countries, with half of the employed in South Asia and two-thirds of those in sub-Saharan Africa stuck in 'working poverty', earning less than $3.10/day (well below UNCTAD's $5/day poverty minimum). (International Labour Organization, 2017).

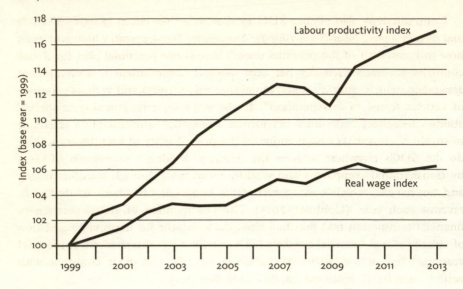

Figure A1.1: Trends in growth in labour productivity and average wage in developed economies (index) 1999–2013

Source: International Labour Organization (2015) Global Wage Report 2014/15: Wages and income inequality, International Labour Office – Geneva: ILO, 2015. P. 8

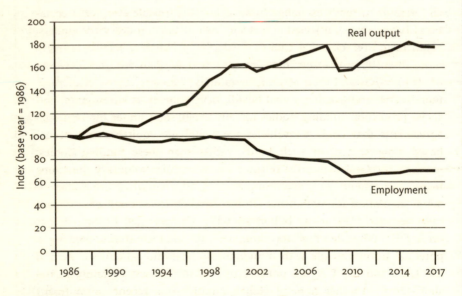

Figure A1.2: US manufacturing output and employment – 1986–2017

Rebased (1986 = 100)

Source: Calculated from primary data sources. Employment data from United States Department of Labour, Bureau of Labour Statistics, available at: https://data.bls.gov/timeseries/CES3000000001; Manufacturing Output data from https://www.federalreserve.gov/releases/g17/ipdisk/ip_nsa.txt

Contradictions also pepper SDG 17: *Strengthen the means of implementation and revitalize the Global Partnership for Sustainable Development*, which addresses how to finance all of the previous ones. There is the perennial plea for donor countries to reach their 0.7 per cent of GNI commitment to development assistance (which, after 47 years, remains mostly unmet) and various promises of various forms of "cooperation". It also calls for strengthening countries' abilities to collect "tax and other forms of revenue" (presumably a reference to royalties), but makes no mention of the progressivity of such taxation. Nor do the SDGs anywhere address the ongoing avoidance or evasion of taxes by transnational companies and wealthy individuals through transfer pricing and tax havens, which costs governments hundreds of billions of dollars in revenue each year. (Cobham, 2015). The one mention of global taxation (a financial transaction tax) that had been the indicator for improved regulation of volatile global financial markets (SDG target 10.5) disappeared in the final version, likely at the behest of the USA, the UK and other countries with vested interests in footloose capital. (See Box A1.3.)

Box A1.3: Global development goals demand systems of global taxation/tax-regulation

As the previous GHW4 pointed out, a financial transaction tax (FTT) on all forms of currency exchange (now technically feasible even for speculation in derivatives), if levied at a rate of just 5 cents on every 100 dollars, could raise over US$ 8.6 trillion a year (McCulloch & Pacillo, 2011) – more than the outside estimates of what is needed to fund achievement of all 17 SDGs and their 169 targets (Ronald Labonte, 2016). Moreover, there are several existing global health, development, environmental and social protection funding bodies already established under international agreements that could be vehicles for a globally equitable and needs-based disbursement of such funds, rather than these funding bodies' (such as the Global Fund's) reliance upon irregular voluntary donations from governments or philanthropies. Ten EU countries are slated to adopt legislation for such a tax (France already levies one) which could raise between US$ 40–47 billion annually. The eventual EU agreement on a FTT offers leverage for campaigns in other countries, creating a potential norm cascade with tremendously healthful potential – even if the USA and the UK are unlikely to join in (at least certainly in the short-term). Another hopeful global initiative is a recent commitment by OECD and G20 countries to create an accounting system whereby transnational corporations pay taxes in the jurisdictions in which they earn their revenue, which should reduce their use of transfer-pricing practices and tax havens (amongst other measures) to avoid taxation.

Echoing the MDG8, SDG 17 also calls for a "universal, rules-based, open, non-discriminatory and equitable multilateral trading system under the World Trade Organization", through "conclusion of negotiations under its Doha Development Round." It is certainly preferable for global trade to have rules than to function anarchically or by a 'beggar thy neighbour' set of rules where might is right (the sort of mercantilist trade rules that some envision Trump as wanting to negotiate or re-negotiate). But there is little evidence to suggest that our current sets of rules have been equitable or that completion of the Doha Round will disproportionately benefit least developed or most low income countries; indeed, the evidence suggests quite the opposite. (Polaski, 2006). 'Equitable' and 'non-discriminatory' make sense only when the universe of economic players are fairly equal, which they are not. This fact is well recognized within the WTO as the 'special and differential treatment' (SDT) that should be accorded to developing countries, and is repeated under SDG target 10.a as one of the means to reduce inequality. But after 20 years of WTO negotiations it is still not legally binding on member countries, and many trade observers doubt that the Doha Round will ever be completed. Even if it were, there remains the conflict between targets 17.14 ("enhance policy coherence for sustainable development") and 17.15 ("respect each country's policy space"), since many analyses of trade agreements (and especially the

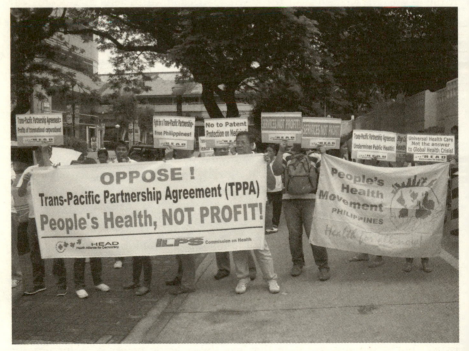

Image A1.3 Trade treaties are major barriers to development: Protests against TPPA in the Philippines (PHM Philippines)

new generation of regional trade and investment treaties) point out how such treaties are the major barriers to countries achieving policy coherence (Blouin, 2007; Koivusalo, Labonte, Wibulpolprasert, & Kanchanachitra, 2013; Labonté, Schram, & Ruckert, 2016), with several agreements likely to be in direct conflict with several SDG health and food-related targets (Ruckert et al., 2017).

The indivisibility of the SDGs

Do these systemic flaws affirm the SDG critics? The answer is both 'yes' and 'no', and pertains to how one approaches the indivisibility of the SDGs, the presumption that all must be acted upon in concert with each other. Stated positively, this presents health activists and civil society groups with potential leverage for what we now call a 'Health in All Policies' (HiAP) approach to government decision-making, or what public health activists labelled 'healthy public policy' during the era of the *Ottawa Charter for Health Promotion*, and 'intersectoral actions for health' when the WHO launched its Commission on the Social Determinants of Health (Nunes, Lee, & O'Riordan, 2016). That such thinking appears to now permeate the highest levels of UN agencies and (nominally at least) their member states gives such an approach a stamp of approval that it lacked in earlier periods. Although health does not hold the same centrality in the SDGs as it did in the MDGs, most of the 17 SDGs deal with societal and ecological determinants of health. The indivisibility of the SDGs, while admonishing states and agencies not to cherry pick from their own personal favourites, poses two significant problems for supportive governments or health activists advocating the SDGs' policy importance. The first, already discussed, is the embedded contradiction between equitable and sustainable development and the insatiable economic growth model of global capitalism, the SDG complaint from the left. The second is that if the SDGs address everything, they risk becoming nothing, the SDG complaint from the right, but one also voiced by some development activists who argue that the SDGs were better suited to the international cooperative decade of the 1990s than the current illiberal era epitomized by Trump (Doane, 2017). In a similar vein, the general lack of explicit accountability measures within the SDGs risks them "becoming everyone's business but no-one's major responsibility... if everyone is accountable in theory, no one is accountable in practice." (Engebretsen, Heggen, & Ottersen, 2017).

Although states' accountabilities under international conventions remain weak, it is still states that are, in human rights parlance, the 'duty-bearers' for the agreements they reach. We may have embraced a new politics of governance (in which state and non-state actors seek common ground on issues) but it remains the state that has the policing power of enforcement, even as the 'market' (private economic actors) retains the financial means to exert undue influence over the state's decisions. It falls upon the amorphous groupings of citizens (civil society) to hold both state and market to account for actions that embody the environmental sustainability and health equity targets of the SDGs. At the same time, it will be hard for many of the world's governments under current global political clouds to focus upon 17 goals and 169 targets. Like the accountability problem, the indivisibility of the SDGs may be sound in theory but wanting in practice. The challenge for health activists is to organize the goals into a shorter priority list as a basis for their accountability advocacy.[4]

The long list of SDG priorities

The SDGs are an effort to combine the health and social development targets of the MDGs alongside those of the post-Rio sustainable development agenda. The relationship between the two is apparent in the vastly more enormous ecological footprint of the world's 1 per cent (and even the top 20 or 30 per cent) compared to the bottom half of humanity (Oxfam, 2015). Almost a decade ago, the UK Commission on Sustainable Development (Jackson, 2009) noted the impossibility of raising the consumption levels of the rest of the world to that of the presently affluent – we do not have enough environmental resources to do so, requiring by some estimates the equivalent of four Earth planets to come even close (McDonald, 2015). We now live in an 'Age of the Anthropocene' in which human actions are determining the trajectories of all the world's ecosystems. Climate change ranks as the immediately most serious, but there are few of our ecosystems that are not under major stress (loss of forest cover, desertification, soil erosion, water depletion, wetland loss and damage, biodiversity loss, species extinctions, fisheries depletions) (Whitmee et al., 2015). There are some signs of positive change, such as increases in the amount of energy being generated from renewable sources.[5] But it is difficult not to lapse into catastrophic terms when viewing the enormity of the environmental damages we humans, our societies and our economies have created, and continue doing so.

Urgent activist priority should thus go to the environmental SDGs, notably SDG 6 on water, 7 on energy, 12 on consumption/production, 13 on climate change, 14 on marine conservation, and 15 on 'terrestrial ecosystems' and biodiversity loss (although it should be noted that many of the other SDGs have environmental targets within them). While important, the environmental SDGs have limitations. The energy goal is primarily concerned with increasing access to "reliable and modern energy services" that would include increasing "the share of renewable energy in the global energy mix" (but with no numerical target).[6] The consumption/production goal includes a target to "rationalize inefficient fossil-fuel subsidies that encourage wasteful consumption...by restructuring taxation and phasing out...harmful subsidies" – although the G20 countries (never mind the rest

Box 1.4: Policy by numbers?

If the policy cliché that what you can't measure doesn't get noticed is true, then health activists need to pay as much attention to the indicators agreed upon for the SDG targets. Although not formally binding, the indicators constitute a form of policy by numbers, or in some instances policy by neglect. Despite the headline importance given to reducing inequalities, for example, there is no mention of the use of Gini coefficients or disaggregated income distribution measures. Instead, the target and indicator for reducing inequality is simply a higher-than-average rate of income growth for the bottom 40 per cent. The MDG lesson-learned of the importance of disaggregated measures appears to be lesson-forgotten in the SDGs. There is no measure for reducing between-country inequalities, and a proposed Inclusive Wealth Index as a complement to GDP was replaced by countries being able to achieve a census "achieving 100% birth and 80% death registration." The indicator for SDG target 8.8 (labour rights) was diluted from the number of ILO conventions ratified to emphasize only "freedom of association and collective bargaining". A proposed indicator for policy coherence (SDG 17.5.1) which referred to constraints on government's policy space within trade and investment agreements or development assistance and loans (usefully specific) was dropped in favour of the "extent of use of country owned results framework," rather obscure and only as applied to development assistance. Many of the other SDG targets had mentioned reductions in inequality as one of their measures; most of these disappeared in the final set. And it was only a concerted advocacy campaign by over 300 health activist groups to overturn a last minute change to one of the indicators for universal health coverage (SDG 3.8) – "number of people covered by health insurance or a public health system per 1,000 population" – which says nothing about affordability of health insurance, back to its original: "Fraction of the population protected against catastrophic/impoverishing out-of-pocket health expenditure" (Lei Ravelo, 2016).

If numbers matter, it is important to ensure that the best ones for health equity and ecological sustainability are the ones used, regardless of the final 'official' and discretionary list.

of the world) have still to agree to a deadline to phase out such subsidies (Denyer, 2016). The climate change goal is the most disappointing, deferring to the United Nations Framework Convention on Climate Change "for negotiating the global response," with the weakly phrased commitments of the Paris Agreement on Climate Change (with much of its language couched in conditional 'woulds' and 'shoulds' rather than forceful 'will' and 'shall') the best on present offer. The climate change SDG, instead, is primarily concerned with building adaptive "resilience" amongst communities, cities and the poor to what seems to be accepted as the inevitable. This does not make health activism on climate change less urgent; only that there is a need for more teeth in its SDG targets and indicators.

The same applies to most of the SDGs, which lose some of their force as their headline intents are translated into measurable targets and suggested indicators (see Box A1.4). Health activists, as with their governments, need to consider each sectoral policy or action implied by one goal or target in terms of how it will support achievement of all the other goals or targets, albeit with an awareness of the fundamental economic flaws within the full set. That being said, where should health activism around the SDGs begin? Suggested below is an initial set (with brief commentary) of the SDGs that are likely to hold the most immediate promise for a healthier, ecologically sustainable life.[7]

Goal 1: End poverty in all its forms Its importance to UN member states is signalled by its position as the first goal, and poverty is certainly the greatest single 'risk condition' for poor health. As earlier noted, Goal 1 requires a meaningful metric and not the World Bank's 'absolute' measure. One of its targets usefully calls for "social protection systems...for all" with an emphasis on the poor and vulnerable, which necessarily demands improved tax measures and, for LMICs, better domestic resource mobilization. It further requires an end to the revenue eroding practices of transfer pricing – a transnational corporate practice to avoid taxes – and tax havens, the persistent of both on which the SDGs are silent.

Goal 2: End hunger, achieve food security and improved nutrition and promote sustainable agriculture Undernourished people cannot be healthy or economically and politically well-functioning citizens. Apart from malnutrition targets, Goal 2 calls for "sustainable food production systems...that increase productivity and production [and] that help maintain ecosystems," emphasizing assistance for small-scale producers. What remains problematic is the emphasis on increasing production (including for "fishers", which challenges one of the targets for Goal 14 on marine resources that cautions the need to "restore fish stocks") without any indication of how this might actually be done.[8] While calling for an end to trade-distorting food export subsidies (something HICs have finally agreed to under WTO rules) there is no mention of trade-distorting domestic production support (which now dominates the practices of countries such as the USA, China, Japan and the EU) and on which the LDCs (least developed countries) are calling for caps and reductions in line with Goal 2's broader intent (ICTSD, 2017).

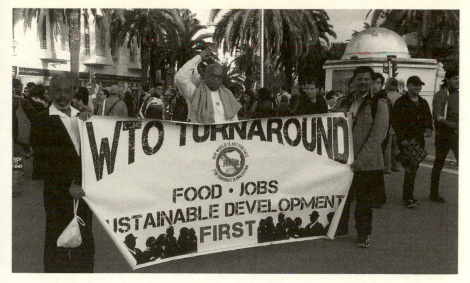

Image A1.4 Trade rules undermine food security: Activists demonstrate at the World Social Forum in Tunis in 2015 (Amit Sengupta)

Goal 3: Ensure healthy lives and promote well-being for all at all ages "Achieve universal health coverage," including "affordable essential medicines and vaccines for all," is important, if weakened by ongoing disagreements over how it be financed (public or private or both), with the private healthcare and financial service sectors of the EU and USA happy to see an enlarged global role for themselves. Also problematic is the continued usage of the term 'coverage' – essentially insurance terminology that allows the possibility of public healthcare services to be outsourced (while continuing to be public financed) to private providers (see Chapter B1). "Universal access to sexual and reproductive health-care services" is equally important for its positive health impacts on women's and children's health, and its ability to keep population growth within ecological limits (see Box A1.5). But most of Goal 3's targets concern reductions in mortality and morbidity rates with little discussion of how these might be achieved, and the risk that Goal 3 becomes 'the' health goal to the neglect of the other SDGs associated with the determinants of health. As former WHO Director-General Margaret Chan expressed, "Universal health coverage…underpins all SDGs and is key to their achievement" (The Graduate Institute Geneva, 2015), a worrying health sector solipsism only slightly expanded by MSF and VENRO (an umbrella group of German NGOs) in their urging of the G20 to give special attention to the health targets of the SDGs (Doctors Without Borders, 2017).

Goal 4: Ensure inclusive and equitable quality education and promote lifelong learning opportunities for all The link between education and good health are

Box1. 5: The population Ponzi scheme

For decades the issue of population planning has been contentious, with both reactionary and progressive arguments calling for efforts to control the size of the human species, which now is the most numerous mammal on the planet and by some numerical distance. Population control has frequently been used by colonizers and elite classes to curb the family size of those they considered inferior, even as feminist and development theorists have argued the importance of guaranteeing the reproductive rights of women often (but not always) emphasizing small family size. Concern over the potential misuse of family planning initiatives exists and is often warranted, but there is broad agreement that the human population cannot continue to expand indefinitely. Yet there is a standard economic argument for continuous population increases that essentially mimics otherwise discredited Ponzi schemes. A Ponzi scheme, named after a fraudulent investor who first dreamt it up, pays investors from capital provided by new investors and not from any real profits. The scheme only succeeds by continually recruiting ever-more new investors, thus expanding the pool of capital to pay the earlier investors, until it eventually collapses (or is found out) with almost all but the scheme's operator(s) losing everything. A dominant demographic argument today mimics the same Ponzi logic. Its argument is that, with population aging, immigration and/or incentives for larger families should be encouraged to re-swell a comparatively shrinking working age cohort (those between 15 and 64 years). The economic rationale is that the taxes collected from the productivity of the working age population is needed to pay for the services and pensions of a proportionately greater and increasing number of elderly. That makes sense, perhaps, for the short-term. But fast forward 40 or 50 years, and the re-swelled working age cohort has itself become elderly (and far more numerous), requiring an ever larger expansion in the base of the working age population. And so on, and on, and on. Like new investors feeding the 'returns' of the earlier and older ones, an ever increasing working age population is assumed necessary to feed the health and social needs of the elderly retired, and to keep the business-as-usual economy growing exponentially. At some point (and we may already have reached it) a continuously expanding pyramidal population base becomes unsustainable on every axis conceivable: economic, ecologic and social.

well-established, particularly for women and girls in low- and middle-income countries (LMICs) (PRB, 2011). The emphasis here needs to be placed on the "quality" of education, and not simply on access. Whether such education leads to greater employment in "decent jobs", another of Goal 4's targets, will depend on how the global over-supply of workers is managed through radically different labour market policies than those erected by the last forty years of neoliberal economics. But it is still better to have a literate and numerate civil society than not, even if un- or under- employed, as that holds some hope for a skilled political change movement. Indeed, without these educational targets Goal 5's aim, *Achieve gender equality and empower all women and girls*, is unlikely to be achieved.[9] An important related educational target emphasizes development of knowledge and skills related to "sustainable lifestyles, human rights, gender equity…and global citizenship" which could help to build a stronger activist base essential to moving governments forward on the SDGs; although the absence of representative global government renders the concept of global citizenship more rhetorical than real.

Goal 6: Ensure availability and sustainable manage of water and sanitation for all No water, no health; poor sanitation, much disease. Goal 6 is the historic mainstay of public health, but its activist prioritization needs to be tempered with some critique. The first target references "affordable drinking water," which could be code for engaging private markets in water supply or user fees for public provision. Recent history in both approaches has not been sanguine for equitable access (Kishimoto, Lobina, & Petitjean, 2015). With diminishing supply and increasing population and agricultural/industrial demand, especially in light of the target to increase agricultural productivity, water access is becoming a source of conflict and a driver of refugee populations. The target "to substantially increase water use efficiency…and ensure sustainable withdrawals and supply of freshwater" is thus central to Goal 6.

Goal 10: Reduce inequality within and among countries Given the impossibility of meaningful poverty reduction through economic growth alone, Goal 10 assumes paramount importance. It targets sustained income growth for the bottom 40 per cent at a rate greater than the national average (which is good as far as it goes), but says nothing about the distortion of accumulating wealth at the top without which inequalities could continue to rise. Importantly it does add 'equality of outcome' to the usual emphasis on 'equal opportunity,' thereby affirming the more difficult of social justice's two main articulations (Labonte, Baum, & Sanders, 2015). The measure for "fiscal, wage and social protection policies" that "progressively achieve greater equality" is the labour share of GDP – of fundamental importance given the gross erosion in this share over the past 40 years of neoliberal economic policies.

Goal 12: Ensure sustainable consumption and production patterns The implication of Goal 12 is more profound than its targets, which recycle most of the tropes of 'sustainable development' that first made their global rounds with the 1987 publication of the Bruntland Report, *Our Common Future* (WCED, 1987). Weak on reducing fossil-fuel subsidies (another sovereign escape clause, "in accordance with national circumstances"), the goal itself needs a syntax inversion: not 'sustainable consumption' (another instance of the consumption noun dominating the sustainable adjective) but 'consume sustainably' (which can only be achieved by reducing current global levels of our material gorging). This recasting of the goal requires a reduction in demand, especially in HICs[10], at a time when conventional economics is calling for an increase in demand to get the growth economy back on track, underpinning again the foundational importance of an appropriately calibrated inequality goal. Consuming and producing sustainably is also inconsistent with Goal 9's different targets and indicators calling for increases in industrialization and industrial employment (making still more stuff for more consumers). Such industrialization increases may be meaningful for LICs (in terms of 'value-adding' for their exported products, think fine chocolate products rather than raw cocoa beans), but would be sustainable only to the extent that there are parallel dramatic decreases in the same in HICs.

This long list of priority SDGs, although forming a base for campaigning and accountability, nonetheless further reveals the permeating 'business-as-usual' model that cripples the utility of the SDGs for meaningful social transformation. But if activists take this near-but-not-quite-fatal flaw into constant consideration in their work, the SDGs still provide us with an imperfect roadmap of a world that just might be liveable into the next century.

The (very) short list of priority SDGs

But even this long list of priority goals could create a cluttered message for health advocates, in which a slew of special interests could drown out the essential transformations needed. This is what happened with the Occupy movement, which became unmoored from its original complaint against the predatory practices of the financialized economy as every social grievance attached itself to the demonstrations and tent cities. If we were to reduce the SDGs to the primary goals, without which none of the others would be likely to succeed even in the short-term, we might consider these three:

1. Ensure quality education for women and girls (which is not to ignore men and boys, but emphasizing women and girls can rapidly advance gender empowerment, one of the best known means to improve health equity).
2. Reduce inequality (which in itself would and should eliminate poverty).
3. Consume and produce sustainably (which requires more equitable global patterns in both, alongside aggregate global reductions, which underpins all of the environmental SDGs).

How, then, do we move forward with this agenda, transforming wondrous words into meaningful actions?

Governance for the SDGs

> We are at a crossroads. One road points to the inexorable rise of authoritarianism, while another opens up a more hopeful cosmopolitan future (Held, 2017).

> There are no non-radical options left before us. (Winship, 2016).

David Held, a scholarly activist, holds out the possibility that we may yet create a global politic in which the lives of each individual, regardless of nationality, are equally valued and accorded equal rights and privileges. That is also the message of the SDGs, and their catch-phrase: "Leave no one behind." Naomi Klein, an activist scholar, is more intensely and immediately critical of the ecological predations of global capitalism, attesting to the incongruity of the SDGs in their assumption that by slight tweaks of the same economic model we can continue to grow and consume our way out of a tragedy of unequal growth and skewed consumption. Both in different ways point to a crisis in contemporary global governance, for it is one thing to campaign for the priority SDGs, but quite another to envision the type of political system or organization that might see to their fruition.

In ethical terms, cosmopolitanism challenges the authoritarianism of today's 'decisionists', who rely upon 'othering' to capture the disenfranchisement of disgruntled citizens. Trump blames the Mexicans, Chinese, journalists and judges, and foments an internationalizing Islamophobia. Modi aims for a Hindu nationalism with similar anti-Muslim undertones. Putin re-creates an imperialist Russia against the rest of the West. Brexit voters see the source of their economic weakening in the EU's bureaucracy. Erdogan plays the separatist terrorist card. For Duterte, drug lords and drug addicts have become the legitimating 'other' for extrajudicial murder. In none of these instances is the inequality intrinsic to a capitalist economy on globalized steroids questioned as a causal agent. That is where Klein's economic critique of neoliberal capitalism comprises the political edge to Held's ethical idealism. This is not to reduce xenophobia (the violent extreme of 'othering') to economic determinism so much as to recognize that economic inequalities have been driving much of the illiberal rejection of the past forty years of a 'hyper-globalization'. The participation of an estimated 4 million worldwide in the women's protest march the day after Trump's ill-attended inauguration was invigorating, with the persistence of such citizen demonstrations of solidarity vital in the days and years to come. But it is perilous for such social activism, in response to the discrimination of right-wing 'othering', to valorize impugned identities (important to do) without also critiquing the economics that underpin their derogation in the first instance.

We do not have a global government and its closest equivalent, the UN system has been under neoliberal assault for decades and is facing its own test of contemporary relevance (O'Grady, 2016). Instead we have 'global governance' – a melange of multi-stakeholder forums with varying degrees of influence and decision-making authority, although with little enforcement powers. Such governance systems can help to set normative agendas, as they have with the headline declarations of the SDGs and the Paris Agreement on Climate Change. Such agenda-setting is not unimportant since, in the struggle for a humanistic (cosmopolitan) political populism to challenge the exclusionary autocratic form on present ascent, it is the visionary claims that constitute the basis of engagement.

The struggle for governance in support of these claims will need to work across government (decision-making) levels, from local to global, if it is to succeed. Such efforts are likely to be easier at local levels, where the indignities of disequalizing neoliberal economics and the exclusionary politics it foments are more apparent, and the 'lived experiences' of environmental fragilities more immediate, can catalyze the often more-responsive and participatory democracies of cities and regions. It is not accidental that municipalities and states have become the loci of opposition to the policies of Trump and the Republican Party in the USA. But, while vital for the opportunity localism allows citizens and civil society organizations to articulate, and to agitate for, a different style of politics and economics embodying the progressive targets of the SDGs, it needs to confront power at the national and global scales. It is at these scales that activism encounters its greatest challenge, in the form of a too-often decision-making capitulation to the interests of elite and powerful individuals and corporations in the guise of multi-stakeholder governance. As governments, public institutions and multilateral UN or affiliated agencies fall under fiscal restraint (the result of years of declines in the share of global economic product going to taxes and the financing of public goods) they rationalize greater engagement with powerful and influential private sector actors. From the WHO's formalization of the participation of 'non-state actors' in its functioning (including the private corporate sector) to the UN's Global Compact with private industry (Adams & Martens, 2015), it is hard to see how such governance will resolve the fundamental contradictions inherent to capitalism that remain implicit (and sometimes explicit, if not in name) in the SDGs.

Thus the larger governance struggle surrounding the SDGs is an older one of constraining the predatory nature of capitalism (neoliberal or otherwise), or seeking its transformation into some different system that respects human rights and that moves rapidly to implement the SDGs (sanitised of their economic contradictions). Simply stated: the headline intent of the SDGs, the most exhaustive and global summary of 'the world we want' yet developed (The World We Want, n.d.), poses an inherent opposition to the premises of global capitalism. As activists mobilize around the SDGs, it is imperative that they continuously bring this contradiction to their populist platforms.

Notes

1 An epigram by the French novelist and critic, Jean-Baptiste Alphonse Karr, published in 1849. Literally: 'the more it changes, the more it stays the same.'

2 This structural conundrum may also explain why creating more consumer 'demand' (through more consumer loans and government stimulus spending) to re-ignite a moribund global economy has become a major concern of the international financial institutions, central banks and many government finance ministries.

3 Similarly, Canada's labour market reported 200,000 new jobs created in 2016, reported as a sign of a fully recovered and rapidly growing economy. Only in passing was it noted that just over 2/3rds of these were part-time, low-paid, insecure and mostly in the service sector (http://www.cbc.ca/news/business/jobs-statistics-canada-january-1.3975643).

4 Similar arguments have been made about the need to prioritize certain 'indivisible' human rights over others, based on ethical reasoning (notably the 'capabilities approach' developed by Amartya Sen and Martha Nussbaum) and an analysis of contradictions within them similar to those within the SDGs.

5 Perhaps because it is less beholden to the oil industry, 'decisionist' China since the 2008 financial crisis has provided proportionately larger sums than most European or North American countries into 'green energy' as part of its economic stimulus program (REF: https://www.theguardian.com/business/2017/jan/05/china-invest-renewable-fuel-2020-energy). One result of this was the relocation to China of a number of US and EU firms producing solar panels or wind turbines, followed by trade disputes over China's (and also India's) 'trade-distorting' subsidies. Despite at least six such trade disputes being initiated against subsidies or local sourcing requirements for renewable energy, there have been no disputes against the estimated $2.9 trillion in government production and consumption subsidies directed towards more health and environmentally destructive fossil fuels.

6 This is not to say that alternative energy sources are free of negative environmental externalities (REF: http://www.theglobeandmail.com/opinion/the-darker-side-of-solar-power/article24649804/; see also: http://svtc.org/our-work/solar/), which only underscores the importance of reducing energy demand, and not merely altering its source. One of the energy targets does call for a doubling in "the global rate of improvement in energy efficiency", although without reference to either an absolute cap on energy supply or a measure of its equitable global distribution.

7 The following section is adapted from Labonté, 2017: Labonté, R., "Health Promotion in an Age of Normative Equity and Rampant Inequality," International Journal of Health Policy and Management (2016), 5(12), 675-82; http://www.ijhpm.com/article_3243_9cfe55f382f6c9876bd955b41b2c9007.pdf

8 Increased production requires technological development (another of SDG 2's targets), begging the question: Where will the huge numbers of people presently earning their livelihoods in agriculture find employment once the low-income world experiences the same productivity miracle as American farmers did over the past two centuries?

9 Goal 5 in its re-statement of "universal access to sexual and reproductive health" importantly references the Beijing Platform for Action, which does recognize the hazards of unsafe abortion and the importance of access to safe abortion in countries where it is legal, a topic on which Goal 3 is curiously silent.

10 Or, as a commentary on the universality of the SDGs, argues, countries must attend not only to progressing through the goals and targets within their own borders, but must ensure that their own actions do not imperil other countries' abilities to meet the targets. This implies taking action commensurate to the degree to which they contribute to the problem globally; and a high level of ambition for HICs in reducing their consumption/production in order for LICs and LMICs to increase theirs

(REF: https://www.iisd.org/blog/reporting-sustainable-development-goals-challenges-oecd-countries-part-2-universality).

References

Adams, B, & Martens, J 2015, *Fit for whose purpose? Private funding and corporate influence in the United Nations*. Bonn, Germany: Global Policy Forum. Retrieved from https://sustainabledevelopment. un.org/content/documents/2101Fit_for_whose_purpose_online.pdf

Bauman, Z 2016, How Neoliberalism Prepared The Way For Donald Trump. Retrieved 23 March, 2017, from https://www.socialeurope.eu/2016/11/how-neoliberalism-prepared-the-way-for-donald-trump/

Blouin, C 2007, Trade policy and health: from conflicting interests to policy coherence. *Bulletin of the World Health Organization*, *85*(3), 169(5)

Bond, Patrick 2015 UN Development Goals Replaced by New "Distraction Gimmicks" | Opinion | teleSUR English. Retrieved March 23, 2017, from http://www.telesurtv. net/english/opinion/UN-Development-Goals-Replaced-by-New-Distraction-Gimmicks-20150925-0033.html

Caldbick, S, Labonte, R, Mohindra, K S, & Ruckert, A 2014, Globalization and the rise of precarious employment: the new frontier for workplace health promotion. *Global Health Promotion*, *21*(2), 23–31. https://doi.org/10.1177/1757975913514781

Cobham, A 2015, 1 June, IMF: developing countries' BEPS revenue losses exceed $200 billion » Uncounted. Retrieved March 30, 2017, from http://uncounted. org/2015/06/01/imf-developing-countries-beps-revenue-losses-exceed-200-billion/

Denyer, S. 2016, 1 July, Richest nations fail to agree on deadline to phase out fossil fuel subsidies – The Washington Post. *The Washington Post*. Retrieved from https://www.washingtonpost. com/world/richest-nations-fail-to-agree-on-deadline-to-phase-out-fossil-fuel-subsidies/2016/07/01/7db563fb-42f0-46c8-bea4-2fcfc0f48c69_story. html?utm_term=.2aad2abf1fd4

Doane, D 2017, 21 January, The global goals need optimism. So how can we meet them in Trump's world? | Deborah Doane | Global Development Professionals Network | The Guardian. Retrieved 8 May, 2017, from https://www.theguardian.com/global-development-professionals-network/2017/jan/21/reality-2017-world-lacks-hope-global-goals-require

Doctors Without Borders 2017, The G20 and global health: A global responsibility to implement the Sustainable Development Goals. Retrieved from http://venro. org/uploads/tx_igpublikationen/Venro-MSF_G20_Positionpaper-final.pdf

Engebretsen, E, Heggen, K, & Ottersen, O P 2017, The Sustainable Development Goals: ambiguities of accountability. *The Lancet*, *389*(10067), 365. https://doi.org/10.1016/S0140-6736(17)30152-6

Farrukah Khan 2016, 13 December, The SDG Story: An Insider Account of How it all Came About. Retrieved 23 March, 2017, from http://impakter.com/sdg-story-insider-account-came/

Held, D 2017, 29 January 29, Broken politics: from 9/11 to the present. Retrieved May 8, 2017, from https://www.opendemocracy. net/david-held/broken-politics-from-911-to-present

Hickel, J 2016, The true extent of global poverty and hunger: Questioning the good news narrative of the Millennium Development Goals. *Third World Quarterly*, 1–19. https://doi.org/10.1080/01436597.2015.1109439

Hicks and Devaraj 2015, The Myth and the Reality of Manufacturing in America. Retrieved 29 March, 2017, from http://projects.cberdata.org/reports/MfgReality.pdf

ICTSD 2017, 2 February, Least Developed Countries Propose New Caps on Trade-Distorting Farm Subsidies at WTO | International Centre for Trade and Sustainable Development. *Bridges*. Retrieved from http://www.ictsd.org/bridges-news/bridges/news/least-developed-countries-propose-new-caps-on-trade-distorting-farm

International Labor Organization 2017, Decent work. Retrieved 8 May, 2017, from http://www.ilo.org/global/topics/decent-work/lang--en/index.htm

International Labour Organization 2017, World Employment and Social Outlook – Trends 2017 – Executive summary – wcms_540899.

pdf. Retrieved March 29, 2017, from http://www.ilo.org/wcmsp5/groups/public/---dgreports/---dcomm/---publ/documents/publication/wcms_540899.pdf

Jackson, T 2009, *Prosperity Without Growth: Economics for a Finite Planet.* London and Virginia: Earthscan. Retrieved from https://www.google.ca/#q=Prosperity+Without+Growth

Karanikolos, M, Mladovsky, P, Cylus, J, Thomson, S, Basu, S, Stuckler, D, ... McKee, M n.d., Financial crisis, austerity, and health in Europe. *Lancet, 381*, 1323–1331.

Kishimoto, S, Lobina, E, & Petitjean, O (Eds.) 2015, *Our public water future: The global experience with remunicipalisation.* Amsterdam, London, Paris, Cape Town and Brussels: Transnational Institute (TNI), Public Services International Research Unit (PSIRU), Multinationals Observatory, Municipal Services Project (MSP), European Federation of Public Service Unions (EPSU). Retrieved from http://www.municipalservicesproject.org/sites/municipalservicesproject.org/files/publications/Kishimoto-Lobina-Petitjean_Our-Public-Water-Future-Global-Experience-Remunicipalisation_April2015_FINAL.pdf

Koivusalo, M, Labonte, R, Wibulpolprasert, S, & Kanchanachitra, S 2013, Globalization and policy space for health, and a HIAP approach. In K Leppo, O Ollila, S Pena, M Wismar, & S Cook (Eds.), *Health in All Policies, Helsinki: Ministry of Social Affairs and Health* (pp. 81–103). Finland: UNRISD.

Labonte, R 2016, Health Promotion in an Age of Normative Equity and Rampant Inequality. *IJHPM, 5*(12), 675–682.

Labonte, R, Baum, F, & Sanders, D 2015, Poverty, justice and health. In R Detels, C Tan, Q Karim, & M Guilliford (Eds.), *Oxford Textbook of Public Health.* Oxford: Oxford University Press.

Labonté, R, Schram, A, & Ruckert, A 2016, The Trans-Pacific Partnership Agreement and health: few gains, some losses, many risks. *Globalization and Health, 12*, 25. https://doi.org/10.1186/s12992-016-0166-8

Lei Ravelo, J 2016, 22 November, CSOs celebrate UHC indicator win. Retrieved 8 May, 2017, from https://www.devex.com/news/csos-celebrate-uhc-indicator-win-89207

McCulloch, N, & Pacillo, G 2011, The Tobin tax:

a review of the evidence. *IDS Research Reports, 2011*(68), 1–77.

McDonald, C 2015, 16 June, How many Earths do we need? Retrieved from http://www.bbc.com/news/magazine-33133712

Mezger, E 2017, 2 February, Europe's Perfect Economy? What The European Working Conditions Survey Tells Us About Germany. Retrieved 8 May, 2017, from https://www.socialeurope.eu/2017/02/europes-perfect-economy-european-working-conditions-survey-tells-us-germany/

Millennium Development Goals and Beyond 2013, We can end Poverty. United Nations. Retrieved from http://www.un.org/millenniumgoals/pdf/Goal_1_fs.pdf

Nunes, A R, Lee, K, & O'Riordan, T 2016, The importance of an integrating framework for achieving the Sustainable Development Goals: the example of health and well-being. *BMJ Global Health, 1*(3), e000068. https://doi.org/10.1136/bmjgh-2016-000068

O'Grady, S 2016, 24 September, Should we axe the United Nations? *Independent.* Retrieved from http://www.independent.co.uk/news/world/should-we-axe-the-united-nations-a7327696.html

Ostry, Loungani, Furceri 2016, Neoliberalism: Oversold? *Finance & Development, Volume 53*, 1–4.

Oxfam 2015, 2 December, Extreme carbon inequality: Why the Paris climate deal must put the poorest, lowest emitting and most vulnerable people first. Retrieved May 8, 2017, from https://www.oxfam.org/sites/www.oxfam.org/files/file_attachments/mb-extreme-carbon-inequality-021215-en.pdf

Oxfam 2017, An Economy for the 99%. Oxfam. Retrieved from https://www.oxfam.org/sites/www.oxfam.org/files/file_attachments/bp-economy-for-99-percent-160117-en.pdf

Polaski, Sandra 2006, Winners and Losers: Impact of the DOHA round on developing countries. Retrieved 30 March, 2017, from zotero://attachment/6303/

PRB 2011, August, The Effect of Girls' Education on Health Outcomes: Fact Sheet. Retrieved 8 May, 2017, from http://www.prb.org/Publications/Media-Guides/2011/girls-education-fact-sheet.aspx

Ross, S 2015, 6 April, Why is productivity an important concept in economics? Retrieved 29

March, 2017, from http://www.investopedia.com/ask/answers/040615/why-productivity-important-concept-economics.asp

Ruckert, A, & Labonte, R 2017, Health inequities in the age of austerity: The need for social protection policies. *Social Science and Medicine*, 1–6.

Ruckert, A, Schram, A, Labonte, R, Miller, B, Friel, S, Gleeson, D, & Thow, A-M 2017, Policy coherence, health and the sustainable development goals: a health impact assessment of the Trans-Pacific Partnership, *27*(1), 86–96.

Shaohua Chen and Martin Ravallion 2012, *Data and methods Global poverty measures Urban-rural poverty measures – GlobalPovertyUpdate-MartinR-SydneyLecture-July2012.pdf*. Retrieved from http://siteresources.worldbank.org/DEC/Resources/GlobalPovertyUpdate-MartinR-SydneyLecture-July2012.pdf

The Economist 2015, Development: The 169 commandments | The Economist. Retrieved 23 March, 2017, from http://www.economist.com/news/leaders/21647286-proposed-sustainable-development-goals-would-be-worse-useless-169-commandments

The Graduate Institute Geneva 2015, 16 November, Margaret Chan: "Universal Healthcare Key to SDG Achievement." Retrieved 8 May, 2017, from http://graduateinstitute.ch/home/relations-publiques/news-at-the-institute/news-archives.html/_/news/corporate/2015/margaret-chan-universal-healthca

The World Bank 2016, Poverty Overview. Retrieved 24 March, 2017, from http://www.worldbank.org/en/topic/poverty/overview

The World We Want n.d., Visualizing People's Voices. Retrieved 8 May, 2017, from http://millionvoices-data.worldwewant2015.org/

United Nations 2015, Transforming Our World by 2030: A New Agenda for Global Action. United Nations. Retrieved from https://sustainabledevelopment.un.org/content/documents/7261Post-2015%20Summit%20-%202%20June%202015.pdf

United Nations Conference on Trade and Development 2013, November, Growth and Poverty Eradication: Why Addressing Inequality Matters. UNCTAD. Retrieved from http://unctad.org/en/PublicationsLibrary/presspb2013d4_en.pdf

Van der Zee, B. 2016, 9 May, The missing development trillions: welcome to the debate, *The Guardian*. Retrieved from http://www.theguardian.com/global-development-professionals-network/2016/may/09/missing-dev

WCED 1987, *Our Common Future*. Oxford: Oxford University Press.

Whitmee, S, Haines, A, Beyrer, C, Boltz, F, Capon, A, de Souza Dias, B F, & Ezeh, A 2015, Safeguarding human health in the Anthropocene epoch: report of The Rockefeller Foundation – Lancet Commission on planetary health. *Lancet*, *386*(10007), 1973–2028.

Winship, M 2016, 4 February, Naomi Klein: "There are no non-radical options left before us" – Salon.com. Retrieved 8 May, 2017, from http://www.salon.com/2016/02/04/naomi_klein_there_are_no_non_radical_options_left_before_us_partner/

Woodward, D 2015, Incrementum ad absurdum: global growth, inequality and poverty eradication in a carbon-constrained world. *World Economic Review, 4*, 43–62.

A2 | 'LEAVE NO ONE BEHIND'
– ARE SDGs THE WAY FORWARD?

In September 2015, the UN General Assembly adopted a resolution on the 17 Sustainable Development Goals (SDGs) of the 2030 Agenda for Sustainable Development, of which Social Development Goal 3 (SDG3) – "seek[ing] to ensure health and well-being for all, at every stage of life" – is an essential part. The SDG document recognizes that health and well-being is part of a global and integrated approach, based on development strategies that preserve the planet, and on socially inclusive and sustainable economic growth. The document pledges that *"No one will be left behind"* and underlines that "[T]his new universal Agenda...seek[s] to realize the human rights of all ...They are integrated and indivisible, and balance the three dimensions of sustainable development: the economic, social and environmental."

The fact that all governments subscribe to such an ambitious plan is important. However, for the SDG goals to be translated into real action the proposed strategies need to be evaluated in terms of the important constraints that have to be overcome to move forward.

To evaluate how this agenda, at least in some essential parts, can be realized by the proposed deadline of 2030, a first and vital step is a reality check. Crucial to that is the proposed comprehensive approach which aims "to address the challenges and commitment effectively", and acknowledges that "eradicating poverty in all its forms and dimensions, combating inequality within and among countries, preserving the planet, creating sustained, inclusive and sustainable economic growth and fostering social inclusion are linked to each other and are interdependent." Moreover, it is important that the need for a commitment "to mak[e)] fundamental changes in the way that our societies produce and consume goods and services", is understood.

How realistic is the proposed strategy for change? Former UN/WHO official Jan Vandemoortele criticizes the SDGs as: "[A]n agenda that sidesteps universal challenges such as growing inequalities", and challenges its proclaimed universal scope. "These omissions are not due to an oversight; they are intentional. Regulating the food industry, financial sector and labor market...do not quite fit within the dominant economic narrative and do not rank high as priorities of most governments". (Vandemoortele, 2016).

An agenda that sidesteps universal challenges such as growing inequalities and obesity cannot claim to be universal in scope. These omissions are not due to an oversight; they are intentional. Regulating the food industry, financial

---

Box A2.1: The SDG agenda

"PEOPLE: We are determined to end poverty and hunger, in all their forms and dimensions, and to ensure that all human beings can fulfill their potential in dignity and equality and in a healthy environment.

"PLANET: We are determined to protect the planet from degradation, including through sustainable consumption and production, sustainably managing its natural resources and taking urgent action on climate change, so that it can support the needs of the present and future generations.

"PROSPERITY: We are determined to ensure that all human beings can enjoy prosperous and fulfilling lives and that economic, social and technological progress occurs in harmony with nature.

"PEACE: We are determined to foster peaceful, just and inclusive societies, which are free from fear and violence. There can be no sustainable development without peace and no peace without sustainable development.

"PARTNERSHIP: We are determined to mobilize the means required to implement this Agenda through a revitalized Global Partnership for Sustainable Development, based on a spirit of strengthened global solidarity, focused in particular on the needs of the poorest and most vulnerable and with the participation of all countries, all stakeholders and all people."

---

sector and labour market—to address obesity and inequality—do not quite fit within the dominant economic narrative and do not rank high as priorities of most governments. Instead, the SDGs conveniently focus on ending extreme poverty and hunger.

In the area of health and well-being for all, the SDGs do offer a more comprehensive framework than the Millennium Development Goals. Nevertheless, to really implement the proposed changes, vested interests will have to be countered, and radical new choices will have to be made. Therefore, this agenda cannot be conducted solely by governments. It must involve social organizations, civil society, academics, community representatives and citizens' assemblies. Without dedicated champions, without a 'struggle for real change', these global targets will remain empty words.

Fundamental flaws and contradictions in the pledge that no one will be left behind

The SDGs were severely criticized when they were proclaimed. *The Economist* called the 169 proposed targets "sprawling and misconceived", "unfeasibly expensive" at US$ 2–3 trillion per year, and so unlikely to be realized that they amount to "worse than useless" – "a betrayal of the world's poorest people" (The Economist, 2015). Moreover, the SDGs were ridiculed as "no targets left behind" during a high-profile meeting of Gates Foundation partners (Paulson, 2015).

In defence of the SDGs it is argued that poverty is a complex problem, and that the elimination of poverty will require much more than charity: It will require comprehensive strategies to reduce inequality, combat climate change, strengthen labour rights and eliminate Western agricultural subsidies. The fundamental challenge, which both major proponents and opponents of SDGs tend to gloss over, is that realizing these goals is 'impossible' without changing the fundamental flaws in the current economic and political architecture of the globe.

The SDG document reflects the emerging comprehensive approach to health and well-being, from attending to healthcare needs at the individual level to addressing health in all its dimensions – social, political, economic and environmental. The document articulates the need to achieve "harmony with nature"; the development of "sustainable patterns of production and consumption"; and a halt to the loss of biodiversity, overfishing, deforestation and desertification.

Such a position, however, is far removed from the current paradigm where pursuit of endless industrial growth is producing poverty, destroying the planet and threatening the basis of our existence. This is where the SDGs are – as some would argue – fatally flawed, because embedded in the SDGs is a fundamental contradiction. The SDGs propose growth strategies that seek to perpetuate the current neoliberal model – ever-increasing levels of extraction, production and consumption. An entire goal, Goal 8, is devoted to export-oriented growth, following the existing neoliberal models (Jason, 2015).

This contradictory relationship to growth extends to the SDGs' approach to global poverty. The Zero Draft promotes growth as the main solution to poverty. But of all the income generated by global GDP growth between 1999 and 2008, the poorest 60 per cent of humanity received only 5 per cent. Jason Hickel, an anthropologist at the London School of Economics, has calculated that without fundamental changes in the globe's economic architecture it would take 207 years to eliminate poverty with this strategy, the global economy would need to expand 175 times its present size (Hickel, 2015).

Clearly this is an impossible aspiration. Even if such immense growth were possible, it would drive climate change to catastrophic levels and rapidly reverse any gains against poverty. The SDGs fail to accept that mass impoverishment is the product of extreme wealth accumulation and overconsumption by a few, which entails processes of enclosure, extraction and exploitation. The SDGs avoid addressing these deeper causes. For example, the problems with the structural adjustment programmes, the greatest single cause of poverty since colonialism, imposed by the World Bank, the IMF and the EU (in Greece) are never mentioned in the SDGs. A vague request to "respect each country's policy space" is made, but, as the Greek crisis reminds us, the world's biggest creditors are not likely to care much for national sovereignty when their finances are at stake.

Instead of tackling this crucial issue, the SDGs do the opposite: Goal 17.10 calls for more trade liberalization and more power for the World Trade Organization, and support for bilateral trade deals — for example, the Trans-Pacific Partnership; Transatlantic Trade and Investment Partnership; and Trade in Services Agreement. And instead of demanding an end to financial speculation that has caused food prices to spike since 2007, pushing 150 million into hunger, the SDGs ask weakly that we "ensure the proper functioning of food commodity markets".

At no moment does the SDG document refer to the need for a strong regulation of the financial markets. Goal 17.13 speaks vaguely of the need to "enhance global macroeconomic stability" through "policy coordination", with no specific targets. Tax evasion and avoidance drain developing countries of US$ 1.7 trillion each year. No word about it. Then there's debt service, which drains another US$ 700 billion per year; instead of demanding cancellation, the SDGs call for "debt financing, debt relief and debt restructuring, as appropriate", which specifically means that debts will not be cancelled (Jason, 2015).

Following the weakening of a nation state driven structure of global governance, as evident from the weakening of the United Nations and its specialized agencies, the World Economic Forum's "Global Redesign Initiative" report proposed a transformation of the UN into a big public–private partnership. The report, *inter alia*, proposes: "Nation states and intergovernmental structures will continue to play a central role in global decision-making. However, those institutions must be adapted to today's needs and conditions if they want to preserve their use and, hence, legitimacy. They must begin by more clearly conceiving of themselves as constituting just part of the wider global

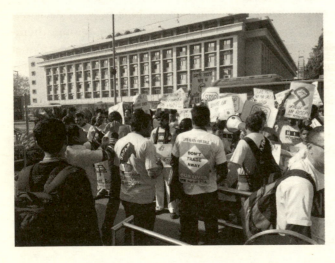

Image A2.1 SDG goal 17.10 supports trade deals: Protests in 2014 in India against regional trade agreement (Delhi Network of Positive People)

cooperation system that the world needs. In fact, they should work explicitly to cultivate such a system by anchoring the preparation and implementation of their decisions more deeply in the processes of interaction with interdisciplinary and multistakeholder networks of relevant experts and actors". The report further argues: "…proposals will be based on the notion of the shared responsibility of all stakeholders for global citizenship. Public–private partnerships will be a core element of future governance systems. In short, this initiative will not necessarily represent a consensus of all stakeholders and individuals participating in it, but will represent the most comprehensive thinking and brainstorming on our global future" (World Economic Forum, 2010).

We can already see global governance being increasingly reoriented to allow direct participation of private actors alongside states (see Chapters D1 and D2). As a consequence democratic representation is weakened in favour of private commercial interests. Given this context powerful interests (rich countries, corporations and private foundations) may well view the SDG process as a step towards the 'multi-stakeholderization' of global governance. We wait for first 'philanthropic entrepreneur' to claim his seat at the UN!

The notion of multi-stakeholder partnerships is embedded in the SDGs. SDG 17 includes the following targets:

"Multi-stakeholder partnerships
- Enhance the global partnership for sustainable development, complemented by multi-stakeholder partnerships that mobilize and share knowledge, expertise, technology and financial resources, to support the achievement of the sustainable development goals in all countries, in particular developing countries
- Encourage and promote effective public, public-private and civil society partnerships, building on the experience and resourcing strategies of partnerships"

In lieu of providing the private sector a seat on the high table of decision-making do the SDGs ask corporations and private investors to commit themselves to binding commitments designed to end poverty and save the planet or propose some accountability mechanisms? Clearly they do not – the SDGs merely 'encourage' corporations to be reasonable! Goal 12.6: "encourage(s) companies, especially large and transnational companies, to adopt sustainable practices and to integrate sustainability information into their reporting cycle".

What the SDGs, perhaps deliberately, fail to acknowledge is that the mindless pursuit of GDP growth is not the solution to poverty, and surely not a solution to the ecological crisis. It is the primary cause. Human progress should be measured in terms of more fairness, more equality, more well-being, more sharing, to the benefit of the vast majority of humanity. The SDGs fail us on this. They offer to tinker with the global economic system in a bid to make it all seem a bit less violent. But this is not a time for tinkering (Schuftan, 2016).

What is sustainable? The elephant in the room

While the term 'sustainable' has become a buzzword in political, economic and development circles, it has become largely meaningless. Few efforts to achieve sustainable development have seriously done so. The suggestion that more people-friendly and environmentally-friendly practices can simply be incorporated into our daily lives to achieve sustainability is not valid. If this world has to move towards sustainability, wealthy nations must massively reduce the extent of material consumption and waste of resources. Gary Leech calls the blindness of this reality "the elephant in the room" in discussions on sustainable development (Leech, 2015).

This is not only about 'willingness'. The driving force of 'our' capitalist production system is profit. And a central capitalist law is the increasing concentration of profit and financial power. In 'Capital in the Twenty-First Century', Thomas Piketty explains that the return to capital is persistently higher than economic growth (The Economist, 4 January 2014). Wealth piles up faster than growth in output or incomes. There can exceptions, when societal counter power (through working class organizations) forces redistribution mechanisms. This was the case in the post–Second World War period in parts of Europe when social struggle in West Europe and the existence of a strong USSR (combined with a period of extraordinary economic growth) led to a more egalitarian interregnum. But, as Piketty explains, this was an exception. And it was the result of a worldwide situation of people's struggles: decolonization of the South, socialism in the East and strong workers' movements in the West.

The need to constantly expand the production and consumption of goods, and the increasing concentration of financial power, is not only in contradiction with sustainable development, it will oppose it 'by all means'. Under uncontrolled capitalism profit comes before people, before the climate, before the planet. Continuing to 'cohabit with the elephant'– based on solemnly proclaimed agreements – means neglecting these facts. Alternative strategies will have to be based on a development of a broad democratic counter-power, in defence of the right to health and well-being for all, in defence of humanity, and in defence of planet Earth.

In this, the realities of wealthy nations (high human development and high ecological footprint) and poor nations (low human development and low ecological footprint) are directly linked. The unsustainably high per capita ecological footprints of wealthy nations, are achieved by wealthy nations consuming other peoples' share of the planet's resources. As a result, the resources of poor countries are exploited not for the benefit of local populations but to satiate the consumption needs of wealthy nations. If we are serious about achieving sustainable development, we have to address this elephant in the room: the better off must dramatically diminish their levels of material consumption, which contravenes the very logic that drives the capitalist system

(Leech, 2015). A failure to implement such systemic change means that all well-intentioned efforts to achieve sustainability will ultimately fail.

The search for a comprehensive approach

For decades, two opposing systems have dominated the health policy debate: the comprehensive healthcare approach, with the 1978 Alma Ata Declaration as its cornerstone, and the profit-making model, emphasizing the role of the private sector. Neoliberal policies create a growing contradiction between increasing health needs and the pursuit of private profits. Market-oriented health reforms pursue the provision of healthcare in a competitive growth model. Not well-being but profit is the primary driving force. The saturation of markets in rich countries leads to pressures towards further liberalization, deregulation and privatization. Not just the 'traditional' economic sectors are included in these programmes; health, education and other social services are also covered in the profit-making model.

Besides ensuring access to care, the right to health includes an adequate strategy towards securing the social determinants of health. A renewed attention to the importance of the social determinants and corresponding strategies for advancing health as a central national objective can be the only way forward. The 2008 report of the Commission on Social Determinants of Health (CSDH) has mentioned that "inequities of power, money and resources have to be tackled" (WHO 2008a). The CSDH has appealed for political action, insisting that "community or civil society action on health inequities cannot be separated from the responsibility of the state to guarantee a comprehensive set of rights and ensure the fair distribution of essential material and social goods among population groups" (Marmot et al., 2008, pp. 1661–69). The strong development of a rights-based approach to health underscores this crucial role of the state in respecting, protecting and fulfilling the right to (the highest attainable state of) health (De Vos et al., 2009, pp. 23–35). Until today this remains a central issue and a largely unfinished business.

In different parts of the world, comprehensive and complementary approaches – embedded in social and cultural traditions – are being developed. An open exchange of aims and objectives and empowering strategies could enrich healthcare concepts, practices and strategies in different parts of the world.

Integrated health and welfare, with priority for 'VIP' clients The Finnish social protection model is supported by a large and strong public sector funded by taxation. Residence-based health services are complemented with a broad social welfare approach, with a relatively high level of various kinds of social benefits. Nevertheless, Finnish health workers acknowledge that even today the challenge is to decrease the differences in health outcomes on the basis of gender and social class. There are insufficiencies with regard to accessibility of services and the coordination of patient care, while loneliness and safety issues at home remain important concerns.

Currently a new integrated social and healthcare model is being tried out, with further integration of health and welfare services through a newly developed 'welfare centre' concept. The aim is to have a single entry point for health and comprehensive well-being, focusing on patient needs; easy access to 'walk-in' quality services; strengthened cooperation and companionship among all professionals; integrated client processes from the first contact, with focus on VIP-clients (defined as the 5 to 10 per cent of the population needing frequent and different kinds of health and social support). This concept is part of a broader 'health in all policies approach' whereby "intersectoral action, healthy public policies and environmental sustainability are identified as central elements for the promotion of health, the achievement of health equity and the realization of health as a human right" (WHO 2013).

Buenvivir, a social philosophy that inspires the South American social movement
The 'buenvivir' (good living) approach proposes that humans are only stewards of the Earth and its resources, and therefore individual rights are subjugated to those of communities and nature.

Ecuador is building on its indigenous past by incorporating the concept of 'sumakkawsay' – or buenvivir – into its approach to development. Rooted in the 'cosmovision' of the Quechua peoples of the Andes, sumakkawsay describes a way of doing things that is community-centred, ecologically balanced and culturally-sensitive. A far cry from the market-is-king model of capitalism, it inspired the recently revised Ecuadorian Constitution, which now reads: "We... hereby decide to build a new form of public coexistence, in diversity and in harmony with nature, to achieve the good way of living."

Buenvivir loosely translates as 'good living' or 'well living'. But for Eduardo Gudynas, a leading scholar on the subject, both these translations sit too close to Western notions of well-being or welfare: "These are not equivalents at all. With buenvivir, the subject of well-being is not [about the] individual, but the individual in the social context of their community and in a unique environmental situation" (Balch 2013).

While concepts and reality might still be two very different things, similar thinking is inspiring other social movements across South America. The link to other indigenous belief systems, such as those of the Aymara peoples of Bolivia, the Quichua of Ecuador and the Mapuche of Chile and Argentina, is explicit. Nevertheless, Eduardo Gudynas clearly states that "it certainly doesn't require a return to some sort of indigenous, pre-Colombian past" and "[i]t is equally influenced by Western critiques [of capitalism] over the last 30 years, especially from the field of feminist thought and environmentalism."

The future starts today

The discussion on the road ahead remains open. Nevertheless, it is clear that change will not occur by itself. It will be the result of the clash of opposing forces, in which we clearly position ourselves on the side of 'well-being for all' and a healthy planet, and against profit for a few. Under which political, economic, social and environmental conditions will health and well-being for all be realizable in the near future? How to ensure strong democratic governments? How to strengthen people's participation at all levels? Under which economic conditions will responsible industries become a 'normal thing'? The debate continues. And we need to mobilize.

References

'All men are created unequal: revisiting an old argument about the impact of capitalism', *The Economist*, 4 January 2014, http://www.economist.com/news/finance-and-economics/21592635-revisiting-old-argument-about-impact-capitalism-all-men-are-created

Balch, O 2013, 'Buenvivir: the social philosophy inspiring movements in South America', *The Guardian*, 4 February, https://www.theguardian.com/sustainable-business/blog/buen-vivir-philosophy-south-america-eduardo-gudynas

De Vos, P, De Ceukelaire, W, Malaise, G, Pérez, D, Lefèvre, P& Van der Stuyft, P 2009, 'Health through people's empowerment: A rights-based approach toparticipation', *Health and Human RightsJournal*, vol. 11, no. 1, pp. 23–35, https://www.ncbi.nlm.nih.gov/pubmed/20845848

Hickel, J 2015, 'It will take 100 years for the world's poorest people to earn $1.25 a day', *The Guardian*, 30 March, https://www.theguardian.com/global-development-professionals-network/2015/mar/30/it-will-take-100-years-for-the-worlds-poorest-people-to-earn-125-a-day.

Jason, H 2015, 'The Problem with saving the world: the UN's new Sustainable Development Goals aim to save the world without transforming it', *Jacobin*, 8 August, www.jacobinmag.com/2015/08/global-poverty-climate-change-sdgs

Leech, G 2015, 'The elephant in the room: capitalism and sustainable development', *Counterpunch*, 16 October, http://www.counterpunch.org/2015/10/16/the-elephant-in-the-room-capitalism-and-sustainable-development>

Marmot, M, Friel, S, Bell, R, Houweling, T A & Taylor, S 2008, Closing the gap in a generation: health equity through action on the social determinants of health', *The Lancet*, vol. 372, pp. 1661–69, https://www.ncbi.nlm.nih.gov/pubmed/18994664

Paulson, T 2015, 'Gates Foundation rallies the troops to attack UN development goals', *Humanosphere*, 6 May, http://www.humanosphere.org/world-politics/2015/05/gates-foundation-rallies-the-troops-to-attack-un-development-goals

Schuftan, C 2016, 'Human Rights: food for the urgent application of a thought', *Human Rights Reader 398. The Social Medicine Portal*, 22 October, http://www.socialmedicine.org/?s=Human+Rights+Reader+398

'The 169 commandments: the proposed sustainable development goals would be worse than useless', *The Economist*, 26 March 2015', www.economist.com/news/leaders/21647286-proposed-sustainable-development-goals-would-be-worse-useless-169-commandments

Vandemoortele, J 2016, 'SDGs: the tyranny of an acronym?' *Impakter*, 13 September, http://impakter.com/sdgs-tyranny-acronym

WHO 2008a, *Closing the gap in a generation: health equity through action on the social determinants of health*, Commission on Social Determinants of Health, http://www.who.int/social_determinants/thecommission/finalreport/en/

WHO 2013, *The Helsinki statement on health in all policies*, The 8th Global Conference on

Health Promotion, Helsinki, Finland, 10–14 June 2013.

World Economic Forum 2010 '*Global Redesign Initiative: A visionary blueprint for meeting the challenges of the 21st century, A collaborative effort of all stakeholders of global society*'. Geneva, Switzerland. http://www.qatarconferences.org/economic/world/GRI_Executive_Summary.pdf

A3 | ADVANCES AND SETBACKS TOWARDS A SINGLE PUBLIC HEALTH SYSTEM IN LATIN AMERICA

In *Global Health Watch* (GHW4) we discussed the overall positive impact on public health after the installation of a number of progressive governments in Latin America (People's Health Movement 2014). These progressive governments were the product of previous social struggles motivated by the discontent against the neoliberal dispensation in several countries in the region. These struggles led to the ascent of several progressive governments which addressed the demand for redistribution policies and managed to somewhat improve the very serious situation of poverty and inequality prevailing in the region. They paved the way for an expansion of democracy, particularly with the emergence of some forms of direct democracy from below (though not uniformly so, especially in the work of trade unions). The new democratic governments managed to establish, to some degree, a set of policies based on social rights and citizenship.

One of the most notable features of these progressive governments was the promotion of a new model of regional integration that substantially changed regional geopolitics. For the first time, the defence ministries of the region met without the tutelage of the USA. The region also saw the creation of the Bolivarian Alliance for the Peoples of Our America (ALBA), the Union of South American Nations (UNASUR), and the Community of Latin American and Caribbean States (CELAC). On the economic front, these governments tried to create instruments of integration such as the Bank of the South (BancoSur).

At the same time, however, these movements and governments were unable to complete the task of dismantling the power of the old oligarchies which were remnants of the previous neoliberal regimes. Generally they also failed to fundamentally alter the previous economic models that were based on external dependency; thereby reproducing patterns of economic growth strongly based on the export of raw materials. Likewise, the proximity of many progressive movements to governments generated some degree of alienation from popular causes. Inexcusable cases of corruption in certain countries also provided avenues for the conservative right to mount attacks on the new governments. This was exacerbated by the fact that in order to survive in government alliances had to be forged with forces linked to the previous neoliberal order – leaving open the possibility that these forces would at some point corrupt, discredit and even betray openly the progressive governments. Further, the failure to honor commitments and the adoption of policies aligned to the previous neoliberal disposition, in some situations, undermined popular unity and had a serious demoralizing effect.

The neoliberal response

After the victory of the democratic movements a conservative offensive, which combined various institutional and insurrectional strategies to destabilize progressive governments, gained prominence. Techniques which turned the media and the economy into strategic battlegrounds were deployed. 'Soft' coups d'état were attempted in Honduras and Paraguay, and then applied on a larger scale in Brazil. In some countries pressure and blackmail were applied from within to neutralize some progressive governments, thus initiating a conservative restoration from within the national context: the most notable case is Peru, where Ollanta Humala – despite having won the elections with a progressive and anti-neoliberal proposal – applied neoliberal policies from the beginning of his government. This has also been the case of Chile and Uruguay, where the Frente Amplio Uruguayo and the Socialist Party of Chile – after being elected to government – have assumed centrist positions, far from their original principles.

The imperialist reaction to the new geopolitical scheme initiated in Latin America was clear and fast, aimed at regaining lost influence, and towards creating the conditions for a conservative restoration in the continent. This is an area of continuity in US foreign policy irrespective of change in government in the USA, with Latin America continuing to be viewed as the 'backyard' of the USA and a natural territory for the exercise of US influence.

It is instructive to note some key arguments advanced in the Geological Survey 2007–2017 of the United States Department of Science and Technology. The study, inter alia, identifies US weaknesses and shortages of strategic resources, particularly of minerals which are indispensable to maintain its military and technological supremacy. Specifically, the study notes that the USA is dependent on imports (of between 50 per cent and 100 per cent of its requirements) for 42 key materials that are indispensable to maintain its level of technological development. Most of these strategic resources are found in abundant quantities in the countries of the Latin American region (U.S. Geological Survey, 2007). The Geological Survey 2007–2017 argues that secured access to strategic resources is linked to national security[1]. Concurrently there has been a growing consensus within UNASUR that regional cooperation is necessary to guarantee the defence of strategic resources (Nolte, Wehner, 2012). The dispute over these strategic resources is one of the fundamental causes of the US effort to regain control of the region. Of course, there are also political reasons: primarily related to threat perceptions in the USA regarding the independent and anti-neoliberal positions advocated by alliances of Latin American countries – for example the opposition to the signing of the Free Trade Area of the Americas (FTAA) agreement from most countries of the region.

In the last few years counter coups have been staged against more than half of the earlier progressive governments of the region. Honduras, Paraguay and Brazil have experienced 'parliamentary coups'; the Left in Argentina suffered an electoral defeat, while Chile and Uruguay succumbed due to their own internal contradictions.

However, in some countries where the conservative restoration has taken place, and neoliberal measures and human rights violations have begun, protests and popular mobilizations are increasing. Thus we are witnessing an intensification of the struggle against neoliberalism. In the medium term a new wave of progressive governments can be envisaged: but the Left in the region need to draw appropriate lessons from the past so that previous errors are not repeated. A key lesson would be to be rid of the illusion that it is possible to redistribute wealth and expand democracy without confronting the power of capital. Progressive governments that come to power on an avowed anti-neoliberal platform need to recognize that their task is not to manage a capitalist State that reproduces itself permanently, but to transform it.

Challenges in transformation of the health system

The mere political decision to establish a universal public health system – egalitarian and with equitable access – is not enough. However, it is the starting point towards building a system that can safeguard the health of the people. Public health is a complex area with multiple dimensions and contradictions which makes it an equally complex arena of political struggle.

All Latin American countries had gone through neoliberal reforms that distorted in some measure their health systems. However, public health systems have been shaped by a different historical process in each country. In Mexico, for example, a public social security system – with its own facilities and salaried personnel – was built in the aftermath of the Mexican revolution. This system was able to provide health services to almost 90 per cent of the population. Public health institutions in Mexico have resisted neoliberal attacks and it has been difficult to dismantle the public system. In contrast in Brazil, despite a constitutional obligation for the State to guarantee the right to health through a public system, public health insurance covers only 25 per cent of the population.

With the significant exception of Cuba, the health sector in the region is subjected to the basic logic of capitalism. Under neoliberal globalization health is now an area where Capital tries to wrest from the State a new terrain for capitalist accumulation, since in economic terms it represents between 6 and 10 per cent of the GDP. On the one hand, there exists the traditional medical-industrial complex (i.e. the pharmaceutical industry, enterprises elated to medical technologies, and service providers). There is now an additional phenomenon – an emerging medical insurance industry which is a new form of Finance Capital (Laurell, n.d.).

Under neoliberalism the health sector was privatized based on the logic that state-run public services are inadequate and inefficient. This led to the prescription that health services must be opened up for market-based competition in order to improve quality and reduce costs. For the followers of this creed, it does not matter that empirical evidence contradicts this dogma. Paradoxically, supranational agencies pressure Latin American governments to adopt the US system of managed healthcare, while the US government has tried to change it because of its high costs (accounting for 19 per cent of the country's GDP), insufficient coverage and poor health outcomes.

The nature of the State, its policies and vision are critical in determining the health policy in a particular country. Broadly two forms of the State currently exist in the Latin American the region: the neoliberal State that seeks to reduce the role of the State in provision of welfare services (such as healthcare) to its citizens, and the Social Democratic State (which we identify here as 'progressive' or 'Leftist'). The latter, as we have discussed earlier, is under a sustained attack from conservative forces that seek to restore the earlier neoliberal policies. Nevertheless the progressive governments in Latin America have made important advances in social policies through the redistribution of wealth. This has also occurred in the realm of public health.

The progressive Latin American governments – Brazil, Venezuela, Ecuador, Bolivia, El Salvador and Argentina – have greatly increased access to health services for those in need. This has been accompanied by redistributive and universal social policies. Health policy in these countries has been based on the idea that it is the State's obligation to guarantee the right to health to all citizens through a public, comprehensive health system financed through public taxation. The specific institutional arrangements to achieve this have varied from country to country depending on the particular situation and the correlation of political forces in each case.

But it needs to be underlined that health is an area of struggle in the process to transform the State. Álvaro García Linera (Vice President of Bolivia) argues that public health is also linked to the ideological struggle for hegemony, and to the scope of the State's institutions. (García Linera, 2013). Mario Testa (Argentinean physician and one of the founders of ALAMES) notes that "the Latin American health specialists are the most frustrated professional group because we know perfectly what we have to do, but we have never been able to do it". He refers to the political-ideological confusion about what constitutes 'good medicine'. The most prevalent notion of 'good medicine' among the public, health professionals and politicians – including those on the left – is of an individual focused system that includes sophisticated technological interventions and state-of-the-art pharmaceutical products[2]. This position ignores the socio-historical determinants of health and disease, ignores the importance of education, promotion, prevention and even clinical

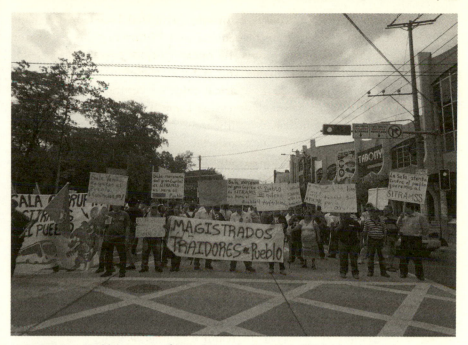

Image A3.1 Health is an area of struggle:Popular struggle in El Salvador against the Constitutional Chamber (Maria Zunega)

knowledge in medical practice. It is an ideology that is assiduously promoted by the medical-industrial-insurance complex.

There still exists a lack of clarity regarding the fundamental understanding that health is not a commodity or a consumer good, and that it does not have a private character; rather it is an attribute of social citizenship and a collective social right. One expression of this lack of clarity is that trade unions have not assumed the role of advocates of collective and social rights, but have negotiated private health insurance (Brazil) or the payment for private services (Venezuela) for their members. At the same time unions have opposed the creation of a single unified public health system, thus leading to persistence of social insurance through payments to a segmented health system.

It should also be noted that some strategies to rapidly expand access to health services have contributed to a new segmentation of the system. This is the case of the 'Barrio Adentro' policy in Venezuela, which was crucial to opening health services to millions of socially excluded people, but simultaneously created a parallel system to existing public services. Another structural as well as political problem is the process of decentralization by which the delivery of health services was handed over to local governments. A problem often encountered is that local governments may lack sufficient resources to guarantee the access to complex or highly specialized health services. Consequently, in some cases local governments have worked against the national health policy by promoting private health insurance and private health services providers due to their lack of resources.

These elements have nurtured an ideological counter-offensive that promotes the idea that the public health system is 'poor healthcare for the poor." In some cases, the legitimacy gained by increasing the span of the public health system has been reversed, particularly because of problems of managing such a large and rapidly expanding system designed to provide comprehensive healthcare services. This counter-offensive has been promoted and supported by the medical/industrial/insurance complex that aligns with forces oppose to the progressive governments.

The mechanisms for capitalist accumulation that still exist within the health sector under progressive governments are sought to be strengthened and expanded in the challenge being mounted against a unified public system. The most common strategy is the expansion of health plans or health insurance that attract patients with shorter waiting times for elective procedures and access to sophisticated medical technologies. This promotes a variety of regressive transfer of resources from the public to the private sector. Another ploy is to introduce new forms of 'public administration' to create internal or external health markets for healthcare services. In both cases, packages of restricted services, mandatory care protocols and quantitative performance measurement are introduced, regardless of their quality. Often these mechanisms are supported by public financing and the private sector is guaranteed a market for their services that is paid for by public revenue. As a result public resources are consumed to finance and support healthcare delivery by the private sector.

Cost of medical care is significantly affected because of the high cost of pharmaceuticals, medical devices and diagnostics. Institutional capacity needs to be developed to regulate the use of technology and its costs. Progressive governments have played an important role in this area by intervening international negotiations and trade agreements and by supporting national production of medicines and medical technologies.

The institutional space is the other major area of struggle for the transformation of the health system to guarantee the right to health. This transformation requires action from within. Public health programs should be constructed as a 'road map'. They must clarify the values, principles and objectives that would guide the transformation and should make their goals and objectives explicit. (Spinelli, 2012). The fundamental role of the Ministry of Health should be to improve health conditions and achieve universal and equal coverage and access to services. Neoliberal policies have led to financial cuts and privatization of public services, thus leading to demoralization in public institutions. While attempting to roll back neoliberal reforms in the health sector, there is a tendency to prioritize the survival of public institutions and the interests of workers. The latter can happen in isolation and not be linked with the role of public institutions in advancing the rights of people who seek healthcare. The challenge is to create a new set of institutional practices rooted in an ethics of public service, and characterized by fair and transparent labour relations. The aim should be to achieve a new institutional agreement through dialogue with workers, and to have a better understanding of the institutional dynamics.

In the process of transforming public institutions the strongest tensions are usually encountered in relation to the interaction with physicians and other health professionals. Physicians tend to consider themselves as the centre of the health system, even though the widespread commercialization and growth of corporate power in the health sector have displaced them from this role. They claim for themselves better working and economic conditions than for the rest of the staff and are reluctant to lose their privileges. The dialogue with them must be centred around the understanding of how the new institutional conditions are threatened by an aggressive commodification of health services. Another priority is a frontal attempt to combat corruption and nepotism in public institutions. Effective administrative measures are necessary as are transparent and accountable practices.

The material and institutional basis upon which of the progressive governments of Latin America tried to build a unified public health system – with universal access to the required health services – was generally very weak. Therefore, the strengthening and expansion of the public institution has been urgent. The new model of care that has been promoted is based on the model of Comprehensive Primary Health Care. However its meaning has not always been fully understood. The new model is not purely technical, but has an important component of transformation of the practices and conceptions of the main tasks related to provision of health services, where popular participation and social control play a central role.

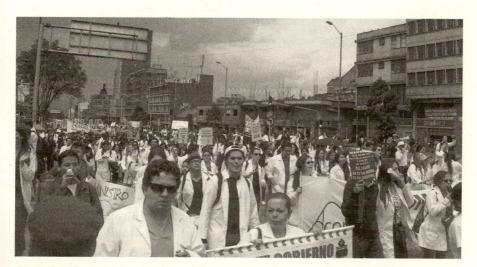

Image A3.2 Popular mobilisation in Bogota, Colombia, for a unified public health system (Mauricio Torres)

All the Latin American progressive governments were supported by sustained and cohesive social and political movements. This is reflected in the fact that the transformations of the public health systems have been accompanied in some countries by the development of institutionalized mechanisms of social control of public health services. Brazil is the most prominent in this respect, where through a constitutional mandate health councils were formed at the municipal, state and national levels. In Bolivia social organizations that have been instrumental in incorporating statutory provisions in the Constitution regarding the integration of a unified public health system. Strengthening and expanding popular participation and social control is, however, a complex path. It involves a process that strives to construct a new concept that replaces the old idea of 'good medicine' and promotes an understanding of health as an essential component of 'good living' – a life that includes dignity and in peace.

The new neoliberal governments and setbacks to the right to health

Among the first acts of neoliberal government that replaced progressive governments in Paraguay, Argentina and Brazil are those aimed at reversing the redistribution processes that led to the improvement of living conditions (particularly wages, education, health and civil liberties). The neoliberal regimes now aimed to disrupt the progress achieved on all fronts. In the health sector the goal is to again promote a market-based health system that includes private care packages informed by the logic of costs and benefits, and mediated by insurance companies, and to restore the development of human resources based on a model which forces workers to compete against each other to obtain the best private or public jobs available in the labour market. Users of the health system are sought to be transformed into mere consumers (purchasers of services) or conditional recipients of public charity funds and thus purchasers of the cheapest health packages.

In Paraguay, user fees for public services which were eliminated by the government of Fernando Lugo, have been re-established. President Cartes' Minister of Health argued that 75 percent of the Paraguayan population does not have any type of insurance and hence the health system must be reorganized. This meant reintroduction of user fees and quotas for limited sections of the population, and a mechanism of insurance to provide 'financial protection' to patients. As in many other countries where Universal Health Coverage (UHC) is being promoted, this will open the way for insurance companies and private service providers to profit from public resources. Under this new scheme, a set of 'benefit' packages are offered to the poor, while full services packages are designed for the rich (who can afford co-payments or co-insurance). The intent is clearly to return to a system that converts public health into a commercial activity, at the expense of people's health.

In Argentina, the progress towards a unified and free public health system during the governments of Néstor and Cristina Kirchner was limited. This was a consequence of the resistance offered by the social security plans managed by the workers' unions as the unions did not want to consolidate a unified and free public health system for the entire population. However there was progress in expanding primary level care and in training doctors – with a community focus and commitment – from less privileged sections in newly created universities and medical schools. When President Macri was voted to power, he issued a decree for the creation of a health insurance system (called CUS) which promoted, as in Mexico, Colombia, Peru, or Chile, a set of 'benefit' packages for the poor which essentially involve transfer of public funds into insurance companies and private service providers.

The use of terms 'insurance' and 'coverage' seeks indicate that provision of healthcare services is a contractual relationship and not a right; when, in fact, since the time of the Ramón Carrillo (Health Minister under President Perón) health has been recognized as a right in Argentina. The decree creating CUS provides a very limited budget that barely covers some benefits and excludes procedures that were earlier available free in the public system. Further, patients will need to prove that they are poor in order to be covered by the insurance package. Responding to these assaults on entitlements a social movement opposing the roll-out of CUS has been formed in Argentina[3].

A similar trend can be seen in Brazil under Temer's presidency. The new government has imposed budgetary cuts on education and health, directed specifically at subverting the SUS (Unified Health System) and public schools. The attack on SUS takes different forms. In an attempt to subvert the system from within, routine administrative measures have been delayed, resulting in shortages of medicines, frequent rotation of municipal health secretaries, lack of information, delay in the payment of wages and privatizations[4]. In the middle of this campaign against the SUS, Temer's government froze public funds for health and education (through an Amendment to the Constitution PEC/241), arguing that the current economic crisis in the country had been caused by an increase in spending on social services. This is a complete fabrication, since public spending on health through the Federal budget has remained constant at 1.6 per cent of GDP from 2002 to 2015, and the relative share of this expenditure of aggregate resources obtained from taxation has dropped from 10.5 per cent to 8.6 per cent in the same period (María Lucia Frizon Rizzoto, 2016).

Besides the PEC/241 amendment, another constitutional modification has been effected: 'The Unbundling of Union Collections Act' allows the government to use 30 per cent of taxes collected, that are supposed to be spent on education, health and social welfare, for other purposes. Estimates suggest that as a consequence of this Act there will be a further drop in public spending on health of 32 billion Reals. The Federal government is also asking the state governments to adopt the same decision at the local level as a condition for renegotiating their debts with the Federal government. In a move similar to what is being proposed in Argentina, the Brazilian Minister of Health, Ricardo Barros, is actively promoting the creation of popular health plans that are 'cheaper' insurance packages with 'benefits' for the poor. These packages will be managed by insurance companies and private service providers. The fundamental intention of these legal reforms is to undermine the universal, equitable and rights-based concept of a Unified Health System (SUS). They represent process of recommodification of public health. These measures are being actively opposed by popular social movements[5].

The changes in Latin American countries are not isolated examples. In many European countries public health systems are being dismantled while resistance mounts in these countries from peoples' and workers' organizations. It is imperative that just as the neoliberal project seeks to globalize its policies, progressive left-wing forces must find a way to globalize their struggles and demands. The political Left can develop a planned strategy of 'globalizing' struggles against the neoliberal assault. This can be done by disseminating the experiences of successful institutional changes, the struggle of health workers to defend public institutions, and the transformation of the approach towards public health to embrace a system that views health as a 'common good' and is based on peoples' demand for equality and premised on popular control of public institutions by social organizations.

Notes

1 The report says: "During the next decade, the Federal Government, industry, and other groups will need to better understand the domestic and global distribution, genesis, use of and consequences of using these resources to address national security issues, manage the Nation's domestic supplies, predict future needs, anticipate as well as guide changing patterns in use, facilitate creation of new industries, and secure access to appropriate supplies." Available at: https://pubs.usgs.gov/circ/2007/1309/pdf/C1309.pdf#page=33

2 See interview with Mario Testa: http://revistaoficio.org/pruebaidep/entrevista-atess-con-dr-mario-testa/

3 See: Área de Salud del Instituto de Estudios sobre Estado y Participación en Salud, *No a la Cobertura Universal de Salud* available at http://atesociosanitario.com.ar/no-a-la-cus-voces-en-defensa-de-la-salud-publica-2/. See: https://www.youtube.com/watch?v=TpAZsWBh86M

4 See: Centro Brasileiro de Estudos de Saúde – Sergipe consulted on 21/11/2016 at http://cebes.org.br/2016/09/nota-do-nucleo-cebes-se-sobre-a-saude-em-aracaju/

5 See: *Manifesto da Frente Mineira em Defensa do SUS e da Democracia* published on 4 August, 2016 at http://cebes.org.br/2016/08/manifesto-da-frente-mineira-em-defesa-do-sus-e-da-democracia/

References

García Linera A 2013, *Democracia, Estado y Nación* La Paz; Asamblea Legislativa Plurinacional. p. 81–116.

Laurell, AC *Contradicciones en Salud: Sobre Acumulación Y Legitimidad En Los Gobiernos Neoliberales Y Sociales De Derecho En América Latina* Saúdeem Debate 38 (103): 873–87.

María Lucia Frizon Rizzoto 2016, *O Cenário depois do Golpe*, Revista Saúde em Debate, Vol. 40, Ed.110, 04/10/2016.

Nolte D, Wehner L 'UNASUR and the New Geopolitics of South America', Paper prepared for the XXIII World Congress of Political Science Madrid, July, 8–12,

2012. http://paperroom.ipsa.org/papers/
paper_10836.pdf

People's Health Movement 2014, 'Social
Struggle, Progressive Governments and
Health in Latin America', Global Health
Watch 4, Zed Books, London. 2014. pp.
59–67. http://www.ghwatch.org/sites/www.
ghwatch.org/files/A3.pdf

Spinelli, H 2012, *El Proyecto Político y Las
Capacidades De Gobierno.* Salud Colectiva
8(2): 107–130

U.S. Geological Survey, 2007, Facing
tomorrow's challenges – U.S. Geological
Survey science in the decade 2007–2017:
U.S. Geological Survey Circular 1309, x +
70 p.

Since prehistoric times, human populations have been on the move, progressively colonizing most of the planet in search for favourable living conditions. Human flows have been the norm, not the exception, across the centuries, spurred and shaped by a myriad of structural and contextual factors, including environmental, economic and social ones.

Substantial attention has been focused on migration in recent years, especially in the context of the acute humanitarian crisis associated with flows of forced migration. This chapter focuses on the structural reasons that underlie migration in a globalised world.

The dimensions of global migration

In 2015, the estimated number of international migrants was 244 million, up from 173 million in 2000 (UNDESA, 2017). Women constitute slightly less than half of all international migrants. In 2005, the number of internal migrants was calculated at around 763 million (Bell &Charles-Edwards, 2013), almost exclusively the result of relocation from rural to urban areas.

Migration continues to be fuelled by a large number of factors interacting in multiple, complex ways. However, over the past four decades, globalization and neoliberal policies have played a particularly significant role as drivers of both internal and international migration, through a variety of direct and indirect mechanisms.

The number of forcibly displaced[1] has increased from 37 million 10 years ago to 65 – the largest number ever since the international community started keeping records (UNCHR, 2017). Approximately one-third of forcibly displaced people are refugees, that is, people who crossed an international border, while the remainder are internally displaced. More than half of all refugees are children. Most recently, conflicts that have resulted in particularly significant refugee movements include, among others, the Syrian civil war (which has produced 25 per cent of all forcibly displaced people globally), conflicts in the Democratic Republic of Congo (3 million people), South Sudan (1.5 million people), Afghanistan (1 million people) and the Central African Republic (0.5 million people). In addition to forcibly displaced people, it is worth remembering that more than 11 million people, worldwide, are stateless. All of these figures are just estimates, usually quite conservative, as counting people on the move has always been especially difficult.

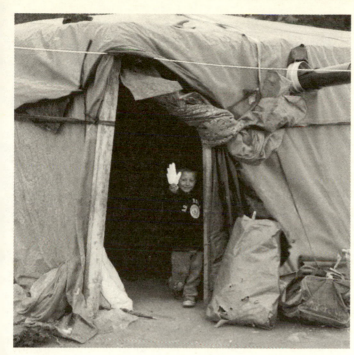

Image A4.1 Young boy at a refugee camp in Turkey (Cem Terzi)

Contrary to the widely held notion that refugees are rehabilitated due to the munificence of developed Northern countries, 85 per cent of all refugees live in low- and middle-income countries (LMICs), up from 70 per cent 10 years ago. By the end of 2014, the country hosting the largest number of refugees was Turkey (UNHCR, 2017).

The complex web of issues that lead to displacement blurs the traditional legal boundaries between migrants and 'refugees' – as defined in the 1951 United Nations Convention Related to the Status of Refugees, signed in Geneva (United Nations, 1951) and subsequently expanded by the 1967 Protocol Related to the Status of Refugees (United Nations, 1967). For most migrants, leaving home and crossing international borders is seldom the result of free choice. People migrate when their current situation leaves them without hope and without the possibility of a secure future for their children and themselves. A distinction is often made between 'voluntary' migrants and refugees to extend the protection of rights of only who are formally recognized as refugees under international law. This is bureaucratized view of this issue: a view that ignores the fact that the lived experiences of refugees and so-called 'economic migrants' are for the most part indistinguishable. Such a view does not address the root causes of migration and displacement. It is not just exceptional events like persecution and conflict that displace people, but also the abysmal conditions of living that a large proportion of the globe's population is subjected to.

Migration theories have evolved over the past century; from those premised on 'push/pull' factors to more nuanced interpretations accounting for the historical, social, economic and cultural forces shaping this phenomenon, as well as for the role played by network ties and transnational identities. In *The Age of Migration: International Population Movements in the Modern World*, Castles, De Haas and Miller (2013) emphasize the complexity, political salience, global nature, and economic and social significance of contemporary migration. Today, migration poses a major challenge to the sovereignty of states, in particular to their ability to regulate movements of people across their borders, and results in diffuse tension, often presented in a dramatic fashion – for example by expressions such as 'Fortress Europe', and reflected in the rhetoric and results of recent elections in North America and Europe.

Globalization and migration

Over the past four decades, globalization and neoliberal economic policies have become one of the most significant forces fuelling migration, if not the most important. Globalization has been defined in many ways. Most definitions, however, stress the nature of globalization as a set of processes that make national borders more permeable to social, political and economic activities; amplify planetary interdependence; and accelerate the circulation of capital, goods, information, innovation and ideas (Held et al., 1999, pp. 483–96). While globalization is a multidimensional phenomenon, the economic dimension lies at its heart in contemporary times.

The origins of contemporary globalization can be identified in a number of political and economic events between the 1970s and 1990s, including the debt crises, the ensuing policies of structural adjustment pursued by high-income countries (HICs) through the International Monetary Fund (IMF) and the World Bank (WB), and the fall of the Berlin Wall, which turned the model of development represented by the USA and its closest allies into the only apparent alternative (Labonte & Torgerson, 2005, pp. 157–79). Contemporary globalization does present novel characteristics, such as its truly universal reach, the size and power of transnational corporations, the unprecedented, if selective, pressure on governments to open their frontiers to the free movement of goods and capital, as the result of enforceable international agreements, and the speed of movement of capital and goods resulting from the application of revolutionary information and communication technologies and travel and transportation technologies (ibid.). Yet, the roots of contemporary globalization are deep and complex, reaching back in history all the way to the European explorations of the late sixteenth century, the progressive colonization of Latin America, India, South East Asia and Africa, and the ongoing pushing of the interests of the 'Global North' in the postcolonial period (Dickinson, 2016). Through the centuries, mercantilism first and capitalism later have progressively pushed their boundaries to seize the planet. The attempt to create a global marketplace is the core endeavour of contemporary globalization.

Over the centuries, the expansion of European interests has consistently resulted in social dislocation and displacement. The process originated in England where, between the late seventeenth century and the first half of the nineteenth century, advances in agriculture, industry, energy and transportation technologies pushed millions of peasants out of rural areas and into industrializing cities. Subsequently the wave hit the New World, producing the largest human migration movement in history that radically disrupted the lives of indigenous people. Traditional subsistence activities and social relations were wiped out and replaced with the structure and mechanisms of the colonial economy. Simultaneously, the need for human resources required to support the economy of plunder enforced by European powers resulted in the forced relocation of 12 million Africans who were brought to the Americas as slaves (ibid.). This wave continues and the process of integration of increasingly large areas of the globe into the capitalist economic market has persisted even after the formal end of the colonial era. Of course, some of the original colonies, the USA in particular, have joined in the race to expand the economic market while local elites in LMICs have consistently allied themselves with the interests of the Global North.

Today, those who find themselves excluded from the decentralized, innovation-based, flexible networks of production, representing the most recent phase of capitalism (Castells, 2000), or at least those among them who have the resources to move in search of a better life, do move. In fact, most migrants still move, either internally or internationally, in search of employment opportunities. Recent International Labour Organization data (ILO 2015) suggests that approximately 72 per cent of all migrants 15 years old or older are migrant workers and, if we include in the count their families, more than 90 per cent of all migrants move in search of employment.

Globalization and neoliberal policies create two tiers of migration. On the one hand, highly skilled professionals are for the most part welcome in High Income Countries (HICs) and sometimes even actively 'poached', as is often the case, for example, with healthcare professionals (Aluttis, Bishaw & Frank, 2014). On the other hand, unskilled workers trying to enter Europe, North America or Australia face old and new barriers and increasingly restrictive immigration policies. These barriers push them to join the legion of 'undocumented' or 'illegal' migrants. This, in turn, strengthens the power of employers and reduces the options available to migrants to demand fair wages and safe working conditions (Dickinson, 2016). Anthropologist Tamara Wilson suggests that one of the aims of increasingly restrictive immigration policies is to keep undocumented immigrant women working in the southern USA separate from the children they left behind in Mexico, therefore decoupling their productive value from their reproductive one (McGuire & Martin, 2007, pp. 178–88). Meanwhile, transnational corporations take advantage of the huge mass of dislocated, unskilled and unemployed workers remaining in LMICs to minimize production costs.

In many ways, the 'age of globalization' and the 'age of migration' coincide. Large numbers of people continue to be impoverished and displaced by policies that encourage privatization, impose financial deregulation, promote regressive taxation, create increasingly significant incentives for transnational corporations and require LMICs to open their borders to imports, creating situations that make local competition unsustainable. Concurrently HICs protect their own markets through tariffs and subsidies on agricultural production (Labonte & Torgerson, 2005, pp. 157–79).

There are indirect ways in which economic drivers of migration act. The imposition of macroeconomic policies that favour local elites tends to promote political instability and conflict or exacerbate pre-existing ones. The history of colonialism and post-colonialism is a history of conflict resulting from increasing destabilization and, often, the direct intervention of HICs interested in maintaining global market mechanisms (Dickinson, 2016). Local and regional conflicts have been a major driver of displacement since immediately after the end of the Second World War, from the Korean war to the Vietnam war, from the countless ethnic conflicts that have raged and continue to rage in Africa to the 'dirty war' fought by the USA in Central America in the 1970s and 1980s,[2] and up to the most recent wars in Iraq and Afghanistan.

In addition, the environmental externalities produced by the dominant model development, characterized by extreme consumerism and increased global trade are reaching unimaginable proportions. Environmental degradation and climate change are already displacing people. As suggested by Butler (2014, p. 1) climate change will "act as a risk multiplier, compounding pre-existing socially and politically-mediated drivers of adverse health consequences, including conflict". The interdependence created by globalization does not guarantee equity and health does not automatically follow wealth. Much of the progress in wealth (and health) has been achieved at the price of environmental destruction and climate change; and the health of people cannot be seen as separate from the health of the planet as a whole. As Hathaway and Boff (2009) have observed, for the first time in the history of humankind all of the major crises we are facing – environmental degradation and climate change, poverty and conflict – are of our own making. As previously discussed, these crises, all contributing to migration and adding to the desperation of the displaced, are the result of the way in which the globalized economy works, and not of isolated 'incidents'.

The discourse on migration: omissions, double standards and exclusions

Not surprisingly, most analysts and commentators steer away from directly addressing the core factors that impact human mobility, resulting, simultaneously, in the suffering of hundreds of millions of people and the political and identity crises we are witnessing today in the 'Western world'. The fact that dramatic global inequities are the prime movers of human dislocation and that these inequities are inextricably related to both historical and contemporary globalization is a reality that is for the most part ignored or underemphasized. As observed by Pécoud (2015) in his analysis of what he calls "international migration narratives", this reality is masked by a dominant approach that aims to bring order to an intrinsically messy and menacing phenomenon, favours based on supposed "global governance" and effectively depoliticizes migration. Pécoud's analysis is a useful starting point for tracing the similarities and links between narratives on migration and some of the central rhetorical constructs of the dominant economic discourse. Both ignore the structural mechanisms linking neoliberalism to global inequities and discount the lived experiences of the excluded and marginalized. A few examples of these links are briefly presented below.

Migration and development Recently, the idea that migration, when supported by appropriate policies, contributes to inclusive and sustainable economic growth and development in both home and host communities has gained momentum, backed by impressive statistics. In 2014, for example, migrants from LMICs sent home an estimated US$ 436 billion in remittances, a 4.4 per cent increase over the 2013 level (World Bank Group, 2016), far exceeding official development assistance and, excluding China, foreign direct investment. These funds are often used to improve the livelihood of families and, sometimes, of communities through investments in health, sanitation, housing, infrastructure and education. It has been emphasized (ibid.) how destination countries can also benefit from migration. Migrants often fill gaps left by critical labour shortages in host countries, create jobs as entrepreneurs, and contribute in terms of taxes and social security resources. As some of the most dynamic forces in society, they can also forge new paths in science, medicine and technology and enrich their host communities by promoting cultural diversity (UNDESA, 2016). The World Bank, for example, considers migration to be a "proven development strategy pursued by agents to maximize their needs and values" (Barnett &Webber, 2010).

This perspective ignores the human and social costs of migration. In addition, it exemplifies one of the most common and pernicious double standards found in the discourse to 'mainstream' migration: as long as it is 'others' who migrate, then migration can be considered as a viable solution! This approach is strongly influenced by the body of literature that, since the 1980s, has emphasized the role of migrants' agency in the decision to resettle. Migrants are not a homogenous group, and their decisions to move usually come at the end of a long and laboured process, are informed by hugely diverse considerations and are often not even individual decisions (Castles, De Haas& Miller, 2013, p. 37). While the issue of agency of migrants in the decision to resettle is not unimportant, what is not accounted for is how extreme poverty, precariousness, insecurity and despair dramatically reduce if not entirely erase the agency of millions of migrants.

Climate change and migration Given the complex relation, the impact of climate change on displacement is a highly contested area (Bowles & Butler, 2014). A number of studies suggest that between 200 million and 1 billion people will be displaced by climate change by the middle of the present century (Christian Aid, 2007; Myers, 2002, pp. 609–13). Even if the most optimistic projections were correct, human movements of this magnitude would have an impact, globally, that is truly difficult to comprehend. To understand the magnitude of the looming crisis we can contrast the projected displacement numbers with the deep social and political crisis that is currently shaking the European Union as a result of the influx of a few million refugees and migrants.

There is a debate regarding which of the two terms, – 'environmental migrants' or 'environmental refugees' – should be used to describe those displaced by climate change. Scholars who favour the term 'environmental migrant' have suggested that calling people displaced by climate change as 'refugees' would damage the interests of *real* refugees. The use of the term 'climate migrant' is part of a discourse that emphasizes migration as an adaptation strategy to climate change, and one that should be encouraged and properly managed. With such an interpretation the notion of adaptation changes from a collective phenomenon, based on political and social transformation of external conditions, to an individual response (Felli, 2013). Climate migration is being promoted as a solution to climate change only to the extent it can be 'managed' through rules, practices and norms. These rules often require that migration be prevented. At the same time the move from the recognition of climate refugees to the management of climate migration shifts the discourse from the arena of international law and human rights to one in which migrants are individuals with an entrepreneurial ethos. Climate migrants are no longer victims in need of justice but entrepreneurs who can lift themselves out of poverty and at the same time contribute to the 'resilience' of their vulnerable communities. 'Vulnerability' is interpreted as a function of people's exposure, and 'resilience' as their individual ability to adapt. Solutions, therefore, are no longer political but individual.

Even if we were to accept migration to be a form of adaptation to climate change, several fundamental questions remain. First, who would migrate? Migration, especially to international destinations, is more likely for those who are better off and better educated. As usual, the most marginalized are left behind and pay for those who leave, as the departure of even a very small proportion of the population can significantly diminish a community's overall social capital, particularly in communities where wealth and education are highly concentrated (Bowles &Butler, 2014).

The second question is about the most likely destinations for climate refugees. Even in scenarios of very severe climate change, it is believed that most movements will occur over short distances, while long-distance migration will occur only when migrants can follow well-established routes (McLeman, 2010, pp. 286–316). From the perspective of the 'Global North' the difference is significant, as migration-related issues are often framed in terms of security[2]. From the perspective of those who have to move and their fundamental human rights, however, there is very little difference. In all cases, they are forced to leave their lives, homes and communities behind. Short-distance displacement might indeed have an even more significant impact on their lived experiences. Most of these movements would be within LMICs, as they are the ones most affected by the extreme consequences of climate change, and short-distance movements would be predominantly from rural to urban areas. Their net result would be increased stress on already limited economic opportunities and infrastructures. Already fragile economies, health systems and entire sectors would be severely compromised and could fail altogether (Bowles and Butler, 2014).

Social costs of migration: fractured families The long-term separation of families, a complex phenomenon of massive proportions, with a clear intergenerational health impact, receives little attention. Human movements of the magnitude we observe today inevitably impact family structures. Economic globalization has affected core relationships of care, such as the separation and reunion of mothers and children (Falicov 2007, pp. 157–71), ostensibly the most problematic form of separation.

The exact number of fractured families is unknown. Yet, there is evidence that the numbers are very large. In China, for example, between 150 and 200 million people are internal migrants who move from rural to urban areas in search of work, while leaving tens of millions of children behind. Often, parents migrate when their children are very small and the separation can last for up to 10 to 15 years (Liu et al., 2010). In the Philippines, it is estimated that a quarter of all children under 18 live separated from their parents (Smeekens, Stroebe and Abakoumkin, 2012, pp. 2250–57). In Mexico, over the past four decades, migration has become the most common cause of 'families without a father', a phenomenon that principally affects poor, rural families (Nobles, 2013, pp. 1303–14).

The main reason parents have to leave their children behind is related to the uncertain nature of migration. Many migrants moving to Europe or North America are unskilled and undocumented. Once in the country of resettlement, they cannot leave again until their immigration status has changed. (Adams 2000, pp. 19–27). Separation may impact all members of the immediate and extended family as well as, often, the communities of origin and of resettlement. Among children left behind, for example, depression and suicidal ideation, anxiety, behavioural problems and substance abuse are all conditions that have been associated with separation (Miller, 2013, pp. 316–23). On the other hand, migrant parents experience a deep and damaging sense of ambivalence with regard to their left-behind children because of the tension between sacrificing their physical presence and having a chance to provide financially for their families (Grzywacz et al., 2006, pp. 85–97).

There is little discussion in academic literature about this phenomenon and as regards interventions in support of fractured families (Cortinois and Aguilera, forthcoming). This is in stark contrast with the rich literature focusing on the impact of separation and divorce on children in Western countries. The tens if not hundreds of millions of families fractured due to long-term internal or international economic migration are, essentially, invisible.

Sometimes, the problem of fractured families is downplayed by saying that these families come from strong traditions of collective care and therefore children left behind can be entrusted to members of the extended family or other community members. In addition, some authors use terms like 'diasporic culture' or 'culture of migration' to describe populations such as, for example, those living in the Caribbean region. Adams (2000, p. 20), at least partially misinterpreting the intentions of Hall (1995) whom he cites, notes that: "Caribbean culture is a diasporic culture, centered around a multiplicity of ethnic groups who identify with an ancestral home outside of the region. Therefore, the trauma of loss and the longing for what has been lost is an inherent part of the culture (Hall 1995). These people are migrant people".

It is difficult to imagine a more ahistorical and fundamentally neocolonial analysis, one that normalizes displacement. It ignores the fact that it was the massive slave trade that forced people to move to the Caribbean region in the first place and that international labour markets are forcing people to move, once again in very large numbers.

Conclusions

Migrants face a triple burden of victimization. First, they suffer the consequences of a model of development that dislocates them and drastically reduces their options, while resulting in ecological mayhem that further disrupts their connection to the land. Second, they are affected by the experiences of precariousness, exclusion, isolation and detention imposed on them by those who benefit, at least in the short term, from that same model of development. And finally, they are hurt by the misconceptions, biases and hypocrisy that distort the largely technocratic and bureaucratized debate on global human displacement.

Notes

1 Forced displacement may be the result of persecution, conflict, repression, natural and human-made disasters, ecological degradation and other causes. Displaced people may remain within the boundaries of their country of origin, therefore becoming internally displaced, or cross international borders, becoming refugees or asylum seekers. The complexity of contemporary migration fluxes is increasingly blurring the distinction between migrants and forcibly displaced people, as briefly discussed later in this chapter.

2 See Curtis, Fussell & DeWaard (2015, pp. 1269–93) and Castles, De Haas & Miller (2013, p. 198) for more on this.

References

Adams, C J 2000, 'Integrating children into families separated by migration: a Caribbean-American case study', *Journal of Social Distress and the Homeless*, vol. 9, no.1, pp. 19–27.

Aluttis, C, Bishaw, T & Frank, M W 2014, 'The workforce for health in a globalized context: global shortages and international migration'. *Global Health Action*, vol. 7, no.1, DOI 10.3402/gha.v7.23611.

Barnett, J & Webber, M 2010, *Accommodating migration to promote adaptation to climate change*, background paper to the 2010 World Development Report, policy research working paper no. 5270, The World Bank, Washington (DC).

Bell, M & Charles-Edwards, E 2013, *Cross-national comparisons of internal migration: an update on global patterns and trends*, Population Division technical papers, 2013/01, United Nations Department of Economic and Social Affairs (UNDESA) Population Division, New York.

Bowles, D C & Butler, C D 2014, 'Socially, politically and economically mediated health effects of climate change: possible consequences for Africa', *South African Medical Journal*, vol. 104, no.8, DOI10.7196/SAMJ.8604.

Butler, CD 2014, 'Climate change and global health: A new conceptual framework – mini review', *CAB Reviews*, vol. 9, DOI10.1079/PAVSNNR20149027.

Castells, M 2000, *End of millennium*, 2nd edn, Blackwell, Oxford.

Castles, S, De Haas, H & Miller, M J 2013,*The age of migration: international population movements in the modern world*, 5th edn, Guilford Press, New York.

Cortinois, A A & Aguilera, M forthcoming, 'Interventions in support of families fractured due to long-term economic migration: a review of the literature'.

Christian Aid 2007, *Human tide: the real migration crisis*, Christian Aid report, Christian Aid, London.

Curtis, K J, Fussell, E & DeWaard, J 2015,'Recovery migration after hurricanes Katrina and Rita: spatial concentration and intensification in the migration system', *Demography*, vol. 52,no. 4, pp. 1269–93.

Dickinson, E 2016, *Globalization and migration: a world in motion*, Rowman & Littlefield, Lanham, M D.

Falicov, C J 2007, 'Working with transnational immigrants: expanding meanings of family, community, and culture', *Family Process*, vol. 46, no. 2, pp. 157–71.

Felli, R 2013 'Managing Climate Insecurity by Ensuring Continuous Capital Accumulation: 'Climate Refugees' and 'Climate Migrants' New Political Economy vol. 18 , Iss. 3, 2013, Routledge

Grzywacz, J G, Quandt, S A, Early, J, Tapia, J, et al. 2006, 'Leaving family for work: ambivalence and mental health among Mexican migrant farmworker men', *Journal of Immigrant & Minority Health*, vol. 8, no. 1, pp. 85–97.

Hall, S 1995, 'Negotiating Caribbean identities', *New Left Review*, vol. 1,no. 209, viewed 24 February 2017, https://newleftreview.org/I/209/stuart-hall-negotiating-caribbean-identities

Hathaway, M & Boff, L 2009, *The Tao of liberation: exploring the ecology of transformation*. Orbis Books, New York.

Held, D, McGrew, A, Goldblatt, D & Perraton, J 1999, 'Globalization', *Global Governance*, vol. 5, pp. 483–96.

ILO 2015, *ILO global estimates of migrant workers and migrant domestic workers: results and methodology —special focus on migrant domestic workers*, International Labour Office, Geneva.

Labonte, R & Torgerson, R 2005, 'Interrogating globalization, health and development: towards a comprehensive framework for research, policy and political action', *Critical Public Health*, vol. 15, no. 2: pp. 157–79.

Liu, L,Sun, X, Zhang, C, Wang, Y & Guo, Q 2010, 'A survey in rural China of parent-absence through migrant working: the impact on their children's self-concept and loneliness', *BMC Public Health*, vol. 10, no. 32.

Lundgren, R I & Lang, R 1989, '"There is no sea, only fish": effects of United States policy on the health of the displaced in El Salvador', *Social Science & Medicine*, vol. 28, no. 7, pp. 697–706.

McGuire, S & Martin, K 2007, 'Fractured migrant families: paradoxes of hope and devastation', *Family & Community Health*, vol. 30, no. 3, pp. 178–88.

McLeman, R 2010, 'Impacts of population change on vulnerability and the capacity to adapt to climate change and variability: a typology based on lessons from "a hard country"', *Population and Environment*, vol. 31, no. 5, pp. 286–316.

Miller, L D 2013, '"I am not who I thought I was": use of grief work to address disrupted identity among Hispanic adolescent immigrants', *Clinical Social Work Journal*, vol. 41, pp. 316–23.

Myers, N 2002, 'Environmental refugees: a growing phenomenon of the 21st century', *Philosophical Transactions of the Royal Society*, vol. 357, no. 1420, pp. 609–13.

Nobles, J 2013, 'Migration and father absence: shifting family structure in Mexico', *Demography*, vol. 50, no. 4, pp. 1303–14.

Pécoud, A 2015, *Depoliticisingmigration: global governance and international migration narratives*, Palgrave Pivot, London.

Smeekens, C, Stroebe, M S & Abakoumkin, G 2012, 'The impact of migratory separation from parents on the health of adolescents in the Philippines', *Social Science & Medicine*, vol. 75, no. 12, pp. 2250–57.

UNDESA 2016, '*International migration report 2015*, United Nations Department of Economic and Social Affairs, New York.

UNDESA 2017, *International migrant stock 2015*, viewed 13 April 2017, http://www.un.org/en/development/desa/population/migration/data/estimates2/estimates15.shtml .

UNHCR 2017, *Figures at a glance*, viewed 13 April 2017, http://www.unhcr.org/figures-at-a-glance.html

United Nations 1951, *Convention relating to the status of refugees(with schedule),signed at Geneva on 28 July 1951*, no. 2545, https://treaties.un.org/doc/Publication/UNTS/Volume%20189/volume-189-I-2545-English.pdf

United Nations 1967, *Protocol relating to the status of refugees, done at New York on 31 January 1967*, no. 8791 https://treaties.un.org/doc/Publication/UNTS/Volume%20606/volume-606-I-8791-English.pdf

World Bank Group 2016, *Migration and development*, World Bank Group, Washington (DC).

SECTION B

**HEALTH SYSTEMS:
CURRENT ISSUES AND DEBATES**

B1 | UNIVERSAL HEALTH COVERAGE: ONLY ABOUT FINANCIAL PROTECTION?

The struggle for health is partly about the struggle for decent healthcare and for functioning health systems that care for sick people and contribute to improving population health. There is much at stake in health system reform, and not just the provision of decent healthcare. The field is intensely contested among various parties (providers, suppliers, insurers and so on) who have a powerful economic interest in the outcomes of the debate. Such interest groups project a policy narrative that proposes 'public interest' logic to their preferred pathways while obscuring their vested interests. Getting a clear picture of the substantive policy issues and choices requires penetrating the fog and reinterpreting the rhetoric.

The pressures for health system reform arise in the systemic problems perceived by different players: community concerns about quality and access,

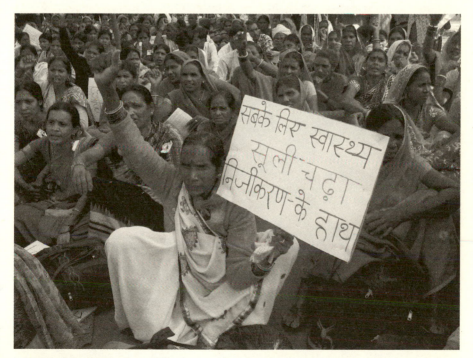

Image B1.1 Community mobilisation can shape health systems: Women in India demonstrate against privatisation of health services (Sulakshana Nandi)

the grievances of providers regarding conditions and remuneration, and corporate concerns about barriers to profitable engagement. These pressures are variously expressed through community mobilization, professional advocacy, research findings, corporate lobbying and bureaucratic task groups. Whether or not change takes place depends on the stability of existing structures and the feasibility of and support for available policy options.

Civil society sentiment and various forms of community mobilization are always part of the dynamic. Effective engagement by community activists involves clear-sighted analysis, a long-range vision for healthcare that can inform policy advocacy around specific opportunities for change, and movement-building in support of both the vision and the specific policy options.

'Universal health coverage' – *slogan de jour*

Universal health coverage (UHC) is the *slogan de jour* in global health systems policy but its meaning is highly contested. At one pole are those, including many World Bank economists, who use the term simply to refer to financial protection: out-of-pocket payment should not be a barrier to accessing services and families should not be impoverished by healthcare costs. According to this view UHC, understood as universal financial protection, can be achieved through different approaches to collecting and pooling funds and paying providers, including through competitive voluntary health insurance and private-sector healthcare delivery. Others, including many WHO officials, accept that financial protection is central to UHC but recognize that having regard to other policy objectives, including quality, equity, efficiency and prevention, adds to the case for tax-based funding, single payer systems, capped programme funding and effective clinical governance. The debate is clouded by politicians such as Margaret Chan, the (former) director-general of the WHO, who has been at pains to present a united front with the World Bank regarding UHC and to paper over the different assumptions about implementation.

Appreciating the different meanings and purposes of the slogan is critical to understanding the politics of the debate, promoting a vision of 'health for all' and mobilizing around specific policy initiatives.

Our purpose in this chapter is to explore the emergence of UHC. The chapter traces some of the political influences and pressures that are at play, defines key policy objectives that are at stake, reviews the evidence regarding how these objectives might be achieved in different settings and formulates political strategies for civil society engagement in the ongoing debates about UHC and health systems development more generally.

We start with an overview of the historical context in which 'universal health coverage' has emerged as the leading slogan in global health system policy debate. We then review the implications of a wider raft of policy objectives, beyond financial protection, for different healthcare financing models. We then explore some perplexing features of the economistic discourse of healthcare financing, focusing particularly on market framing, the commodification of the healthcare relationship, the metaphor of 'purchasing' and the ubiquitous 'benefit package'. We then step back in terms of scale and locate the debates around healthcare financing within the context of economic globalization and the neoliberal project. Finally we review what is known about the dynamics of health systems development and how policy generalizations find their way into institutional structures on the ground. Our purpose in this final section is to contribute to discussion within civil society about how popular movements can drive healthcare reform.

The emergence of UHC

The history of global health system policy debates can be traced in terms of the salient themes and slogans that have characterized each period.

There is no clear slogan that can be associated with the early years of the WHO. Rather, there was a continuing tension between the advocates of 'social medicine' and those of 'disease-specific programmes', notably malaria, smallpox and polio. This was the period of the Cold War and the WHO Secretariat was closely scrutinized by the USA, the largest donor. The replacement of Brock Chisholm as director-general by Marcelino Gomes Candau in 1953 symbolizes the marginalization of the health system policy by specific disease-control programmes.

The WHO was pushed into paying closer attention to health systems during the 1970s, in part by the then Soviet Union wanting to demonstrate the benefits of its Semashko model (Litsios, 2002, pp. 709–32) and in part by the Christian Medical Commission advocating what was to become, through the 1978 Alma-Ata Conference, 'primary healthcare' (Litsios, 2004, pp. 1884–93). However, the global economy at the end of the 1970s was confronted by global stagflation, leading in the early 1980s to the debt crisis, with the emergence of 'structural adjustment' as a driver of health system policymaking (largely public-sector disinvestment). With the support of the Rockefeller Foundation, primary healthcare (PHC) morphed into 'selective primary healthcare' and under the newly appointed James Grant the United Nations International Children's Emergency Fund (UNICEF) retreated to GOBI (growth monitoring, oral rehydration, breast feeding and immunization) (Cueto, 2004, pp. 1864–74). However, the 1980s are remembered more as 'the lost decade' rather than for selective primary healthcare.

In an attempt to re-legitimize structural adjustment, the World Bank produced the 'Investing in Health' report in 1993, which argued for stratified health insurance and private/voluntary healthcare delivery (The World Bank, 1993). The report pressed for a safety net for the poor, based on a minimal, tax-funded 'benefits package'. This minimalist model included provisions for selected 'cost effective' 'interventions', including vaccination, insecticide-treated bed nets and nutritional supplementation, but did not provide for the diagnosis and treatment of the millions suffering from AIDS/HIV. However, by the mid-1990s the benefits of anti-retroviral treatment for AIDS/HIV had been demonstrated and stoked the rights-based demand for access to treatment (Fee & Parry 2008, pp. 54–71) and the minimalist model of investing in health receded into history.

Gro Harlem Brundtland (director-general of the WHO, 1998–2003) sought to return the focus of global health policy to health systems with the 'World Health Report 2000'. This report was strongly influenced by World Bank thinking and sought to establish a framework that naturalized the role of private providers and private health insurance in healthcare delivery. The report was accompanied by a league table of national health systems based on questionable concepts, methods and data. The report did not reflect well on either the WHO or its director-general.

The rise and rise of the treatment access movement (Robins, 2010, pp. 651–72) represented a setback for the neoliberal project. It was forced to address the demand to find the resources to ensure treatment access, and also to respond to the widespread delegitimation of the Trade-Related Aspects of Intellectual Property Rights (TRIPS) agreement ('T Hoen, 2009) and the associated drive for trade liberalization (Smith, 2002, pp. 207–28). A striking reflection of this popular delegitimation was the adoption in December 2001 by the Ministerial Council of the World Trade Organization (WTO) of the Doha Declaration on the TRIPS Agreement and Public Health, which affirmed that 'the TRIPS Agreement does not and should not prevent Members from taking measures to protect public health' and reaffirmed 'the right of WTO Members to use, to the full, the provisions in the TRIPS Agreement, which provide flexibility for this purpose' (WTO Ministerial Council, 2001).

The need to shore up the legitimacy of the neoliberal regime was addressed with the Millennium Development Goals (MDGs), the greatly increased flow of resources and the flourish of new 'global health initiatives' (GHIs), led by the Global Fund to Fight Aids, Tuberculosis and Malaria (GFATM), Unites States President's Emergency Plan for AIDS Relief (PEPFAR), GAVI, the Vaccine Alliance and Bill & Melinda Gates Foundation (BMGF) (Sanders, n.d.). (See Chapters D2 and D4.)

Within a few years into the new millennium the flaws of this regime were becoming evident: multiple top-down vertical initiatives increased the administrative burden on ministries of health, fragmented health systems in vertical silos and a brain drain from national health systems into those vertical silos. In response to these adverse consequences, a new slogan, 'health systems strengthening' (HSS), emerged. This was in part a recognition that weak health systems were a major barrier to the effective application of the increased flow of resources, but it also reflected a recognition of the fragmenting effect of vertical global programmes and the cost of coordination locally (High-Level

Taskforce on Innovative International Financing for Health Systems 2008; WHO, 2007).

When Margaret Chan took over the leadership of the WHO after the death of Lee Jong-Wook in May 2006, she announced a return to comprehensive primary healthcare (WHO, 2006), but over the next few years it became evident that her passion was not going to inspire a large-scale diversion of resources from the vertical programmes into PHC-inspired health systems strengthening and certainly not a return to Alma-Ata.

Meanwhile, a parallel movement for universal coverage was developing within the WHO. The WHO's Executive Board in April 2004 considered the report on 'Social Health Insurance' (WHO 2004a), which introduced the elements of healthcare financing (revenue collection, funds pooling, resource allocation/purchasing), noted the broad choice of tax-based versus social insurance-based revenue collection and then proceeded to explore the conditions for a social insurance approach to healthcare financing. The report was returned to the Executive Board in December 2004 with the same title 'Social Health Insurance' but substantially redrafted (WHO, 2004b). The focus was now on healthcare financing more generally and with the policy goal of universal health coverage much more prominent. Social health insurance was no longer presented as the preferred option.

The USA's response in the Executive Board was explosive.

"Dr Steiger (United States of America) said that he was disappointed with the deep-seated bias shown in WHO, including the Executive Board, against private enterprise. All proposals embodied a statist approach and reflected a presumption that the private sector's motives were questionable, on subjects such as infant formulas, pharmaceuticals and food. In the '3 by 5' initiative, for instance, there was little mention of the private sector or of the advantage that could be taken of the many non-state providers. The report regrettably reflected that bias. There was no comprehensive description of the full range of public and private options for comprehensive health insurance for all.
The Secretariat, and the relevant documentation, ought to make clear the advantages of private providers, such as responsiveness to patients, flexibility, innovation and efficiency. Subsidies to purchase private insurance could achieve equity in a mixed system, and every government needed a reasonable overall regulatory regime. WHO should continue its work on the subject but propose a broader range of schemes and mixes that would expand coverage and minimize problems such as those mentioned by the previous speaker. The range should include the private and public systems, and blends of the two, depending on a country's political and economic realities, while striving for efficiency and sustainability". (WHO, 2005a)

The draft resolution prepared by the WHO Secretariat was substantially modified in response to the US tirade (and adopted as EB115.R13). When the revised paper A58/20[1] and resolution were considered again at the World Health Assembly (WHO, 2005b) the US delegate was again insistent about competitive health financing and mixed service delivery.

> "Mr Abdoo (United States of America) endorsed the goal of comprehensive health insurance. All Member States would benefit from a robust discussion of how to strengthen health-care coverage. It would be useful for the Secretariat to provide a report on the various possibilities for achieving universal coverage, including market-based approaches. Member States and the Secretariat should give due consideration to the benefits of a private system that could focus direct government resources where they were most needed. Those benefits included individual choice, reduction in tax burdens, flexibility, innovation and efficiency. Subsidies to purchase private insurance could achieve equity in a private system. Further, government systems had several disadvantages: greater bureaucracy, higher taxation, long waiting times, rationing of care and less efficiency, thereby decreasing access to and quality of health care; they were also difficult to sustain in the face of growing demand, ageing populations and increasing costs. Countries required competitive financing and delivery systems that were responsive to health-care needs and made the most of advances in medical science and technology. Member States would therefore be best served by the provision of data on the broadest possible range of options, private and public systems and mixes of the two, that would expand coverage and minimize out-of-pocket payments while achieving efficiency, transparency and sustainability and be adaptable to meet their specific political, socioeconomic and health situation. The public and private sectors both had critical roles to play". (Ibid.)

During the debate, Thailand, Kenya and the UK proposed significant changes to the draft resolution forwarded from the 115th Session of WHO Executive Board while the USA sought to change all references to universal health coverage to universal insurance coverage. In the end it was decided to adopt the resolution forwarded from the Executive Board with the addition of a paragraph about reviewing progress on implementation and all of the other issues raised at the 58th Session of World Health Assembly. The issue was scheduled for discussion the following year but when it was reviewed at the 59th Session of the WHA in May 2006 there was no discussion of any of the amendments! As a major donor to the WHO, the strength of the US position must have been somewhat intimidating for the WHO Secretariat.

It is not likely that the health financing experts at the WHO would have received any support from the World Bank, at this time, led as it was by Paul Wolfowitz (previously undersecretary for defence under George W. Bush). The prevailing attitude within the World Bank is reflected in two reports on private health insurance, both co-authored by Alexander Preker (Preker, Sheffler & Bassett, 2007; Preker, Zweifel & Schellekens, 2010). The 2010 report argues for a strong emphasis on private voluntary health insurance so that "private means can make a significant contribution to public ends".

"It is the poor and most vulnerable that are at greatest risk due to lack of protection against the impoverishing effects of illness. The research for this volume shows that, when properly designed and coupled with public subsidies, health insurance can contribute to the well-being of poor and middle-class households, not just the rich. And it can contribute to development goals such as improved access to health care, better financial protection against the cost of illness, and reduced social exclusion. Opponents vilify health insurance as an evil to be avoided at all cost. To them, health insurance leads to overconsumption of care, escalating costs—especially administrative costs—fraud and abuse, shunting of scarce resources away from the poor, cream skimming, adverse selection, moral hazard, and an inequitable health care system. Today many low-and middle-income countries are no longer listening to this dichotomized debate between vertical and horizontal approaches to health care. Instead, they are experimenting with new and innovative approaches to health care financing.

Health insurance is becoming a new paradigm for reaching the Millennium Development Goals (MDGs). They emphasize the need to combine several instruments to achieve three major development objectives in health care financing: 1) sustainable access to needed health care; 2) greater financial protection against the impoverishing cost of illness; and 3) reduction in social exclusion from organized health financing instruments. The use of insurance was recommended to pay for less frequent, higher-cost risks and subsidies to cover affordability for poorer patients to higher-frequency, lower-cost health problems".

The World Bank and the major GHIs were subjected to a certain amount of prodding at this time through the High-Level Taskforce on Innovative International Financing for Health Systems[2] (September 2008 to May 2009), which was set up in response to concerns about the fragmenting impact of the vertical GHIs and their impact on the balance of healthcare spending.

"Development assistance for health (DAH) has more than doubled since 2000 and has played a major role in making these gains. However, without more effort to build stronger national health systems in the 49 poorest countries, each year half a million women will continue to die from preventable complications in pregnancy, a quarter of a million adults will die from HIV and up to 11 million unplanned pregnancies will occur. And if the current financial crisis persists, these numbers will be even worse. The World Bank estimates between 200,000 and 400,000 additional children may die every year—between 1.4 and 2.8 million before 2015. Progress is impeded by insufficient funding, poor use of resources, and fragmented and largely unpredictable financing flows. Low-income countries currently spend only USD 25 per capita on health; of this USD 10 comes from out-of-pocket payments and only USD 6 from DAH. More than 50 per cent of DAH provided directly to countries is allocated to infectious diseases, while less than 20 per cent is invested in basic health-care services, nutrition and infrastructure". (High-Level Taskforce on Innovative International Financing for Health Systems, 2008)

The World Bank was further challenged in July 2012 with the appointment of Jim Yong Kim as its president, on the nomination of President Barrack Obama. Kim's background in Partners in Health, a US non-governmental organization, was well known, as was his support for primary healthcare and a social-justice approach to health policy. In his speech to the World Health Assembly in May 2013 (WHO 2013), Jim Kim said:

"Thirty-five years ago, the Alma Ata Conference on Primary Health Care set powerful moral and philosophical foundations for our work. The Declaration of Alma Ata confirmed the inseparable connection between health and the effort to build prosperity with equity, what the Declaration's authors called 'development in the spirit of social justice.

The fragmentation of global health action has led to inefficiencies that many ministers here know all too well: parallel delivery structures; multiplication of monitoring systems and reporting demands; ministry officials who spend a quarter of their time managing requests from a parade of well-meaning international partners. This fragmentation is literally killing people. Together we must take action to fix it, now".

Notwithstanding his recognition of Alma-Ata, the main focus of Jim Kim's speech was on universal health coverage, which he clearly identified as including both financial protection and health systems strengthening. However, he made no reference to the challenges of integrating private finance and private providers in his vision of ensuring "that everyone in the world has access to affordable, quality health services in a generation".

Meanwhile Margaret Chan was also moving her rhetoric from her earlier celebration of primary healthcare to an increasing focus on universal health coverage. In her acceptance speech in November 2006 (WHO 2006) there were five mentions of PHC and one of universal access. In the following year, in the director-general's report to the World Health Assembly (WHO, 2007) there were six mentions of PHC and one each of universal coverage and universal access. Fast-forwarding to the director-general's report of May 2012 (WHO, 2012), there were three mentions of PHC, five mentions of universal coverage, two of universal health coverage and one of universal access.

PHC versus UHC While there is some overlap in terms of the policy specifics, the differences in emphasis between the PHC and UHC approaches are significant. The Alma-Ata discourse involves a focus on building and supporting the primary healthcare sector and envisages a prominent role for community health workers and community involvement in planning, accountability and prevention. The PHC approach envisages primary healthcare practitioners working closely with their communities on the social and environmental determinants of health as well as in healthcare development. This implies a dominant role for public-sector providers because private-sector providers are demonstrably unable to realize the broader principles of PHC in their practice. By contrast, the UHC discourse (the WHO version) starts with a focus on financial protection and argues explicitly for public, single payer *financing* (not care). It includes a commitment to health systems strengthening and the importance of primary care but treads lightly around community involvement and the role of private providers.

Jeffrey Sachs (2012, pp 944–47) presented a cogent set of arguments for public-sector provision of primary healthcare in low-income countries. He cited, first, the incentives for private providers to inflate costs, second, the strong tendencies of private providers to congregate in wealthier communities and, third, the reasons of efficiency and governance. Sachs's position is complicated because he is a strong advocate for the 'minimum benefit package' model, based on specified cost-effective interventions. However, it is unrealistic to expect publicly owned and delivered primary healthcare to restrict its service delivery to such highly specified programmes. By contrast, the advocates of

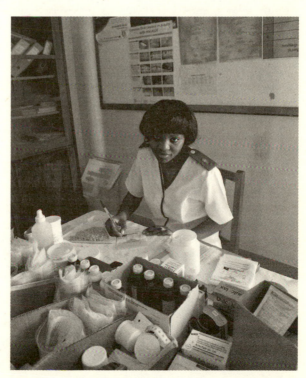

Image B1.2 Health worker at a public facility in Namibia (Eric Miller)

health insurance claim that the 'purchase' of specified health services through a restricted publicly subsidized benefit package can focus public (and foreign) funding on the priority 'interventions' and poor communities. The corollary of this is that payment for all other services is entirely out of pocket, which fails the financial protection objective unless it is linked to voluntary health insurance that is quite inequitable.

In 2010 the WHO's World Health Report focused on healthcare financing and universal health coverage, including a return to Resolution A58.33 from 2005. While the report is understandably cautious, it affirms some important principles: abolish user charges at the point of service; a small number of big pools, preferably a single national pool, is more equitable and sustainable than many different pools; equity, efficiency, quality and prevention in service delivery matter and are affected by resource allocation/purchasing mechanisms (in particular fee for service); effective governance is the key to improving efficiency and quality.

In July 2012 Jim Kim inherited a project at the World Bank, the Universal Health Coverage Series, which distinguishes very clearly the Bank's approach to UHC from that of the WHO's. The concluding report from the series was published in 2013. The astonishing thing about this report (Giedion, Alfonso & Díaz, 2013), indeed the whole project, was that it explicitly refrained from considering quality, equity or efficiency. In methodological terms the project sought to correlate funding arrangements in 22 countries (and one US state) with their 'outcomes', conceptualized as access, financial protection and health status. The authors acknowledged that "other relevant outcomes might also be analyzed, such as quality, equity, and efficiency. However, to keep the study manageable, we selected just three—access, financial protection, and health status—given their immediate relation to UHC and their importance."

The assumption that health status is an appropriate indicator of universal health coverage is most unusual. While effective healthcare with universal access will contribute to population health gain, it is small compared with effective action on the wider social determinants of health. A focus on access and financial protection, without regard to quality, efficiency or equity, has the effect of discounting the importance of health system capacity and side-stepping the WHO's arguments about single payer financing and strong health system governance.

Notwithstanding the flying rhetoric of Jim Kim at the WHA in 2013, it appears that the warm collaboration between the World Bank and WHO obscures some very significant differences in approach, exemplified by Preker's enthusiastic defence of competitive voluntary health insurance and the decision of Giedion, Alfonso and Díazto to exclude quality, equity and efficiency from the scope of their study of 'the impact of universal coverage'. Understanding the pragmatism behind this unholy alliance is absolutely necessary to participating strategically in healthcare financing debates and the politics of implementation.

From a financial protection perspective (preventing cost barriers to access and healthcare impoverishment) both tax-based financing and various insurance arrangements (including a subsidy for the poor) may be viewed as comparable strategies. However, in terms of equity they are not comparable: competitive health insurance markets provide different products for different income strata and offer different benefit packages according to ability to pay. Certainly they do not provide for equitable redistribution of resources through pooling across income levels.

The competitive health insurance market in the USA illustrates this particularly well. Insurance plans for low-income workers are more likely to have tight utilization control, high deductibles, primary care fund-holding, and restricted benefit packages, including restrictions on choice of providers. Plans for high-income earners are likely to have looser utilization controls, fee for service reimbursement and more generous benefit packages (Gabel, 1999, pp. 62–74; Hellander and Bhargava, 2012, pp. 161–75). WHO technical papers have repeatedly emphasized the need for a compulsory rather than voluntary approach to revenue generation and for a few large pools rather than many smaller pools (Kutzin, 2014).

Why and emphasis on public provision of care is important From a purely financial protection perspective, service delivery through public or private or mixed providers may be comparable. However, they have very different implications for quality, equity, efficiency (technical and allocative) and prevention (which makes the exclusion by Giedion Alfonso and Díazof quality, equity and efficiency from the World Bank's UHC Series all the more regrettable)[3].

In the World Health Report of 2010, the WHO cites estimates of healthcare efficiency to the effect that up to 40 per cent of healthcare expenditure globally may be wasted. In a very useful background paper Chisholm and Evans (2010) summarize the sources of inefficiency (Table 1) and assemble the evidence for this estimate.

TABLE B1.1: Sources of inefficiency in healthcare provision

Healthcare workers	Inappropriate or costly staff mix
Medicines	Underuse and overpricing of generic drugs
Medicines	Irrational use of drugs
Medicines	Substandard or counterfeit drugs
Healthcare products	Overuse of procedures, investigations and equipment
Healthcare services	Suboptimal quality of care and medical error
Healthcare services	Inappropriate hospital size
Healthcare services	Inappropriate hospital admissions or length of stay
Health system leakages	Corruption and fraud

Source: Chisholm and Evans (2010)

Clearly, promoting efficiency in the management of funds and in service delivery is of critical importance to universal health coverage. In an open-ended competitive voluntary health insurance scheme there is a constant tension between premium levels and payments to providers and this can be extremely expensive to manage. In single pool, single payer systems (as in, among others, the UK, France, Italy, Canada and Australia) the cost of collection and disbursement is much less. Different modes of provider payment also have implications for efficiency. Although there are no specific modes of payment that create a perfect incentive environment for all types of service providers, efficiency can be promoted by adapting particular modes of payment for particular types of service and avoiding open-ended financing commitments. What are critical are: first, the information systems which monitor service delivery (Chaudhry et al., 2006, pp. 742–52); second, the management systems which constrain or redirect resource flows; and third, the capacity to innovate as needed (Sparkes Durán & Kutzin, 2017). An organized and accountable approach to all three requirements is more practicable with public-sector providers supported by single payer financing, in comparison with a much more arm's-length relationship between the financial stewards and private health insurance funds and private providers.

Allocative efficiency is also an important policy goal, incorporating the distribution of resources across geography, workforce, institutions, services and programmes. Resource flows should be directed to those regions, workforce categories, institutions and programmes where more outcomes can be achieved for the same investment. There is a range of tools for redistributing resource flows in a purchasing environment, including technology assessment, varying prices, capping programme expenditures, regulation and subsidy, but they require excellent information systems and can be difficult to manage. The hovering of private practitioners around wealthier communities is one of the most reliable (and understandable) findings in health systems research and represents an almost insurmountable problem for regulators. Government funders/regulators working with public sector providers also face challenges in promoting allocative efficiency but have significant advantages in terms of the capacity to effect such adjustments (Gao et al., 2011, pp. 655–63).

The same is true of quality and safety. Clearly, perverse incentives impacting on quality and safety can be identified in both public and private healthcare delivery. Arguments for the inherent advantages of different modes of provision tend to get bogged down in competing examples or high-level theorization of different incentive environments. A more useful approach may be to focus on the challenge of regulating for quality and safety. A useful paradigm for thinking through such regulatory challenges is the idea of 'clinical governance' (Hammond, 2010, pp. 1–12). Clinical governance is a complex multi-component endeavour that calls for good information systems, competent governance and management, and the deliberate cultivation of patient centredness and

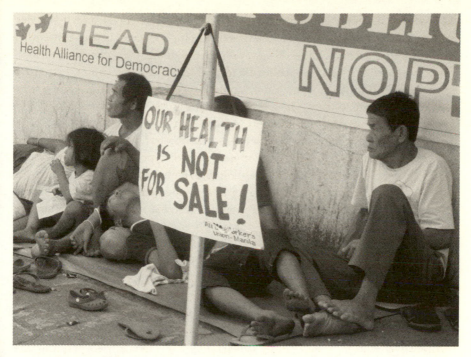

Image B1.3 Health workers in Manila agitate against privatisation of a public hospital (M3M)

continuous improvement. The evidence relating different modes of provider payment to the effectiveness of clinical governance is scanty (Brand et al., 2012, pp. 483–94). However, the autonomy and privacy of private ambulatory practice (as compared with community health centre practice) certainly limits the scope for measurement, peer review, regulatory initiatives and appropriate professional development. Likewise, the commercial relationship between private hospitals and their visiting private practitioners militates against the kind of monitoring and stewardship that can be achieved in more hierarchically organized healthcare institutions.

Finally, consider prevention (encompassing individual services such as screening and vaccination, and community programmes such as young mothers' groups), action on environmental hazards and action on the wider social determinants of health (employment, education and infrastructure). The minimal benefit package does not include advocacy alongside communities and in the absence of a benefit most private practitioners regard such engagement as way beyond their remit. However, there are many contemporary examples (TWHA and PHM, 2017) as well as iconic projects guided by the Alma-Ata Declaration (Newell, 1975), which have enabled clinicians to feed their experience and expertise into community action.

At this point in our discussion we can identify three questions that may guide the rest of our analysis. These are:

- What lies behind the World Bank's wilful exclusion of quality, efficiency, equity and prevention, from their analyses of healthcare financing?
- What sense can be made of the unholy alliance of the World Bank and WHO to proselytize their ideas about UHC?

How might community activists, including progressive practitioners and academics, engage in this snakepit?

The economistic mindset

We start with some reflections on the disabilities associated with the conventional economics paradigm in which every social problem, it would seem, must be framed in terms of market relations so that the tools of economics can be brought to bear on the discussion. In prevailing policy discussions of UHC, this framing is reflected in the commodification of 'service', the tortured metaphor of 'purchasing', and the construction of priority-setting purely in terms of technology assessment (and benefit packages).

The problems with the commodification of healthcare services are partly about the specification and standardization of the 'commodity', but more profoundly about the extraction of the act of service provision from the human relationships within which it takes place. Every service takes place between one or more clinicians and the patient and their family. The service that is to be included in the benefit package only makes sense in terms of the wants and needs of the patient (and family and community): diagnostic, prognostic, therapeutic, emotional and social. The first principle in redesigning healthcare for quality (Institute of Medicine, 2001) is that 'Care is based on continuing healing relationships'. To specify and price this service without regard to the clinical relationship discounts the values that make healthcare important. To contract with providers for the delivery of services that are divorced from the clinical relationship renders meaningless any provisions regarding accountability for outcomes. A marketplace in which providers compete to deliver specified services for specified prices in completely unspecified contexts is a weak mechanism for promoting efficient, quality healthcare.

The metaphor of purchasing (See also Box B1.1) invites further reflection on the economistic mindset. Neoliberal economists rail against 'big government' and the perversions of the 'principal–agent relationship'. In this context the principal is the citizen and the agent is the parliament/bureaucracy. The argument is that government is not sufficiently accountable to the citizen and pursues its own interests but that transforming government services into markets where services are commodified, priced and bought and sold (for example, vouchers for education) returns sovereignty to the principal (citizen). However, the purchasing metaphor, as applied to health insurance or the 'purchaser–provider split', involves a surrogate purchaser, be it the health insurance plan or the purchasing agency. In this case the accountability of the agent (health insurer) to the principal (the patient) is weak. The neoliberal solution lies in a competitive market for health insurance so that consumer sovereignty can be restored through 'choice'. The purchasing paradigm and the market template have no solutions to the continuing challenge of information asymmetry (regardless of who the purchaser is).

What is ignored by the purchasing metaphor (and practice) is the relationship (between patient and family with clinicians) and the context (including the judgement about the need for a particular programme of interventions and the care with which those interventions are carried out). Healthcare is co-produced, not just by patient/family and clinicians but also by the myriad of support functions and personnel. In accordance with the principle of 'total quality management', the outcomes of the clinical programme (efficiency as well as quality) depend on the whole system. The purchasing metaphor renders the periphery of this complex system invisible.

The economistic mindset is nowhere more evident than in policy discussions of priority-setting, which is commonly constructed purely in terms of technology assessment: evaluating the cost-effectiveness of a diagnostic test or a drug or surgical procedure. The application of such findings will inform a decision about entitlement (including the 'intervention' in the benefit package) and about price setting (in terms of reimbursement). Priority-setting, structured around the benefit package, assumes health insurance-based financing. Technology assessment has an important role to play in shaping clinical practice, but not all resource allocation choices can be reduced to a 'benefit package' design. In the context of administered systems of healthcare, such as public-sector hospitals, resource allocation choices are made in the context of budgeting, and promoting allocative efficiency involves evaluating the prospective outcomes of different choices with respect to programme funding. This approach enables a much broader range of considerations in determining priorities.

The macroeconomic imperative

Debates over healthcare financing are embedded in wider tensions about the management of the global economy. The 1980s debt crisis (and the retreat from primary healthcare to GOBI) reflected a major change in the trajectory of the global economy, from the 'long boom', following the Second World War, to an era of slower growth but accelerated globalization and financialization. The assumptions underlying 'investing in health' were not about healthcare at all. They were about managing the instabilities and vulnerabilities of global capitalism in the 1990s and ensuring that the poor countries knew their place in that system. The MDGs and the associated flush of resources through the GHIs were as much about relegitimizing economic globalization following Jubilee 2000, the Treatment Action Campaign and the Battle of Seattle, as they were about 'development'.

Box B1.1 The drive for 'Strategic Purchasing'

Strategic Purchasing' ('SP') has been advocated as a healthcare financing measure which is central to improving health system performance and making progress towards universal health coverage (UHC). The World Health Report 2000 unveiled a full-section on 'Strategic Purchasing' used interchangeably with 'active purchasing'. It argued for the move from 'Passive Purchasing' to 'Active or Strategic Purchasing'. 'Passive purchasing' implies following a predetermined budget or simply paying bills when presented. 'Strategic purchasing' involves a continuous search for the best ways to maximize health system performance by deciding which interventions should be purchased, how, and from whom' (WHO, 2000). The World Bank's advocacy has been explicitly focused on contracting private sector for healthcare provisioning (World Bank, 2004).

It has been argued that just having more money for health will not ensure universal coverage, unless it is spent more efficiently – therefore, the call for health systems to seek greater 'value for money'. 'Selective Contracting' is a central feature of 'SP' as a mean to improve efficiency. Providers – 'public' or 'private' are to be contracted based on who offer the best 'value for money' in terms of prices and quality. 'SP' is essentially seen as means to harnessing energies of the private sector for public health goals (Palmer, 2000).

The theoretical assumptions behind the concept of 'SP' are based on the logic of the market and assumes that 'SP' will lead to greater competition and greater choice for users by making the money follow the patient. It seeks to incentivise performance through 'contracts' and assumes that information systems can be created to allow the 'Purchaser' as well as the patients to pick the best amongst the 'providers' and to measure their results and quality. It argues for autonomy for 'purchaser' and 'provider' and thereby separation of these two roles (Mathauer, 2015). This is influenced by the 'New Public Management' discourse of the 1980s that asked governments to enter into contracts with their own hospitals, so as to use 'contract' as a mode of governance and fund allocation and to bring in efficiency by creating 'internal markets' (Lewis, 1996).

Much of the discourse on 'SP' shows public systems of provisioning in poor light and government directly providing services by allocating budgets is seen by the proponents of 'SP' as the central problem in efficient delivery of healthcare. Direct provision is judged to be inefficient and branded as 'passive purchasing', and it is proposed that it be replaced with 'active or strategic purchasing' through 'selective contracting' (Mathauer, 2015).

The transformation of NHS in England is an early example of 'purchaser-provider split', which followed the path of 'marketisation' which in turn opened the gates of 'privatisation' of a large chunk of its health-care provisioning (Fillippon, 2016). Many countries with well-functioning health systems based on public provisioning, including the Scandanavian countries, introduced 'internal markets' by separating the purchaser and provider roles. Literature on their experience suggests that the promised gains in efficiency rarely happened and any gains were not attributable to marketization or contracting (Robinson, 2003). New Zealand introduced the 'purchaser-provider split' and after experience of a decade, decided to revert back (Cumming, 2016). The evidence from LMICs is limited and does not really show any significant successes of 'SP' in improving equity or quality.

References:

Cumming J 2016, 'Commissioning in New Zealand: learning from the past and present'. Aust J Prim Health. 2016;22(1):34-9. doi: 10.1071/PY15164.

Filippon J et al. 2016, 'Liberalizing" the English National Health Service: background and risks to healthcare entitlement'. Cad Saude Publica. 2016 Aug 29;32(8):e00034716. doi: 10.1590/0102-311X00034716.

Lewis J 1996, 'The Purchaser/Provider Split in Social Care: Is It Working?' Social Policy Administration. Volume 30, Issue 1 March 1996 Pages 1–19 http://onlinelibrary.wiley.com/doi/10.1111/j.1467-9515.1996.tb00478.x/full

Mathauer I 2015, 'Setting the scene: Moving towards UHC through strategic purchasing of quality health care', 29 June 2015, Department of Health Systems Governance and Financing, World Health Organization

Palmer N 2000, 'The use of private-sector contracts for primary health care: theory, evidence and lessons for low-income and middle-income countries'. Bulletin of the World Health Organization, 2000, 78 (6) 829

Robinson M 2003, 'The Australian Budgeting System: On the Cusp of Change'. Discussion Paper No. 165 December 2003. Queensland University of Technology, Australia. http://eprints.qut.edu.au/314/1/WP_Robinson_Cooperation.pdf

WHO 2000, 'World Health Report 2000', WHO

WHO n.d., 'passive to active purchasing' http://www.who.int/health_financing/topics/purchasing/passive-to-strategic-purchasing/en/

World Bank 2004, 'Health Financing for Poor People, Resource Mobilisation and Risk Sharing' World Bank, 2004

The ascendancy of UHC was partly a response to the failures of narrow vertical disease-focused GHIs and the need for a more comprehensive approach to healthcare financing. However, UHC really took off following the global financial crisis in 2008 when continued liberalization of trade, increasing economic integration and the runaway financialization of the global economy were being widely questioned. Again the dance of legitimation is a useful trope: the legitimacy of the global regime came into question and hence the need to address the more egregious criticisms of that regime.

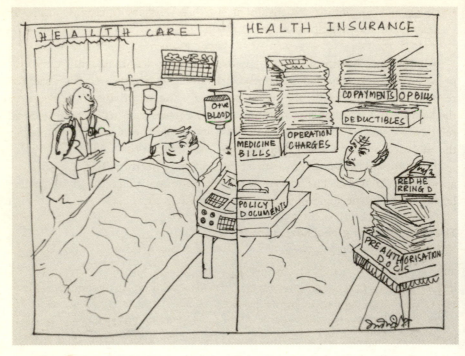

Image B1.4 An economistic mind-set promotes health insurance (Indranil Mukhopadhyay)

This background is crucial to understanding the gulf between the recommendations of the WHO's healthcare financing experts and the economists of the World Bank, and the struggle of Margaret Chan and Jim Kim to establish the (apparent) unity of the WHO and the World Bank around the slogan of UHC and the focus on financial protection.

The global financial crisis reflected the looming overhang of global productive capacity over aggregate demand. For a decade global consumption had been supported by debt, and by China and Germany buying US bonds to prevent their own currencies from appreciating while keeping the US dollar strong and the US consumer buying. The economic policy priorities in the wake of the global financial crisis were to:

- refinance the banks through imposing austerity
- open new markets for private investment (including healthcare and health insurance markets)
- contain taxation so as to reduce the corporate tax burden (and release resources for shareholder dividends) and force governments to create space for the privatization
- render inequality acceptable by providing safety nets for the poor (rather than adopting policies that would reverse widening inequality)

- encourage continuing expansion of trade in services (including trade in healthcare and health insurance).

The WHO's healthcare financing experts work within a culture that is preoccupied with improving population health and healthcare. They are not responsible for managing the world economy. The World Bank's experts on the other hand work within a culture that has to be seen to have answers in relation to healthcare (and other sectors) while playing its role in managing the global economy for the transnational capitalist class.

The differing mandates of the two bodies align perfectly with their respective approaches to UHC. The imperatives of institutional politics and leadership legacy underlie the logic of an apparent united front.

The pragmatics of global health governance

The saga of UHC provides a window on the dynamics of global governance in the present period. This is not merely of academic interest; it is of immediate and practical importance for activists who are struggling to achieve UHC within a 'right to health' framework.

The dynamics of global health governance can be described at different levels, from individuals, to institutions, to systemic forces.

The role of individuals and political parties is real but limited. The outstanding examples in this story were the election of Obama, the appointment of Jim Kim as president of the World Bank and subsequent appointments at the World Bank. It may be also that Margaret Chan's adoption of the UHC motif in part reflected an aspiration to leave behind her a recognizable legacy like Halfdan Mahler did with primary healthcare and Gro Harlem Brundtland with the Framework Convention on Tobacco Control.

The institutional level of analysis highlights further influences such as:

- the differing mandates and cultures of the two organizations, as discussed
- the dependence of the WHO on the large donors, including in particular the World Bank, BMGF and Rockefeller Foundation, the USA and Europe;
- the overt bullying by the USA directed towards containing the technical advice of WHO's healthcare financing experts
- the institutions and culture of conventional economics and their role in framing the health policy discourse
- political institutions at the national level, including ministries of finance and various elite formations.
- Beyond specific institutions are the large-scale political or systemic forces that are clearly at play in the saga of UHC. These include:
- the subprime mortgage collapse, including the bloated financial sector (which was its genesis), the cost of bailing out the banks and the resistance of the banks to effective regulation

- the demands of the transnational corporations (TNCs) for lower taxes and their power to extort tax concessions through the promise of investment, jobs and foreign currency
- the pressures for liberalizing trade in services: for example, from the financial sector for trade in financial services (including health insurance) and various middle-income countries who see increasing economic returns from trade in health services, including both medical tourism and remittances
- the dance of legitimation; the social movements and ideological industries that contend over the prevailing sentiment regarding the legitimacy of the global regime and the pressure for policy concessions as needed to assuage sagging perceptions
- the rise in xenophobia (and demagoguery) associated with economic stagnation and insecurity, a significant dampener on expressions of wider solidarity.

Activist strategies for healthcare reform need to drive change at all three levels.

How health systems develop

The final feature of the UHC discourse that needs to be highlighted is the mechanistic and top-down understanding of policy implementation that permeates the technical literature. This was particularly well reflected in the World Health Report in 2010, which frames the 'agenda for action' in terms of a crude version of the 'policy cycle' (assessment, strategy development, implementation, evaluation and so on).

Whether they are based in Washington or Geneva, policy experts providing technical advice to governments see themselves as dissociated from the ebbs and flows of institutional stability within their client countries. Indeed, if you are providing advice to whole categories of countries it seems to make sense to subsume the barriers of the real world into the processes of 'assess',

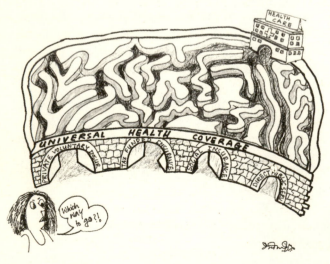

Image B1.5 Different interpretations of UHC (Indranil Mukhopadhyay)

'strategize' and 'implement', rather than acknowledge the different political realities with which advocates for reform must deal.

An alternative narrative of health systems development might focus more on the incremental nature of the development and the ways in which episodes of incremental reform are dispersed across time and across different parts of the system. As particular institutional domains unfreeze, often quite unpredictably, and new 'windows of opportunity' open, localized reforms can be effected if the perceived problems, the circulating policy options and the political winds are aligned (Kingdon, 1984).

The concept of incremental health systems development, with dispersed reform initiatives determined by opportunity, practicable policies and sufficient consensus, raises questions about coherence across this sequence of dispersed policy reforms. Certainly, examples are common of incoherent health systems development where particular reform initiatives are determined only by localized political pragmatism. What can give coherence to a sequence of reforms is a common vision of 'the health system we want'. In this case policy formation and political consensus are shaped by a shared vision that across space and time gives a degree of coherence to the accumulation of more specific initiatives.

Constructing the processes of health system reform as a sequence of dispersed opportunities for incremental reform has important implications for activists. It can be difficult to predict when or where windows of opportunity for health system reform will open. For this reason there is a strong case for working on a whole-of-system basis to project a whole-of-system vision and create a policy environment that is conducive to strategic health system reform. This strategy assumes that no matter where or when the opportunities arise, appropriate policy ideas for this sector will be circulating; the various constituencies will be ready to support change; and there will be a broadly shared vision in place that will help to align the various dispersed reform initiatives.

Notes

1 See http://apps.who.int/gb/archive/pdf_files/WHA58/A58_20-en.pdf

2 See https://www.internationalhealthpartnership.net/en/about-ihp/past-ihp-meetings/high-level-taskforce-for-innovative-international-financing-of-health-systems/

3 By way of contrast see Morgan, Ensor & Waters (2016, pp. 606–12).

References

Brand, C A, Barker, A L, Morello, RT, Vitale, MR, Evans, S M, Scott, I A, Stoelwinder, J U & Cameron, PA 2012, 'A review of hospital characteristics associated with improved performance', *International Journal for Quality in Health Care*, vol. 24, no. 5, pp. 483–94, DOI 10.1093/intqhc/mzs044.

Chaudhry, B, Wang, J, Wu, S, Maglione, M, Mojica, W, Roth, E, Morton, S C & Shekelle, PG 2006, 'Systematic review: impact of health information technology on quality, efficiency, and costs of medical care', *Annals of Internal Medicine*, vol. 144, no. 10, pp. 742–52, DOI 10.7326/0003-4819-144-10-200605160-00125.

Chisholm, D& Evans, DB2010, *Improving health system efficiency as a means of moving towards universal coverage*, World health report background paper 28, World Health Organization.

Cueto, M2004, The origins of primary health care and selective primary health care', *American Journal of Public Health*, vol.94, no. 11, pp. 1864–74.

Fee, E& Parry, M2008, 'Jonathan Mann, HIV/ AIDS, and human rights', *Journal of Public Health Policy*, vol. 29, pp. 54–71, DOI10.1057/ palgrave.jphp.3200160.

Gabel, JR1999, 'Job-based health insurance, 1977–1998: the accidental system under scrutiny', *Health Affairs*, vol. 18, no. 6, pp. 62–74, DOI10.1377/hlthaff.18.6.62.

Gao, J, Moran, E Almenoff, P L, Render, M L, Campbell, J & Jha, AK2011, 'Variations in efficiency and the relationship to quality of care in theveterans health system', *Health Affairs*, vol. 30, no. 4, pp. 655–63, DOI10.1377/hlthaff.2010.0435.

Giedion, U, Alfonso, E A, & Díaz, Y2013, '*The impact of universal coverage schemes in the developing world: a review of the existing evidence*', Washington, DC.

Hammond, S2010, 'Clinical governance and patient safety: an overview', in Haxby, E, Hunter, D & Jaggar, S (eds), *An Introduction to clinical governance and patient safety*, Oxford University Press, pp. 1–12.

Hellander, I & Bhargava, R2012,'Report from the United States: the US health crisis deepens amid rising inequality – a review of data, fall 2011', *International Journal of Health Services*, vol. 42, no. 2, pp. 161–75, DOI10.2190/HS.42.2.a.

High-Level Taskforce on Innovative International Financing for Health Systems 2008, *More money for health, and more health for the money*, https:// www.internationalhealthpartnership. net/fileadmin/uploads/ihp/Documents/ Results__Evidence/HAE_results__lessons/ Taskforce_report_EN.2009.pdf>

Institute of Medicine (US) Committee on Quality of Health Care in America 2001, *Crossing the quality chasm: a new health system for the 21st century*, National Academies Press,Washington, DC.

Kingdon, JW1984,*Agendas, alternatives, and public policies*, University of Michigan, Boston.

Kutzin, J2014, *Health financing for UHC: why the path runs through the finance ministry and PFM rules*, paper presented at the Fiscal Space, Public Finance And Health Financing, Montreux, http://www.who.int/ health_financing/events/1_kutzin_d1s1_hf_ for_uhc_fiscal_pfm.pdf?ua=1

Litsios, S2002, 'The long and difficult road to Alma-Ata: a personal reflection', *International Journal of Health Services*, vol. 32, no. 4, pp. 709–32, https://doi. org/10.2190/RP8C-L5UB-4RAF-NRH2

Litsios, S2004, The Christian Medical Commission and the development of the World Health Organization's primary health care approach', *American Journal of Public Health*, vol.11, pp. 1884–93, http:// ajph.aphapublications.org/doi/pdf/10.2105/ AJPH.94.11.1884

Morgan, R, Ensor, T & Waters, H2016,'Performance of private sector health care: implications for universal health coverage',*The Lancet*, vol. 388,no. 10044, pp. 606–12, http://dx.doi.org/10.1016/S0140-6736(16)00343-3

Newell, K W (ed.) 1975, *Health by the people*, WHO, Geneva.

Preker, A S, Sheffler, R M, & Bassett, MC2007 *Private voluntary health insurance in development : friend or foe?* http://hdl. handle.net/10986/6641

Preker, A S, Zweifel, P & Schellekens, OP2010, *Global marketplace for private health insurance: strength in numbers*, The World Bank,Washington, DC.

Robins, S2010, '"Long live Zackie, long live": AIDS activism, science and citizenship after apartheid', *Journal of Southern African Studies*, vol. 3, pp. 651–72, DOI10.1080/0305707042000254146.

Sachs, JD2012,'Achieving universal health coverage in low-income settings', *The Lancet*, vol. 380, no. 9845, pp 944–47.

Sanders, Dn.d., *Global health initiatives: context, challenges and opportunities, with particular reference to Africa*, WHO Collaborating Centre for Research and Training in Human Resources for Health http://www.who.int/healthsystems/ reference_Africa.pdf

Smith, J2002, 'Globalizing resistance: the Battle of Seattle and the future of social movements',in Smith, J & Johnston, H (eds.), *Globalization and resistance: transnational dimensions of social movements*, Rowman & Littlefield, Lanham and Oxford, pp. 207–28.

Sparkes, S, Durán, A, & Kutzin, J2017, *A system-wide approach to analysing efficiency across health programmes*, http://www.who.int/health_financing/documents/system-wide-approach/en/

'T Hoen, E F M 2009,*The global politics of pharmaceutical monopoly power, drug patents, access, innovation and the application of the WTO Doha Declaration on TRIPS and Public Health*, AMB Publishers, Diemen.

The World Bank 1993, *World development report: investing in health*, The World Bank, Washington, DC.

TWHA & PHM 2017, *Manual 'building a movement' – case studies*, https://twha.be/manual-building-movement-case-studies

WHO 2004a, *Social health insurance, report by the secretariat*, 29 April, http://apps.who.int/gb/archive/pdf_files/EB114/B114_16-en.pdf

WHO 2004b, *Social health insurance, report by the secretariat*, 2 December, http://apps.who.int/gb/ebwha/pdf_files/EB115/B115_8-en.pdf

WHO 2005a, *Executive Board 115th session, summary records*, 17–24 January, http://apps.who.int/gb/ebwha/pdf_files/EB115/B115_REC2-en.pdf#page=91.

WHO 2005b, Fifty-eighth World Health Assembly, summary records of committees, reports of committees, 16–25 May, Geneva, http://apps.who.int/gb/ebwha/pdf_files/WHA58-REC3/A58_REC3-en.pdf#page=193

WHO 2006, *Dr Margaret Chan director-general elect speech to the first special session of the World Health Assembly*, 9 November, http://apps.who.int/gb/archive/pdf_files/WHASSA1/ssa1_div6-en.pdf>.

WHO 2007, *Address by Dr Margaret Chan, director-general to the sixtieth World Health Assembly*, 15 May, http://apps.who.int/gb/archive/pdf_files/WHA60/A60_3-en.pdf

WHO 2012, *Address by Dr Margaret Chan, director-general, to the sixty-fifth World Health Assembly*, 21 May, http://apps.who.int/gb/ebwha/pdf_files/WHA65/A65_3-en.pdf

WHO 2013, *Sixty-sixth World Health Assembly*, 19 July, http://apps.who.int/gb/ebwha/pdf_files/WHA66/A66_DIV4-en.pdf

WTO Ministerial Council2001, *Doha declaration on the TRIPS Agreement and Public Health*, https://www.wto.org/english/thewto_e/minist_e/min01_e/mindecl_trips_e.htm

Community-controlled primary healthcare (PHC) services are governed by a board of management consisting of community members, allowing high-level community inputs into service planning, delivery and evaluation. The history of community control in PHC predates the World Health Organization's Alma-Ata Declaration on Primary Health Care (WHO 1978). The Alma-Ata Declaration laid out the key aspects of PHC, which were being implemented in many nations, to provide a vision for achieving health for all by the year 2000: namely, the provision of comprehensive PHC to promote health and prevent disease, as well as the provision of curative and rehabilitative services that address existing ill health.

The Alma-Ata Declaration "requires and promotes maximum community and individual self-reliance and participation in the planning, organization, operation and control of primary health care". The Alma-Ata Declaration also argued for a new world economic order to counter the massive growth in the power and influence of the transnational corporations, which were weakening the power of citizens to take action in support of their health. The subsequent WHO Ottawa Charter for Health Promotion (WHO, 1986) heavily emphasized the need for enabling community power and control in order to promote health. The People's Charter for Health[1] (2000) was grounded in the need for citizens' involvement in all aspect of healthcare, stressing that "Strong people's organizations and movements are fundamental to more democratic, transparent and accountable decision-making processes."

Health systems and services have implemented community participation in ways that are often not as democratic as envisaged in the People's Charter for Health (Rifkin, 2009, pp. 31–36; Rifkin, Lewando-Hundt and Draper, 2000). The continuum and typologies of community participation in health services show how community inputs can range from tokenistic efforts and consultations to seek community views to structural participation, as in the case of community-controlled services, where the community has real power to control the scope of participation, and affect service decisions and planning (Arnstein, 1969, pp. 216–23; Baum, 2015; Oakley, 1989). Across the continuum, the terms used to describe the different levels of community participation differ. This acknowledges that different community participation efforts vary in the extent to which they truly realize the democratic control of health services.

While efforts at the consultative end of the spectrum are largely concerned with ensuring the acceptability of health services, community control has the more ambitious goal of providing space for community power to control healthcare, to increase the community's control over its own health and to improve the responsiveness of the health service to the local community (Freemanet al., 2016a, pp. E1–E21). Internationally, this goal continues to be blocked by, and is always hard won against, the opposing force of entrenched corporate and private sector interests in the health field (Mackintosh et al., 2016, pp. 596–605; Mooney, 2012). In the face of the current trend towards privatization of healthcare services, revisiting and revitalizing the community control of health services is more relevant than ever.

The Alma Ata Declaration was informed by many case studies of grassroots healthcare programmes in China, Cuba, India, Indonesia and elsewhere, which stressed participation, local flexibility and responsiveness, the use of community health workers and less professional dominance (Cueto, 2004, pp. 1864–74; Rifkin, 2003, pp. 168–80). In Australia, one of the pre-Alma-Ata pioneers of comprehensive PHC and community control has been the Aboriginal Community Controlled Health Organizations (ACCHOs).[2] Briefly, ACCHOs were first established in the 1970s as a response to the Aboriginal and Torres Strait Islander peoples' poor access to health services and the discriminatory practices in mainstream healthcare (Torzillo, et al., 1992). Currently in 2017, there are about 150 Aboriginal community-controlled organizations in Australia, serving between a third to a half of the total Aboriginal and Torres Strait Islander population (Dwyer, et al., 2011, pp. 34–46). The principle at the heart of the ACCHOs is that Aboriginal and Torres Strait Islander communities should be in control of their own health and healthcare (Bartlett and Boffa, 2001, pp. 74–82). Aboriginal community-controlled health services "are initiated, planned and governed by boards elected from the local Aboriginal community" (National Aboriginal Community Controlled Health Organisation, 2011, p.1), though some organizations started as government services with the control then transferring to the community (South Australian Department of Health, 2010).

Alongside ACCHOs, multidisciplinary community health services with community boards emerged in Australia in the early 1970s under the federal community health programme (Australia. Hospitals and Health Services Commission. Interim Committee, 1973). Community health services developed in Canada (Abelson and Lomas, 1990, p. 575), the USA (Ulmer, et al., 2000) and elsewhere, working in a manner consistent with the Alma-Ata vision of comprehensive PHC. The present chapter considers the evidence for the benefits of community control, with specific reference to ACCHOs and community health centres.

Evidence for the benefits of community control in ACCHOs

The great extent of health inequities and the barriers to health service access faced by Aboriginal and Torres Strait Islander peoples in Australia have been well documented (Australian Institute of Health and Welfare, 2011; Australian Institute of Health and Welfare, 2015). The lack of equity has occurred in the context of ongoing colonization due to which mainstream health services are often not culturally safe, reproduce unfair power relationships, are not in accord with Aboriginal and Torres Strait Islander perspectives on health and well-being, and fail to address the inequities of such social determinants of the peoples' health as income, access to transport, and racism and discrimination (Freeman, et al., 2014, pp. 355–61). Indigenous peoples in Canada, New Zealand and Australia have all emphasized the centrality of self-determination to health and well-being, and the need for indigenous community-governed health services (Lavoie and Dwyer, 2016, pp. 453–58).

In Australia, the ACCHOs were a result of grass roots Aboriginal and Torres Strait Islander-led activism, identifying community-controlled health services as the solution to the problem. Given this, it is unfortunate that the innovative approaches and unique contribution to indigenous health of Aboriginal community-controlled health organizations are too often neglected in PHC studies. It is typical for research studies to rely on quantitative comparisons between mainstream PHC and ACCHOs, despite the very different models of care and the populations served (Dwyer, et al., 2015). The results of such studies are mixed, but often indicate that ACCHOs achieve clinical curative or chronic condition management outcomes similar to mainstream PHC (general

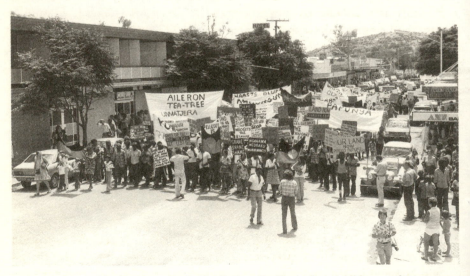

Image B2.1 Public demonstration in Alice Springs, leading to the establishment of Congress, 1973. (Central Australian Aboriginal Congress)

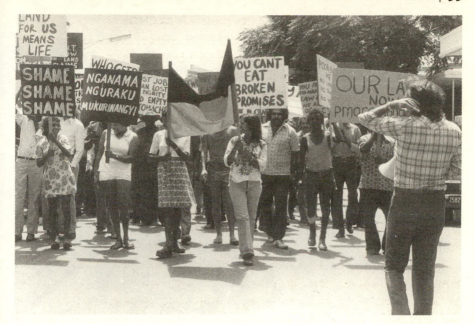

Image B2.2 ACCHOs were a result of grass roots Aboriginal-led activism. (Central Australian Aboriginal Congress)

practice) despite having a more complex and disadvantaged caseload (Aboriginal Health & Medical Research Council, 2015; Dwyer et al., 2015; Mackay, Boxall and Partel, 2014). This is in itself a very strong finding, but does not still take into account the more comprehensive suite of activities the ACCHOs engage in, such as community development, advocacy and health promotion.

A study of a community-controlled health service, the Central Australian Aboriginal Congress Aboriginal Corporation, in the Northern Territory, found that in addition to primary medical care, the Congress exhibited strengths in comprehensive PHC over and above those in the other PHC models in the research study, including the following (Freeman et al., 2016b, pp. 93–108):

- more comprehensive multidisciplinary services, with a wide range of allied health disciplines, along with visiting specialists to provide services out of the Congress clinics
- a wide range of strategies to engage with and seek inputs from the community, including the community board: the only example of structural participation in the research, which allowed the community to set the scope and nature of their participation
- considerable efforts to ensure accessibility of services, through the provision of a mix of appointments and drop-ins, transport service, outreach services and home visits, employment of local Aboriginal staff and respect for local cultural protocols

- greater orientation towards health promotion and addressing the social determinants of health, while meeting the strong demand for curative services, including collaborative advocacy on alcohol supply reduction measures, early childhood services and community health education.

The Central Australian Aboriginal Congress Aboriginal Corporation drew its name from Mahatma Gandhi's Congress Party, and to this day has a quote on him its website that is often attributed to him (CAAC 2017):

"Our clients are the most important visitors on our premises.
They are not dependant on us.
We are dependent on them.
They are not an interruption on work.
They are the purpose of it.
They are not an outsider to our business.
They are part of it.
We are not doing them a favour by serving them.
They are doing us a favour by giving us the opportunity to do it."
Gandhi [*sic*]

A number of health services in Australia have been transferred from state government management to community control, providing an opportunity to examine what benefits community control may bring. In the Northern Territory, where some key research has been done, once health services were transferred to Aboriginal community control, a range of benefits were observed: there was an increased focus on health promotion, greater employment of local people, a greater focus on culturally safe care and improved community participation (Dwyer et al., 2015). Adequate resourcing of community-controlled health services is also critical: the Central Australian Aboriginal Congress benefited from an AUD 30 million per annum budget, and when the health services in the Northern Territory transitioned to community control, this came with an increase in budget. However, the findings still highlight how community control appears to allow a more comprehensive PHC vision to bloom, in line with the Alma-Ata Declaration.

These findings reflect other international experiences of indigenous community-controlled health services. In Canada, indigenous community-controlled health services have been largely services transferred from federal government management (Lavoie and Dwyer 2016, pp. 453–58). In one study (Lavoie et al., 2010, pp. 717–24), it was found that the First Nation community health services, which transitioned from government control to community control, achieved a 30 per cent reduction in hospital utilization rates for ambulatory care sensitive conditions (those conditions for which PHC is most well placed to prevent hospitalization). The benefits were greater the longer the services had been under community control, and the authors concluded the positive health benefits were due to self-determination. In the USA, some organizations have been transferred to community ownership from the Indian Health Service. There is not enough research on the benefits or performance of these organizations, though there is some evidence that community-controlled services focus more on prevention and local needs than do federal services (Rainie et al., 2015, pp. 1–24).

In Australia, the Redfern Statement, signed by over 50 Aboriginal and Torres Strait Islander and non-indigenous organizations, called for a change in policy and government relationships on Aboriginal and Torres Strait Islander health to transform inequitable power relationships and support self-determination (National Congress of Australia's First Peoples et al., 2016). The achievements of Aboriginal community-controlled health services in Australia and internationally provide evidence for the importance of self-determination and increased power and control as determinants of indigenous health.

Evidence for the benefits of community control in community health centres

Another leading model of community-controlled PHC is community health centres, found in many countries, including Australia, Canada and the USA. In Australia, these centres have their roots in the Federal Community Health Program (National Hospital and Health Services Commission Interim Committee 1973), although this programme only lasted three years and left the different states and territories to run community health centres in their own way. Two states, South Australia and Victoria, have particularly strong histories of vibrant community health sectors based on a comprehensive PHC approach (Legge et al., 1996, pp. 22–26). Legge et al., (ibid.) emphasize the importance of community participation, particularly the power of community control, in achieving good comprehensive PHC practice. Critically, a comprehensive PHC approach allows the melding of professional approaches to health that focus on diseases and risk factors with community approaches that are more likely to focus on living conditions and community capacity to work to improve health. This potential is supported by a 1992–1993 survey of South Australian boards of community health centres, which found that two of the three functions board members were most involved in were "deciding philosophy and policies" and "deciding which issues the health service should address" (Laris, 1995).

Since the period that Laris (ibid.) and Legge et al. (1996) have studied, there has been in South Australia and other states and territories a state policy move away from comprehensive PHC (though less so in Victoria). Community boards in South Australian services were abolished in 2004, with power shifting to the central health department by 2006. A series of neoliberal restructures and changes to South Australian PHC have been documented, and indicates the threat that neoliberalism, with its narrow focus on outputs and control of staff through managerialism, poses globally to community control of health services and to comprehensive PHC generally (Baum et al., 2016, pp. 43–52).

Community health centres also have a strong history in Canada, where the implementation of this model has varied from province to province. Some have community governance structures, while others do not. A survey conducted by the Canadian Association of Community Health Centres (2013) of over 200 centres across Canada found that those with community governance were more likely to undertake work that addressed social determinants of health and health equity: for example, programmes and advocacy about food security, racism, housing and homelessness, poverty and income security, and refugee health services. Again, this demonstrates a link between community control of health services and the ability to enact the comprehensive Alma-Ata vision of PHC. In the USA, community health centres service 22 million people, primarily those with low income, who are uninsured or have low English proficiency (Li et al., 2016, pp. 356–70). These, too, are community- governed, and have a focus on prevention and the social determinants of health, including access to healthy food, employment, housing and education (National Association of Community Health Centres, 2012).

Conclusion

Community control has the potential to democratize health services. Implementing the approach throughout health systems would help realize the original Alma-Ata dream of health or all: through community perspectives that complement and strengthen professional views of health; through community management to take responsibility for the health of the local community in such a way as to foster action on the social determinants of health; by responding to local needs, supporting accessibility and building community capacity for health.

Community control offers more relevant, effective and efficient healthcare than corporatized, for-profit care. Involving citizens in the management of health services is likely to make them strong advocates for non-commercialized healthcare and provide a counter voice to the powerful corporate voices baying for more chances for profit. For indigenous peoples, it also provides greater self-determination and control over health and healthcare, and more culturally respectful services that take into account holistic, indigenous conceptions of health and healing.

Community control will contribute to decolonization, which is essential to restoring indigenous people's health and well-being. Of course it is also a central mechanism in the achievement of comprehensive PHC as envisioned in the World Health Organization's Alma-Ata Declaration – a vision that was immediately challenged by a more selective, technical view of PHC and which continues to be challenged in an era of neoliberalism, austerity and the privileging of biomedical and commercialized models of health. The value of community control in combating these threats to comprehensive PHC and health for all is as relevant, and as urgent, as ever.

Notes

1 The People's Charter for Health is a statement of the shared vision, goals, principles and calls for action that unite all the members of the PHM coalition... [A] widely endorsed consensus document on health since the Alma-Ata Declaration,... [it] was formulated and endorsed by the participants of the First People's Health Assembly held at Dhaka, Bangladesh in December 2000. http://www.phmovement.org/en/resources/charters/peopleshealth

2 The ACCHOs were the subject of a chapter in *Global Health Watch 4*. See *Global Health Watch 4*, http://www.ghwatch.org/sites/www.ghwatch.org/files/E9.pdf

References

Abelson, J & Lomas, J 1990, 'Do health service organizations and community health centres have higher disease prevention and health promotion levels than fee-for-service practices?'*Canadian Medical Association Journal*, vol. 142, no. 6, p. 575.

Aboriginal Health & Medical Research Council 2015, *Aboriginal communities improving Aboriginal health: an evidence review on the contribution of Aboriginal Community Controlled Health Services to improving Aboriginal health*, Aboriginal Health & Medical Research Council, Sydney.

Arnstein, S R 1969, 'Ladder of citizen participation', *Journal of the American Institute of Planners*, vol. 35, pp. 216–23.

Australia. Hospitals and Health Services Commission. Interim Committee1973, *A community health program for Australia: a report from the National Hospitals and Health Services Commission Interim Committee*, Canberra.

Australian Institute of Health and Welfare 2011, *Access to health services for Aboriginal and Torres Strait Islander people*, Cat. no. IHW 46, Australian Institute of Health and Welfare, Canberra.

Australian Institute of Health and Welfare 2015, *The health and welfare of Australia's Aboriginal and Torres Strait Islander peoples*, Cat. no. IHW 147, Australian Institute of Health and Welfare, Canberra.

Bartlett, B & Boffa, J 2001, 'Aboriginal community controlled comprehensive primary health care: the Central Australian Aboriginal Congress', *Australian Journal of Primary Health*, vol.7,pp. 74–82, DOI10.1071/PY01050.

Baum, F 2015,*The new public health*, 4th edn, Oxford University Press,Melbourne.

Baum, F, Freeman, T, Sanders, D, Labonté, R, Lawless, A & Javanparast, S, 2016, 'Comprehensive primary health care under neo-liberalism in Australia', *Social Science & Medicine*, vol. 168, pp. 43–52.

CAAC 2017, *Client services*, Central Australian Aboriginal Congress, viewed 26 February 2017 http://www.caac.org.au/.

Canadian Association of Community Health Centres 2013, *CHCs organizational survey*,viewed 2 February 2016, http://www.cachc.ca/2013survey/.

Cueto, M 2004,'The origins of primary health care and selective primary health care', *American Journal of Public Health*,vol.94, pp. 1864–74.

Dwyer, J, Lavoie, J, O'Donnell, K, Marlina, U, & Sullivan, P 2011, 'Contracting for indigenous health care: towards mutual accountability', *Australian Journal of Public Administration*, vol. 70, no. 1, pp. 34–46, DOI: 10.1111/j.1467-8500.2011.00715.x>.

Dwyer, J, Martini, A, Brown, C, Tilton, E, Devitt, J, Myott, P & Pekarsky, B 2015, *The road is made by walking: towards a better primary health care system for Australia's First Peoples – summary report*, The Lowitja Institute, Carlton.

Freeman, T, Baum, F E, Jolley, GM, Lawless, Edwards, T, Javanparast, S & Ziersch, A 2016a, 'Service providers' views of community participation at six Australian primary healthcare services: scope for empowerment and challenges to implementation', *The International Journal of Health Planning and Management*, vol. 31, pp. E1–E21, Doi: 10.1002/hpm.2253.

Freeman, T, Baum, F, Lawless, A, Labonte, R, Sanders, D, Boffa, J, Edwards, T & Javanparast, S2016b,'Case study of an Aboriginal community controlled health service in Australia: universal, rights-based, publicly-funded comprehensive primary health care in action', *Health and Human Rights Journal*, vol.18, pp. 93–108.

Freeman, T, Edwards, T, Baum, F, Lawless, A, Jolley, G, Javanparast, S & Francis, T 2014, 'Cultural respect strategies in Australian Aboriginal primary health care services: beyond education and training of practitioners', *Australian and New Zealand Journal of Public Health*, vol. 38, no. 4, pp. 355–61, DOI: 10.1111/1753-6405.12231.

Laris, P1995, 'Boards of directors of community health services', in Baum, F (ed.), *Health for all: The South Australian experience*, Wakefield Press, Adelaide.

Lavoie, J G & Dwyer, J 2016, 'Implementing indigenous community control in health care: lessons from Canada', *Australian Health Review*,vol.40, no. 4, pp. 453–58, DOI: http://dx.doi.org/10.1071/AH14101.

Lavoie J G, Forget, E L, Prakash, T, Dahl, M, Martens, P & O'Neil, J D 2010, 'Have investments in on-reserve health services and initiatives promoting community control improved First Nations' health in Manitoba? '*Social Science & Medicine*, vol. 71, no. 4, pp. 717–24.

Legge, D, Wilson, G, Butler, P, Wright, M, McBride, T & Attewell, R 1996, 'Best practice in primary health care', *Australian Journal of Primary Health*,vol.2, no. 1, pp. 22–26.

Li, V, McBurnie, M A, Simon, M, Crawford, P, Leo, M, Rachman, F, Cottrell, E, Dant, L, Oneha, M & Weir, R C 2016, 'Impact of social determinants of health on patients with complex diabetes who are served by national safety-net health centers', *The Journal of the American Board of Family Medicine*, vol. 29, no. 3, pp. 356–70.

Mackay, P, Boxall, A & Partel, K 2014, *Relative effectiveness of aboriginal community controlled health services compared with mainstream health service*,Deeble Institute/ Australian Healthcare and Hospitals Association, Canberra.

Mackintosh, M, Channon, A, Karan, A, Selvaraj, S, Cavagnero, E & Zhao, H 2016, 'What is the private sector? Understanding private provision in the health systems of low-income and middle-income countries', *The Lancet*, vol. 388, no. 10044, pp. 596–605, DOI10.1016/S0140-6736(16)00342-1.

Mooney, G 2012, *The health of nations: towards a new political economy*, Zed Books, London.

National Aboriginal Community Controlled Health Organisation 2011, *An overview*, National Aboriginal Community Controlled Health Organisation, Canberra.

National Association of Community Health Centres 2012, *Powering healthier communities: community health centers address the social determinants of health*, National Association of Community Health Centres, Bethesda.

National Congress of Australia's First Peoples et al. 2016,*The Redfern statement*, http://nationalcongress.com.au/wp-content/uploads/2017/02/The-Redfern-Statement-9-June-_Final.pdf.

Oakley, P 1989, *Community involvement in health development: An examination of the critical issues*, World Health Organization, Geneva.

Rainie, S, Jorgensen, M, Cornell, S, & Arsenault, J 2015, 'The changing landscape of health care provision to American Indian nations', *American Indian Culture and Research Journal*, vol. 39, no. 1, pp. 1–24.

Rifkin, SB2003, 'A framework linking community empowerment and health equity: It's a matter of CHOICE', *Journal of Health, Population, and Nutrition*, vol. 21, pp. 168–80.

Rifkin, S B 2009, 'Lessons from community participation in health programmes: a review of the post Alma-Ata experience,' *International Health*, vol. 1, no. 1, pp. 31–36, DOI 10.1016/j.inhe.2009.02.001.

Rifkin, S B, Lewando-Hundt, G & Draper, AK2000, *Participatory approaches in health promotion and health planning: a literature review*, Health Development Agency, London.

South Australian Department of Health 2010, *Aboriginal Health Care Plan 2010–2016*, Statewide Service Strategy Division, Adelaide.

Torzillo, P, Rainow, S, Pholeros, P, Tunkin, W & Vartto, K1992, 'Extending community health services', in Baum, F, Fry, D & Lennie, I (eds), *Community health: policy and practice in Australia*, Pluto Press, NSW.

Ulmer, C, Lewis-Idema, D, Von Worley, A, Rodgers, J, Berger, LR, Darling, EJ&Lefkowitz, B 2000, 'Assessing primary care content: four conditions common in community health center practice', *Journal* of Ambulatory Care Management, vol. 23, no. 1, pp. 23–38.

WHO 1978, Declaration of Alma-Ata, international conference on primary health care, USSR, 6–12 September, World Health Organization, Alma-Ata.

WHO 1986, Ottawa Charter for health promotion, First International Conference on Health Promotion, 21 November, Ottawa.

Introduction

In the mid-1960s a group of progressively-minded New York activists came together to found the Health Policy Advisory Center or Health/PAC as it came to be called. It was a time of intense activism in New York as poor communities took to the streets demanding improved services and were emboldened to actually take over Lincoln Hospital in the Bronx (known locally as 'the butcher shop').[1]

Following a 1967 'exposé-analysis' written by one of the authors of this chapter (Robb Burlage), Health/PAC began publishing a monthly bulletin offering a 'New Left' perspective on health. Three years later in 1970, John and Barbara Ehrenreich published a book-length critique of US healthcare based on the Health/PAC article, titled *The American Health Empire*.

The medical–industrial complex

In November 1969, Health/PAC first used the phrase 'medical–industrial complex' (MIC) as a way of characterizing the US health system. The term was a spin-off from President Eisenhower's farewell address in 1961, during which he discussed the dangers of the "military–industrial complex".

Health/PAC's use of the term 'MIC' incorporated the perception that healthcare was moving away from a system built on individual doctors and small community hospitals; healthcare was becoming more and more the 'business' of large academic centres that Health/PAC characterized as medical empires. These medical empires were constructed around a central (private, academic) hospital and outlying satellite (city) hospitals, serving mainly poor communities. The idea of a medical empire incorporated the understanding that the healthcare system had a colonial nature. The satellite hospitals' role was to service the evolving Academic Medical Centers.

The utility of a concept Most analyses of the US healthcare system attribute its failures to one of two problems. Either the US system is portrayed as an over-regulated market that escapes 'market discipline' or it is presented as a fragmented 'non-system'. *The American Health Empire* offered an alternative explanation: The problems of US healthcare were due to its focus on profit: "Health is no more a priority of the American health system than safe, cheap, efficient, pollution-free transportation is a priority of the American automobile industry." (Ehrenreich B and Ehrenreich J, 1970) This was a key insight for two reasons: First, it pointed out that the essential problem with the health system was the commodification of health and the idea that health was an economic good. Second, true reform would have to dismantle this model. Decades of modest reforms did little to improve poor performance on the part of the overall system.

Parsing out President Eisenhower's speech on the military–industrial complex In his 1961 speech, President Eisenhower first introduced the concept of the military–industrial complex with these words: "In the councils of government, we must guard against the acquisition of unwarranted influence, whether sought or unsought, by the military industrial complex. The potential for the disastrous rise of misplaced power exists and will persist[2]."

Eisenhower's speech was essentially concerned with the threat to government posed by the enormous power of the defence industry and the military. He discussed three entities: the military (an organ of the state), the defence industry (private corporations) and the councils of government (the US Congress).

Eisenhower's concern – the co-optation of the state for private ends – was similar to that of *regulatory capture*, which occurs when "a regulatory agency, created to act in the public interest, instead advances the commercial or political concerns of special interest groups that dominate the industry or sector it is charged with regulating"[3].

A 'market-driven' healthcare system During the early days of the Trump administration, the Republicans sought (unsuccessfully) to sell their idea of a 'market-driven' healthcare system. Markets, they argued, would bring down costs and improve quality. In the words of Republican Speaker Paul Ryan: "The 'Patients' Choice Act of 2009' transforms healthcare in America by strengthening the relationship between the patient and the doctor; using choice and competition rather than rationing and restrictions to contain costs; and ensuring universal, affordable healthcare for all Americans[3]". As we examine the US healthcare system, it will become clear that the idea that markets (choice and competition) improve healthcare is not based on any 'really existing' experience.

A conservative critique of the MIC Although Health/PAC had conceived the concept of a medical–industrial complex, mainstream outlets typically associate this idea with the late Dr Arnold Relman, who wrote an article in the *New England Journal of Medicine* (*NEJM*) in 1980 called "The new medical–industrial complex". Relman came from an aristocratic Boston medical culture and was not primarily interested in radical change in the healthcare system. But he was concerned about the "large and growing network of private corporations engaged in the business of supplying health services to patients for a profit—services heretofore provided by non-profit institutions or individual practitioners". Relman was concerned that the increase in 'for-profit' activities within medicine posed difficult conflicts of interest for individual physicians, while polluting the rational scientific independence of health research. (Relman, 1980).

Relman also offered a cogent critique of the 'healthcare marketplace'. First, he noted that for many people health was a human right and not a 'good' that could be bought and sold in a market. Second, he argued that most people who needed care were insured either by their employers or the government; this meant they did not directly pay for care and were thus insulated from the real costs. Thus, "the classic laws of supply and demand do not operate because health-care consumers do not have the usual incentives to be prudent, discriminating purchasers". Finally, he pointed out that most healthcare decisions were actually made by doctors whose decisions could involve real conflicts of interest, such as a tendency to do unnecessary testing in a fee-for-service system (ibid).

Relman did not mention one of the key practical problems with market-based health systems: their lack of transparency. Currently, US hospital charges are hard to find, difficult to interpret and seem to follow no particular logic (Brill, 2013). There is little chance this will change in the near future.

These critiques are important for those of us who wish to de-commodify human health and suffering, but they held little force in a healthcare system that was expanding rapidly. Yet we can see how all the problems mentioned by Relman are manifest in our current healthcare 'marketplace'.

Meet the MIC: major players

We can use these ideas to better understand the current system and its problems, in terms of the main players of the healthcare industry and parts of the government involved in the provision of healthcare.

According to statistics from the Organization for Economic Cooperation and Development (OECD), from 2015 the USA has been spending approximately US$ 9,451 per capita on health, representing some 16.9 per cent of the US GDP (OECD, 2017). Most countries spend far less. On average, OECD countries spend about 8.9 per cent of the GDP on health, so that US expenditures (in terms of GDP percentage) is *nearly double the OECD average*. It is not the case that US healthcare outcomes (which are largely dependent on social and economic conditions) are better than those of other countries. Furthermore, even after the implementation of the Affordable Care Act, millions of Americans were unable to afford health insurance and/or healthcare

The large amount we pay for healthcare reflects the role of profit within the healthcare system and we can identify the big players here by following the money. They include, among others, the health insurance companies, the pharmaceutical companies, the government players, for-profit long-term care services and the medical elites.

The insurance industry Health insurance companies collected some US\$ 635 billion in 2015 (Insurance Information Institute 2017). Yet many have questioned exactly what social benefit these companies provide. In theory, a robust insurance market will drive down costs and improve quality. But it is not clear that this is happening. Instead we see the insurance market consolidating via mega-mergers into a small group of 'too big to fail' health companies. Much of what the Affordable Care Act did was subsidize the private insurance system.

By 2014, 83 per cent of health insurance was provided by one of four companies: Cigna, Aetna, United Healthcare and Anthem (The Commonwealth Fund 2017). Subsequently, the field attempted further consolidation. United Healthcare merged with Humana (and adopted its name). Aetna then attempted to purchase the resulting company. Cigna and Anthem then announced a merger plan, which was stopped by the courts on anti-trust grounds.

Such mergers exemplify what happens in open markets. Rather than competing, companies find it safer to merge with competitors. The end result is a few very big companies who have no interest in a price war. This is just the opposite of the supposed benefits of the market.

The pharmaceutical industry: legal extortion In 2016 US pharmaceutical sales reached US\$ 425 billion (Bloomberg, 2016). Current estimates are that the pharmaceutical industry will have international sales of US\$ 1.4 trillion by 2020 (IMS Institute for Healthcare Informatics, 2015). In the past few years we have seen a new model of pharmaceutical sales that verges on extortion; it is a part of what some have called 'the flagrant-extortion economy' (Chocano, 2017).

This transformation is illustrated by Valeant Pharmaceuticals. The story begins in 2004 when activist-investor Bill Ackman teamed up with the CEO of Valeant Pharmaceuticals, J. Michael Pearson. Pearson argued that most of the money spent on research and development (R&D) would ultimately not result in a useable drug. He suggested a different strategy. First, they would slash Valeant's R&D department, purchase patents from other pharmaceutical companies (or merge with them), and hike up the prices on the newly acquired medications which had patent protection. He also came up with an idea to incorporate Valeant as a Canadian firm; this would allow them to avoid high US corporate tax rates.

The result was massive increases in the prices charged for Valeant drugs. Glumetza (a diabetes drug) saw a price jump from US\$ 520 to US\$ 4,600. Other companies took advantage of Pearson's strategy and also raised their prices. The result is that patented drugs have seen astonishing price increases; prices for patented drugs are estimated to have increased 18 per cent each year since 2010 (Kacik, 2017).

This strategy turned the idea of a healthcare market in the USA on its head. The market now became a vehicle for using a monopoly to accumulate riches. Rather than respond to this crisis by regulating prices – something the US government could legally do – the Obama administration criticized the industry but took no action. Valeant would ultimately fail because it overextended itself. As noted by James Surowieki (2016) writing in *New Yorker Magazine*, "Valeant has been less like a drug company than like a super-aggressive hedge fund that just happened to specialize in pharmaceuticals." We don't know how many people died because they could not afford the exorbitant costs of their drugs.

But this lack of price protection for patients is nothing exceptional. The Medicare programme, which accounts for about 30 per cent of all national healthcare spending, is *specifically prohibited* from negotiating prices with the drug companies.[5] This prohibition (called the 'non-interference clause') reflects the power of the pharmaceutical companies as well as Republican arguments that price negotiations would 'expand the role of government' (Cubanski and Neuman, 2017).

There may be more mundane reasons why the Congress has not allowed Medicare to negotiate prices with Big Pharma. Big Pharma is one of the largest lobbies in Washington, DC. Data provided by OpenSecrets.org (2016) shows that in 2016 companies that produced pharmaceutical and health products spent US$ 246 million on lobbying. This largesse was spent on 315 clients by some 1,125 lobbyists; there are only 534 members of Congress. In 2016 Paul Ryan alone would benefit from US$ 395,000 in lobbying gifts.[6]

In addition to receiving lobbying money, many representatives hold large investments in healthcare companies and thus have a direct financial interest in reducing taxes and fees for the pharmaceutical industry. Unfortunately, under current congressional rules this is entirely legal (Glawe, 2017). As Mark Twain said, "We have the best Congress money can buy."

Academic Medical Centers Columbia University was the model used by Health/PAC for its concept of a medical empire, and the centre of the empire was a large academic hospital. It utilized 'colonized' city hospitals as a source of profit and 'teaching material' (that is, patients who could be used for teaching or research purposes). The division between 'centre' and 'periphery' (to use the language of colonialism) was reflected in the colour of the patients – mainly white at Columbia's Presbyterian Hospital and mainly black at Harlem Hospital. It is worth pointing out that nearly five decades after Heath/PAC raised this as an issue, New York's elite hospitals continue to cater to white clientele with private insurance (PNHP, 2017). In 2016, Columbia reported US$ 5.2 billion in total revenues of which US$ 100 million went to charity care; this all the while being tax-exempt as a 'not-for-profit'.

Columbia Presbyterian has received major funding from the state (primarily to conduct research and teaching) as well as from philanthropy and private industry. The hospital also exercises significant political power. In 2010, this power allowed the university to profit from the state's right of eminent domain to evict an entire community that stood in the way of a planned university expansion (Bagli, 2010).

In a de-industrialized New York City, economic activity centres on the so-called FIRE economy (finance, insurance and real estate). Elite representatives of the FIRE economy – particularly finance – make up the Universities Board of Trustees and place it centrally within a nexus of power in New York (Columbia University, 2017).

Academic Medical Centers have been central, particularly in metropolitan areas, in the creation in the last decade or so, of so-called 'health systems' as hospitals merge and morph into 'networks'. The NYC metro-region, encompassing more than 10 million people, has about a half-dozen of these 'health systems'.

Public hospitals In many large US cities, there is typically one municipal hospital, which is responsible for providing 'charity' care to those in need. They are essentially the provider of last resort for those patients who do not have insurance. New York City runs 11 public hospitals under a federal administration that is hostile to them. They operate in a system that is deeply fiscally challenged. Nonetheless, these public hospitals are an important source of care, particularly for the half-million 'undocumented immigrants' who live in New York City.

The healthcare workforce The healthcare workforce is represented by a variety of professional societies. These would include the American Academy of Pediatrics, the American Medical Association, the American Academy of Family Practice, the Society of General Internal Medicine and the American Public Health Association (to name just a few). These organizations are often (but not always) somewhat conservative; after all, they represent individuals who are privileged in American society. This has led to patterns of thought and behaviour that were quite inadequate to respond to the recent Republican attack on the healthcare system.

Many of them are victim to something akin to 'regulatory capture', by partnering with private entities who dwarf them in size and do not work in favour of the public's health. For example, for many years the website of the American Academy of Family Practice (AAFP) offered educational material with the Coca-Cola logo; this has now been removed, but the AAFP remains largely dependent on funding from Pharma (AAFP, 2016).

Unions Heathcare unions – particularly nurses' unions such as the New York State Nursing Association and the California Nurses Association/National Nurses United – have been in the forefront of progressive activism, showing a far more sophisticated approach to political advocacy than most professional medical societies. Medical schools tend to inculcate values of hierarchy and an avoidance of social issues, which are seen as 'political'. Physicians' unions are relatively rare and often represent doctors associated with a particular institution or public hospitals.

Major governmental players The US government is heavily involved at various levels, both in providing direct healthcare services and in healthcare research. Much of this activity involves interaction with other areas of the MIC.

CMS: Centers for Medicare and Medicaid Services: The CMS was created in 1977 to manage Medicare (primarily services for the elderly and disabled) and Medicaid (a joint federal state programme to provide healthcare to the poor). It later assumed control of the Children's Health Insurance Program (CHIP), which provides insurance for children up to age 18. Thus, CMMS touches people at all stages of life.

Medicare has been one of the great successes of the US healthcare policy. Currently, Medicare covers 55 million Americans (about 15 per cent of the population), is widely popular and has administrative costs of only 2 per cent (Archer, 2011). Private insurance companies, in contrast, are mandated to keep administrative costs to less than 20 per cent! Unfortunately, this creates a perverse incentive for the insurance companies to inflate prices. A hospital bill for US$ 100 allows for overhead expenses of US$ 20. If the bill is US$ 200, the insurance company can now pocket US$ 40 in overheads.

Medicare faces a number of challenges as the US population ages. It is under attack from conservative Republicans who just don't like the idea of federal financing for healthcare and would like to see Medicare turned into a voucher programme. In response to these pressures, Medicare has been mandated to provide supplemental insurance (sometimes called Medi-Gap or Medicare Advantage) policies to people who can afford them. The experience of these private programmes has not been good. They have used a variety of strategies to cherry-pick the healthiest Medicare recipients and work to channel off resources from the larger system.

The Medicare Advantage programme has also been plagued by fraud on the part of the insurance companies. Recent allegations from a whistleblower suggest that United Health Group overbilled Medicare Advantage to the tune of 'hundreds of millions' or even 'billions of dollars' (Walsh, 2017). In short, the USA loses enormous sums of money to failed privatization programmes and to the grossly inflated overhead costs of the private insurers.

Military health care and Veterans' Administration: The military health system in the USA has two major programmes for civilians. One, originally called CHAMPUS and now referred to as TRICARE, was primarily for the families of soldiers and covered between 2.6 to 9 million people (Harvard University, 2007). An additional 8.9 million veterans are served by the Veterans' Administration (VA) system, which includes 150 hospitals and 820 community-based outpatient clinics (Alba, 2014).

The VA is unique in America in that it represents a truly socialized health system in which care is delivered by a government entity at no charge. During the early 2000s the VA was seen as one of the best run hospital systems in the country, due in part to a national electronic medical record. More recently, there have been scandals related to fraudulent reporting by clinical directors under pressure to meet appointment deadlines.

Some have argued that when one puts together all the different groups receiving some form of government subsidy for their healthcare, more than half of healthcare dollars are coming from the federal government. A variety of sources suggest that eliminating the private insurance system would free up resources now spent on bureaucracy and allow for healthcare to be provided to all Americans without increasing taxes or fees (PNHP, 2016).

The National Institutes of Health: The National Institutes of Health (NIH) is the premier medical research centre in the USA. It is composed of 27 specialized institutes and centres. In the past two decades, the NIH budget has been a contested topic in Washington. The current budget is US$ 34 billion. But this is the result of a 22 per cent drop in NIH funding from 2003 to 2015. The Trump administration had proposed an additional US$ 1.2 billion cut this year and a further US$ 5.8 billion reduction for 2018.

For profit and not-for-profit: is there really a difference? One of the striking features of the current MIC is the way in which the lines between 'for-profit' and 'not-for profit' have become blurred. John Ehrenreich (2016) has noted

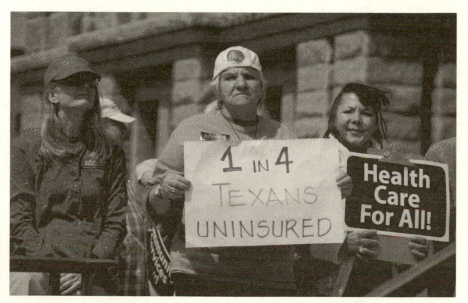

Image B3.1 Participants in rally in support of Medicaid in Texas (www.flickr.com/photos/26672416@N00/8532545606 by 'Texasimpact'; License: CC BY-SA 2.0, https://creativecommons.org/licenses/by-sa/2.0/)

that "Non-profit organizations [have become] larger...now some 10 [per cent] of the American population is working for a non-profit—but the non-profits behave more and more like for-profit businesses."

Becoming a not-for-profit allows institutions to avoid taxes and yet continue to operate as businesses.[7] Given the generous tax breaks afforded to not-for-profits, corporations see profit and not-for-profit as two complementary forms of doing business.

The medical elites and the MIC We can see the MIC personified in a group of elite physicians who serve multiple roles in the MIC. We will take the example of Dr Victor Dzau to illustrate the role played by these elite doctors.

Dr Victor Dzau is chairman of the National Academy of Medicine (NAM), part of the National Academy of Sciences. The NAM is a private, non-governmental organization, which advises the US government on health-related matters. The NAM reports are important documents, which are generally well respected. Dzau, himself, is a graduate of McGill Medical School, was on the faculty at Harvard Medical School, conducted important research in cardiology and was an advisor to the NIH and its directors.

In 2004 he took a position as president and chief executive officer of the Duke University Health System (DUHS). Questions then began to emerge about his compensation. In 2010 a group of Divinity students at Duke protested the high salaries paid to the Duke leadership. They singled out Dzau who had received a US$ 983,654 bonus on top of his salary; his final compensation was US$ 2.2 million (Health Care Renewal, 2010). By 2014, his salary was reported to be US$ 8 million (Cai, 2016).

If this seems to be a lot of money, it's because it is. Particularly, for a university that is nominally a non-profit.[8] But it is also in line with the salaries paid to other heads of health systems; in New York City multi-million dollar salaries seem to be the norm (Vincent and Klein 2015).

After he was tapped for the position to head the National Academy of Medicine, it would emerge that Dzau had sources of income beyond his university salary. He sat on the board of directors of three health-related companies: Medtronics, Alnylam Pharmaceutical and Genzyme. More disturbing yet was that he also sat on the Pepsi Board. These board positions provided Dzau with an additional US$ 1 million in compensation in 2009.

These board positions pose difficult questions in terms of professional ethics. By being on the board he was supposed to defend the interests of the Pepsi stockholders. What about his responsibilities to the patients at Duke? Why was he making such an exorbitant salary at a nominally *'not-for-profit institution'*? Before joining the NAM, Dzau would resign from these board positions but the troubling questions remain: Who is he working for at the NAM? The public's health? The Pepsi stockholders? Or simply himself?

This ability to move between the business world and medicine is not unique to Dzau. A study published in the *British Medical Journal* in 2015 examined 446 US healthcare corporations traded on NASDAQ during 2013. Of these, 41 per cent reported at least one director affiliated with academic medical and research institutions. These 'dual' directors received a median compensation of US$ 193,000 annually and owned a median of 50,699 corporate shares (Anderson, Good and Gellad, 2015).

Conclusions

International ramifications: The MIC is not limited to the USA. Pharmaceutical companies are well distributed internationally and US insurance companies have made some inroads into overseas markets. There are now international hospital chains. Much of the battle internationally is over who controls the World Health Organization (WHO) and what its role should be (see chapter D1). In this battle, we see the international expression of the trends and tactics described in this chapter (ARTE, 2016).

The US experience as a cautionary tale: Despite all claims to the contrary healthcare does not make a good commodity and 'market place solutions' have been a failure in the USA. This is not a viable model for a robust, efficient healthcare system that protects the public's health. Privatization does not make things better: it just parasitizes the public systems.

How we think about things matters: We constantly hear that the USA has a 'non-system'. But the MIC concept allows us to take the big view and to understand how the profit motive corrupts the healthcare system. It needs to be understood as a systemic problem, not one of corrupt individuals and bad government. (Although there is plenty of both around.)

If one thinks that healthcare is primarily about health, changing the system becomes a nightmare. Understanding that it is primarily about profit provides a far richer approach. Remember the adage: Follow the money.

Unions matter: Many (if not most) healthcare workers are motivated by a desire to help others and are frustrated by the barriers of our current system. Healthcare unions have played an important role in progressive change in the USA and they should be supported.

It's not about the money, stupid!: Because profit is at the heart of our healthcare system, healthcare reform is all about money and financing. But money and financing are only part of healthcare and they obscure other important matters. How do we deal with racial disparities in health and healthcare? How do we create a vibrant primary care system? How can we reduce the cost of iatrogenesis? Some things are simply more important than money and they should not be ignored.

Notes

1 This chapter is based in part on an article titled 'The Medical industrial complex in the age of financialization', to be published by Monthly Review Press in the fall of 2017 as part of a book on the healthcare system. We note that many members of Health/PAC remain active in teaching and mentoring a new generation of activists in New York.

2 See text of speech: http://avalon.law.yale.edu/20th_century/eisenhower001.asp

3 See: Regulatory capture: https://en.wikipedia.org/wiki/Regulatory_capture

4 See: Patients' Choice Act 2009, http://paulryan.house.gov/healthcare/pca.htm#sthash.jOpscqzV.dpuf./

5 Other federal programmes, such as Medicaid and the Veterans' Administration, are allowed to negotiate with the drug companies.

6 It is interesting to note that Hillary Clinton received US$ 2 million from health lobbyists; this was far more than any other member of Congress.

7 See the example of the American Shipping Bureau (NPR, 2012).

8 People remark that the two highest paid university employees are the basketball coach and the head of the University Medical Center.

References

AAFP 2016, *Board of directors Report E to the 2016 congress of delegates*, http://www.aafp.org/dam/AAFP/documents/about_us/congress/BoardReportE-AAFPNonDuesRevenue2016.pdf

Alba, M 2014, NBC News, http://www.nbcnews.com/storyline/va-hospital-scandal/va-numbers-how-big-it-who-uses-it-n1101771

Anderson, T, Good, C B & Gellad, WF 2015, 'Prevalence and compensation of academic leaders, professors, and trustees on publicly traded US healthcare company boards of directors: cross sectional study', *British Medical Journal*, vol. 351, https://doi.org/10.1136/bmj.h4826

Archer, D 2011, *Medicare is more efficient than private insurance*, Health Affairs Blog, 20 September, http://healthaffairs.org/blog/2011/09/20/medicare-is-more-efficient-than-private-insurance/

ARTE 2016, *The WHO: in the clutches of lobbyists?* www.arte.tv/en/videos/061650-000-A/the-who-in-the-clutches-of-lobbyists

Bagli, C V 2010, 'Court upholds Columbia campus expansion plans', *The New York Times*, 24 June, http://www.nytimes.com/2010/06/25/nyregion/25columbia.html

Bloomberg 2016, *Prescription drug spending hits record $425 billion in U.S.*, https://www.bloomberg.com/news/articles/2016-04-14/prescription-drug-spending-hits-record-425-billion-in-u-s

Brill, S 2013, 'Bitter pill: why medical bills are killing us', *Time*, 20 February, https://www.uta.edu/faculty/story/2311/Misc/2013,2,26,MedicalCostsDemandAndGreed.pdf

Cai, K 2016, 'University tax forms show differences in top administrators' salaries', *The Chronicle*, 14 July, http://www.dukechronicle.com/article/2016/07/university-tax-forms-show-differences-in-top-administrators-salaries

Chocano, C 2017, 'From Wells Fargo to Fyre Festival, the scam economy is entering its baroque phase', *The New York Times Magazine*, https://goo.gl/jUhHm8

Columbia University 2017, *The trustees of Columbia University*, http://secretary.columbia.edu/trustees-columbia-university

Cubanski, J & Neuman, T 2017, *Searching for savings in Medicare drug price negotiations*, http://kff.org/medicare/issue-brief/searching-for-savings-in-medicare-drug-price-negotiations/

Ehrenreich B and Ehrenreich J 1970, The American Health Empire: Power, Profits and Politics, Random House, New York, 1970

Ehrenreich, J 2016, *Third wave capitalism: how money, power, and the pursuit of self-interest have imperiled the American dream*, Cornell University Press, Ithaca, NY.

Glawe, J 2017, *Pro-Trumpcare Republicans owned millions in health-care stock*, Daily Beast, 24 May, http://www.thedailybeast.com/articles/2017/05/24/pro-trumpcare-republicans-owned-millions-in-health-care-stock?source=email&via=mobile>

Harvard University 2007, *Health care delivery covered lives—summary of findings*, https://www.hks.harvard.edu/m-rcbg/hcdp/numbers/Covered%20Lives%20Summary.pdf>.

Health Care Renewal 2010, *Duke divinity students protest pay of chancellor for health affairs*, 6 December, http://hcrenewal.blogspot.com/2010/12/duke-divinity-students-protest-pay-of.html>.

IMS Institute for Healthcare Informatics 2015, *Global medicines use in 2020*, https://s3.amazonaws.com/assets.fiercemarkets.net/public/005-LifeSciences/imsglobalreport.pdf

Insurance Information Institute 2017, *Insurance industry at a glance*http://www.iii.org/fact-statistic/industry-overview

Kacik, A 2017, 'Surging price of branded drugs squeezing healthcare providers' bottom lines', *Modern Healthcare*, 4 May, http://www.modernhealthcare.com/article/20170504/NEWS/170509935

NPR 2012, *Some nonprofits look suspiciously like for-profits*, National Public Radio, 14 November, http://www.npr.org/2012/11/14/165093535/some-nonprofits-look-suspiciously-like-forprofits

OECD 2017, *Health spending (indicator)*, viewed 18 May 2017,DOI10.1787/8643de7e-en.

Opensecrets.org 2016, *Pharmaceuticals/health products*, https://www.opensecrets.org/industries/recips.php?cycle=2016&ind=h04>

PNHP 2016, Who is PNHP? Physicians for a National Health Program, http://www.pnhp.org/

PNHP 2017, *Hospitals in New York City segregated by race and insurance status: new study*, 2 February, http://www.pnhp.org/news/2017/february/hospitals-in-new-york-segregated-by-race-and-insurance-status-new-study

Relman A S, 1980 'The New Medical-Industrial Complex' N Engl J Med 1980; 303:963-970 October 23, 1980 DOI: 10.1056/NEJM198010233031703

Surowiecki, J 2016, 'The roll-up jacket', *New Yorker Magazine*, http://www.newyorker.com/magazine/2016/04/04/inside-the-valeant-scandal

The Commonwealth Fund 2017, *Evaluating the impact of health insurance industry consolidation: learning from experience*, http://www.commonwealthfund.org/publications/issue-briefs/2015/nov/evaluating-insurance-industry-consolidation

Vincent, I & Klein, M 2015, 'This guy makes $10M a year to head a nonprofit', *New York Post*, 29 November, http://nypost.com/2015/11/29/nonprofit-chief-makes-eye-popping-10-million-a-year/

Walsh, M W, 2017, 'Scheme tied to UnitedHealth overbilled Medicare for years', *The New York Times*, 16 February, https://www.nytimes.com/2017/02/16/business/dealbook/unitedhealthcare-improperly-took-money-from-medicare-suit-says.html

Public health in South Africa in the 1930s and 1940s

In the late 1930s and early 1940s progressive new thinking around public health, community medicine and family practice emerged in South Africa. Pioneering doctors, notably Sidney and Emily Kark, understood the social, economic and environmental roots of ill health and disease and the importance of active community participation and inter-sectoral coordination in health promotion.

At Pholela, a rural setting where the migrant labour system forced local men to work on the distant mines, the Karks employed and trained local community health workers (health assistants) who compiled detailed maps drawn from the local population. These became the foundation for the first population census in the area, which compiled information from 887 inhabitants of the 130 homes adjacent to the health centre. Its report highlighted the need for village planning in basic sanitation, soil erosion and nutrition.

The geographic area of work was expanded annually, and a yearly household health census administered by the health assistants was introduced. Health and agricultural workers worked closely together to reduce malnutrition and improve the soil (Yach and Tollman, 1993, pp. 1043–50). They called this community-oriented primary healthcare (COPHC). COPHC linked community development with primary medical care, with community epidemiology as its base.

The home visit, and not the clinic, became the basis for activity. Health assistants compiled detailed records of home visits. Preventive and curative healthcare merged into "a more comprehensive outlook best described by the title of social medicine" (Digby, 2008, pp. 485–502). The results were remarkable: crude mortality rate decreased from 38.3 per 1,000 in 1942 to 13.6 per 1,000 in 1950; infant mortality dropped from 275 to 100 per 1,000; and the incidence of severe malnutrition fell. These improvements were accompanied by increasing interest and active cooperation on the part of the people served by the project (Kark and Cassel, 1952).

In 1942, the government established the National Health Services Commission (NHSC) with Sidney Kark as technical adviser (Yach and Tollman, 1993,pp. 1043–50). The NHSC's mandate was to make recommendations for an organized health service to ensure "adequate medical, dental, nursing and hospital services to all sections of the people" (Jeeves, 2005, pp. 87–107).

Two years later, the NHSC report declared that the health of the people was "far below what it should be and could be". It blamed this upon poverty and on primitive health and educational facilities. It proposed a single national health service (NHS) for all, funded by progressive taxation. Healthcare delivery was to be done by teams of doctors, nurses and auxiliary personnel mandated to preserve and promote health, moving away from reliance on curative medicine. Furthermore, it was held that the reform of the health system alone would achieve little if the country did not address the underlying social causes of disease (ibid., p.91).

The 'basic unit' of the system would be the community health centre rather than more hospitals, providing personal health services for all the people "as a citizen's right...according to needs rather than means". Four hundred centres were proposed under twenty regional health authorities, each covering roughly 25,000 people. The pioneering Pholela project served as a model (Digby, 2008, pp. 485–502).

The NHSC's idea of a single national health system, based on community health centres, challenged the existing thinking in both South Africa and Britain. It came up against a range of powerful vested interests. Powerful provincial health departments insisted on control over large central hospitals; the Medical Association of South Africa insisted on the right to private practice. The government resisted drafting legislation necessary to establish the system. Health centres that were established never received enough resources to realize their potential and remained marginal. The window of opportunity to establish a national health service closed when the racist National Party won the 1948 election on an Apartheid ticket.

Health civil society during apartheid and in the 1990s

By the mid-1980s the apartheid health system had established 14 very patchy official Departments of Health (DoH) across the country. Under the divide and rule policies of apartheid, each so-called 'independent homeland' (*bantustan*) had its own puppet government with its own DoH. In addition, the rest of the country (the 'main' South Africa) needed three separate governance structures and health departments – one for each defined racial group without a homeland: Whites, Coloureds and Asians. The health centres established after the NHSC report had been "reduced to a cheap option for black health care" (Marks, 1997, pp. 452–59).

Growth and achievements of health civil society during apartheid The 1980s spawned massive internal civil society resistance to apartheid. This included the rise of a progressive health and social services movement representing both professional groupings and community-based projects. Though the organizations were united in opposition to apartheid, there were intense ideological debates among them. For example, the National Medical and Dental Association

(NAMDA), established by doctors and dentists to oppose the collaborationist Medical and Dental Associations of South Africa, was seen by other oppositionist health worker organizations as elitist and perpetuating divisions between professionals and non-professionals (Picket et al., 2012, pp. 403–05).

Through the 1980s and into the 1990s, the focus of struggle shifted from opposition to apartheid towards developing health policy for the future. Though there was an expressed commitment to the broad developmental inter-sectoral PHC approach among all the organizations, there were tensions between those who favoured a centralist, top-down approach and those committed to a community-based bottom-up approach.

In 1990, the apartheid government revoked its ban on the African National Congress (ANC) and released Mandela and his comrades from prison. As the ANC prepared itself to govern, it incorporated the core of the health policy work of the anti-apartheid health movement into its 1994 Health Plan. Meanwhile, the labour movement under the Congress of South African Trade Unions (COSATU) pressurized the ANC to adopt the broad Reconstruction and Development Programme (RDP) "to meet the basic needs of people: jobs, land, housing, water, electricity, telecommunications, transport, a clean and healthy environment, nutrition, health care, and social welfare".

After a landslide victory in the 1994 election, the ANC formed the first democratic government with a human rights–based constitution. Health activists looked forward to a new health system based on PHC, while the RDP would take care of the social determinants of health. Many key activists moved from civil society into government.

The current South African health crisis

This optimism proved to be short-lived. Twenty-three years later, seven decades after the birth of COPHC, South Africa is in the midst of a major health crisis. For an upper middle-income country, health outcomes are a long way from where they could, and should, be. Figure B4.1 shows health (as life expectancy) in relation to wealth (GDP per capita) for most of the world's countries in 2015. In general, population health is better in rich than in poor countries – most fall on a band running from bottom left (poor and unhealthy) to top right (rich and healthy). South Africa does not fall within that health–wealth band: for example, poorer countries like Bangladesh, Kenya, Ghana and Rwanda – countries poorer than South Africa – have better health outcomes. It should be noted that average numbers like these hide inequality, a major cause of poor health. South Africans experience a massive quadruple burden of disease attributable to four categories of disease:

- HIV/AIDS, tuberculosis and other infections
- high maternal and child mortality
- high levels of violence and injuries

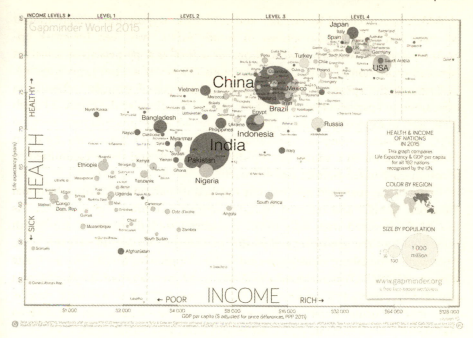

Figure B4.1: Health life expectancy vs wealth (per capita GDP)

Source: Based on a free chart from www.gapminder.org (Gapminder, 2017)

- escalating non-communicable (lifestyle) diseases such as obesity, heart disease, diabetes and cancer.

The social determinants of health (SDH) – adequate sanitation and housing, decent and safe work, clean environment and a healthy food environment – remain highly stratified by race and class. Income inequality is among the highest in the world, with a Gini coefficient of 0.7.

How South Africa got here is a dismal testament to the devastating and dehumanizing legacy of apartheid and the prevailing power of vested interests and opportunists, the malignant, insidious influence of rampant corruption, the abandonment of the RDP in 1996 in favour of a neoliberal macroeconomic policy ironically termed the Growth, Employment and Redistribution (GEAR) programme, as well as the marginalization of active, informed citizenship following the deliberate disbanding of the vibrant civil society networks.

The HIV epidemic and developments in health civil society

After a promising start under President Mandela, the presidency of Thabo Mbeki between 1999 and 2008 was characterized by AIDS denialism and the refusal by his health minister, Manto Tshabalala-Msimang, to develop and implement anti-retroviral (ARV) treatment programmes in the public sector. A key study indicates that more than 330,000 lives or approximately 2.2 million person-years were lost as a result. Thirty-five thousand children were born with HIV by not implementing a mother-to-child transmission prophylaxis program with nevirapine, resulting in an additional 1.6 million lost person-years. The total lost benefits of ARVs (anti-retroviral medicines) are at least 3.8 million person-years for the period 2000 to 2005 (Chigwedere et al., 2008, pp. 410–15).

Developments in civil society The Mandela era marked the marginalization of progressive civil society, including social movements in health, as many activists moved into government and others felt that the struggle had been won and was over.

The AIDS denialism of the Mbeki era sparked the re-awakening of social movements in health with the launch of the Treatment Action Campaign (TAC) in 1998 to "campaign for access to treatment for all South Africans by raising public awareness and understanding about the availability, affordability and use of HIV treatments". Though initiated by a small group of activists, the TAC soon established chapters in many regions of the country. Though its membership consisted mainly of black and poor people with HIV, it included many others, including academics, professionals and faith groups, who joined because they were social activists and identified with the cause. The TAC's campaign methodology included civil disobedience, street demonstrations, literacy programmes, publications and court action.

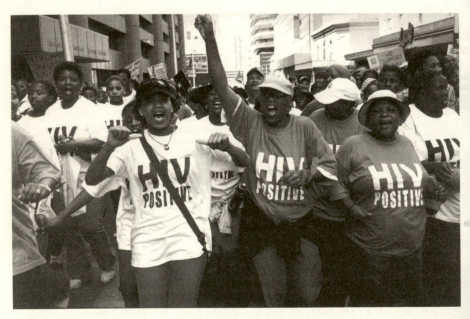

Image B4.1 March to Parliament by TAC in 2003 (Louis Reynolds)

The TAC had several victories by combining mass mobilization and litigation. In April 2001 it and its overseas allies, particularly the AIDS Coalition to Unleash Power (ACT UP) in the USA, pressured the Pharmaceutical Manufacturer's Association (PMA) and its supporters in the US government to withdraw a lawsuit against the South African government for importing cheaper generic ARVs. In 2002, the TAC won recognition for the right of pregnant women to access an anti-retroviral drug, nevirapine, at all public health facilities capable of providing a PMTCT (prevention of mother-to-child transmission) service.

Finally, after more than a decade of denialism, the government agreed to a plan to distribute ARVs to people living with HIV/AIDS in late 2003. There is no doubt that TAC's multi-strategy campaigning had a pivotal role in this about-face.

The ARV treatment roll-out started in April 2004, and it is now the largest ARV programme in the world, with more than 20 million people tested and almost 4 million on treatment. The rapid improvement in both underfive mortality and life expectancy since 2005 is largely attributable to this programme, since neither the improvements in the SDH nor in the general quality of care can account for this (Figure B4.2).

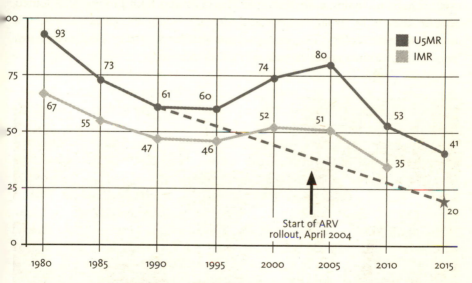

Figure B4.2: Trends for U5MR and IMR in South Africa between 1980 and 2015

Source: CHERG/WHO/UNICEF for distribution of causes of neonatal and under-five deaths (Liu et al., 2014). An updated version is available in Liu et al. (2016, pp. 2151–61).

Notes:
U5MR = under-five mortality rate
IMR = infant mortality rate
The dotted line shows the approximate trajectory the country should have followed to meet the U5MR target of 20 (indicated by the star); the solid line shows the trajectory that was followed instead. The arrow shows when the anti-retroviral programme started

The rise and success of the TAC campaign occurred in a period when influential external donors – notably the Global Fund to Fight AIDS, Tuberculosis and Malaria (GFATM) and the US President's Emergency Plan for AIDS Relief (PEPFAR) – started funding HIV/AIDS activities undertaken by a range of 'service delivery' non-governmental organizations (NGOs), which have come to dominate the health civil society in the past 15 years. Such NGOs employed large numbers of lay health workers known variously as treatment/adherence supporters, counsellors, home-based carers and so on, who now collectively make up the approximately 70,000 community care workers (CCWs) in the country.

This NGO-ization of health civil society is not confined to South Africa. It reflects the changed nature of donor funding under neoliberalism – namely, the directing of substantial funding through private and non-government recipients in a climate of cuts in public spending by the state under austerity.

The National Health Insurance project

The current health system mirrors inequalities in society, with a modern, urban-based and specialist-dominated private sector accounting for 50 per cent of total spending, and with approximately 50 per cent of general practitioners and over 70 per cent of medical specialists serving about 16 per cent of the population.

In December 2007, the ruling ANC resolved to establish a National Health Insurance (NHI) scheme to achieve universal health coverage (UHC) and realize the state's constitutional obligation to deliver healthcare with financial protection to all. The proposed National Health Insurance Fund (NHIF), financed predominantly from progressive taxation, will purchase healthcare for all from "accredited public and private providers".

In preparing for the NHI, the health department has attempted to strengthen the public health sector through the implementation of a policy termed the Re-engineering of Primary Health Care (RPHC). The RPHC comprises three streams: Ward-based Outreach Teams (WBOTs) based on community health workers (CHWs) to strengthen community-based services; a school health stream; and District Clinical Specialist Teams with a focus on maternal and child health. The RPHC has initially been implemented at 11 pilot sites to test the model.

The WBOTs are key to achieving improved coverage of households and ensuring basic PHC activities, including addressing local SDH. Success depends crucially on recognition and affirmation, by both the health authorities and local health professionals, of the central role of the CHWs in achieving health for all.

Community care workers and community health workers The NHI provides an opportunity to integrate the current 70,000 CCWs into the formal health

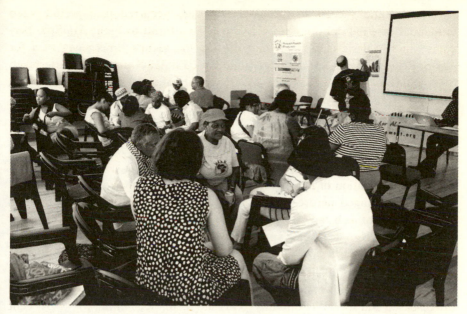

Image B4.2 Community health workers at a workshop organised by PHM (Louis Reynolds)

system as community health workers or as part-time workers operating at the household level. They represent an important health resource for providing and extending key but simple health interventions to vulnerable and underserved populations.

Yet in most of the pilot sites, the CCWs lack basic information about the NHI and are not included in consultation or integrated properly into programmes. In South Africa, there is currently no standardized training or employment of the CCWs. Despite this, thousands are working in vulnerable communities helping to address the need caused by South Africa's massive burden of disease and the failure of our ailing health system.

Many CCWs work as volunteers, others for a stipend from NGOs, a few through health departments. Where wages are paid, they range from ZAR800 to 2,000 per month (US$ 60 to 150). Payment is often erratic and dependent on the current budget of the employing organization, and most of the CCWs are employed through temporary annual contracts that may or may not be renewed. Because their work is not formally recognized, they have no associated benefits and almost no occupational health and safety training. In addition to the potential risk of communicable diseases, the CCWs are exposed to tremendous personal risk, including violent muggings, sexual assault and exposure to the domestic and community violence endemic to many South African communities. They often walk alone from house to house when they are called upon for help and have no protection and often little support from local health facilities.

In other countries, the CHWs perform a wide range of essential functions in the community management of important prevalent diseases like HIV and TB. Given appropriate training, support and recognition, they can recognize and start early treatment of life-threatening conditions like pneumonia, diarrhoea, acute malnutrition and malaria. They can also promote maternal, neonatal and child health.

The NHI plan grossly underestimates the number of CHWs that will be needed. Currently, each CHW is expected to cover 250 households. Given the burden of disease and given that many households are crowded, this is impossible and unsustainable. Furthermore, the scope of practice of the planned CHWs is confined to undertaking household registration and providing information and advice. The CCWs provide very basic home-based care.

The optimal arrangement, given South Africa's burden of disease and its size, would be a combination of CHWs who would undertake the more complex tasks of curative care and personal prevention, with CCWs performing the laborious and time-consuming home care of the sick and bed-ridden. Increasing the total number of community-based workers would have the additional advantage of creating employment for women, thereby promoting improved household income and health benefits, especially for children,

During the anti-apartheid struggle CHWs played a key role in community mobilization for improved social and environmental conditions as well as better medical care. To realize the potential for CHWs to lead actions to address SDH will require a radical shift in thinking. A truly democratic government should welcome and support this notion.

The broader health worker crisis The current austerity policies and tight limits to public spending under neoliberalism have led to inadequate allocation of financial resources to the public sector. A freeze on posts for health workers has led to shortages of professionals, excessive workloads, long shifts and intolerable working conditions, especially in rural areas.

This poses enormous risks to patients as well as health professionals themselves. Recently a 25-year-old doctor fell asleep and crashed while driving home after a long shift, killing herself and critically injuring two others, one of whom died later. This incident brought to light that young doctors face many risks due to austerity. The impact of such neoliberal policies is not confined to South Africa – austerity has also led to protracted doctors' strikes in Kenya and Zimbabwe resulting in much unnecessary suffering and even avoidable deaths.

A critical perspective on South Africa's health reforms

The possibility that South Africa will soon achieve health for all and universal health coverage appears bleak. On the one hand, the state is paralysed by strife within the ruling ANC and seems unable to make rapid progress towards reducing inequality, addressing the social causes of ill-health and establishing an equitable health system. On the other, powerful vested interests in lucrative private healthcare are using this weakness to lobby for what amounts to a nationwide public–private partnership.

Evaluations conducted at the 11 NHI pilot sites to date are, on the whole, disappointing. Dysfunctional facilities, poor management and leadership, and inadequate human resources for health (HRH) are key problems. At a broader level, the risk of the NHIF being maladministered or looted is high in the current climate of rampant corruption and state capture by rich and powerful conglomerates.

The NHI risks aggravating urban-rural inequity. NHI accreditation will be less demanding for urban than rural facilities where HRH are scarce and government has not been able to address the situation. Furthermore, private providers are overwhelmingly urban.

This situation calls for active and informed citizenship on a massive scale to mobilize for health. Recently the People's Health Movement, the Treatment Action Campaign and Section 27 (a prominent advocacy organization focused on Section 27 of the Constitution, which entrenches relevant socioeconomic rights) hosted a National Health Assembly of civil society. Provincial Assemblies in all nine provinces have paved the way.

The aim of this coalition is to develop a broad social movement in civil society to campaign for the right to health for all. The central role that the TAC played in bringing sense to our approach to the HIVAIDS pandemic showed how citizen action can bring about change from below However, these problems could be overcome with powerful civil society mobilization to ensure greater investment, especially in more HRH, appropriate training and leadership, and ending corruption in both public and private sectors.

References

Chigwedere, P, Seage, GR III, Gruskin, S, Lee, T H & Essex, M 2008, 'Estimating the lost benefits of antiretroviral drug use in South Africa', *Journal of Acquired Immune Deficiency Syndromes*, vol. 49, no. 4, pp. 410–15 http://journals.lww.com/jaids/Abstract/2008/12010/Estimating_the_Lost_Benefits_of_Antiretroviral.10.aspx

Digby, A 2008, 'Vision and vested interests: National Health Service reform in South Africa and Britain during the 1940s and beyond', *Social History of Medicine*, vol. 21, no. 3, pp. 485–502.

Gapminder 2015, *Gapminder World Poster 2013* https://www.gapminder.org/downloads/gapminder-world-poster-2013/

Jeeves, A 2005, 'Delivering primary care in impoverished urban and rural communities: the Institute of Family and Community Health in the 1940s', in Dubow, S and Jeeves, A (eds), *South Africa's 1940s: worlds of possibilities*, Double Storey, Cape Town, pp. 87–107.

Kark S L, Cassel J 1952, The Pholela Health Centre: a progress report. South African medical journal, 1952

Liu, L, Johnson, HL, Cousens, S, Perin, J, Scott et al., 2016, 'Global, regional, and national causes of child mortality: an updated systematic analysis for 2010 with time trends since 2000', *The Lancet*, vol. 379, no. 9832, pp.2151–61, http://dx.doi.org/10.1016/S0140-6736(12)60560-1

Marks, S 1997,'South Africa's early experiment in social medicine: its pioneers and politics', *American Journal of Public Health*, vol. 87, pp. 452–59.

Pick, W, Claassen, J W B, Le Grange, CA &Hussey, GD2012, 'Health activism in Cape Town: a case study of the Health Workers Society', *The South African Medical Journal*, vol. 102, no. 6, pp. 403–05, viewed 10 April 2017, http://www.samj.org.za/index.php/saj/article/view/5624/4208

Yach, D & Tollman, S M 1993,'Public health initiatives in South Africa in the 1940s and 1950s: lessons for a post-apartheid era', *American Journal of Public Health*, vol. 83,no. 7, pp. 1043–50.

B5 | THE 'NEW' KAROLINSKA HOSPITAL: HOW PPPs UNDERMINE PUBLIC SERVICES[1]

Conservative economists often berate low and middle-income countries (LMICs) for their failure to pursue neoliberal reforms while restructuring healthcare services. The failures are sought to be explained as being caused by inefficient and corrupt financial and administrative systems in these countries. However evidence indicates that neoliberal reforms in restructuring healthcare services, such as Public Private Partnerships (PPPs), are inherently flawed and represent a transfer of public resources to the private sector and do not lead to any increased efficiencies. In this chapter, we illustrate this by tracing the story of the 'new' Karolinska hospital in Stockholm.

The Stockholm County Council (SCC), at the beginning of this millennium, unveiled plans for a 'world class' hospital in the city – the new Karolinska hospital. While renovating the existing hospital would have cost 4-5 billion SEK – Swedish Krona (approximately US$ 500 million) (Ennart and Mellgren, 2016, p. 64), the plan to build a new hospital was projected to cost billions of crowns more. The project was conceived as a PPP. This chapter traces the process through which the project was conceived, and is being implemented.

Vision of a new Karolinska

The provision of healthcare services in Sweden is divided between the central government, 20 county councils and 290 municipalities. The county councils are responsible for provision of primary and secondary healthcare services and representatives to the councils are elected every four years. Healthcare is financed by municipal taxes, contributions from the central government and modest user-fees.[2] The Karolinska hospital is the largest hospital in Stockholm with approximately 15,000 employees and is closely linked to the top medical university in Sweden – the Karolinska institute.[3] The vision of the 'new' Karolinska included that of a hospital with deeper ties between clinical care and research. The SCC proposed a PPP to finance and construct the new hospital – an approach that had not been tried in Sweden earlier.[4]

The PPP involved contracting a private company to finance, construct and maintain the hospital and in exchange the company was to receive an annual payment from the public authority. It was claimed that as the financial arrangements would be finalized in advance, delay in project implementation would cost the company, and this would act as a check on time overruns (Bordeleau C 2014). The SCC agreed to go ahead with the project on receipt of three competitive bids from private contractors. However, the city council received only one bid.[5] The city council hired Gullers, a private consultancy firm, to provide guidance regarding if the project should continue. The city council was strongly advised not to proceed (Ennart H and Mellgren F 2016 p.82). Doubts were raised regarding the project's financial viability as the contracted private entity would need to raise loans at a higher rate than what the government could if the latter were directly involved in managing the project. In spite of such doubts the SCC accepted the bid received. In 2010 an agreement was signed by the council with Skanska (a multinational construction and development company based in Sweden) and the British investment fund, Innisfree. Together they created the 'Swedish Hospital Partners (SHP)', a venture company that was to guarantee satisfactory completion of the project.

From the inception of the project it was clear that the council's decision was driven by a neoliberal ideological bias which had 'faith' in the 'efficiency' of the private sector.

Hidden costs and secrecy

During the final negotiations between SCC and Skanska and Innisfree, several important changes were made in the contract that dramatically in-creased costs. The contract, as initially conceived, was broken down into over a hundred additional contracts over and above the main contract. These included, for example, work related to construction of the laboratory, offices for the administration, medical equipment and the telecommunication system. This method of systematically extracting parts out of the initial agreement and creating additional contracts is a well-known ploy in PPPs. In typical PPPs costs increase with every additional contract while the process becomes less transparent. In the case of the Karolinska hospital council members and officials negotiating the agreement had very limited capacity to scrutinise the calculations provided by Skanska, thus making it impossible to negotiate better terms.[6]

The entire deal has been shrouded in secrecy. The agreement itself was designated as 'confidential' both before and after it was signed. This confiden-tiality clause related to the agreement extended to members of the SCC, who risked high legal penalties if they discussed the agreement with experts or the media. The terms of the agreement have become available very gradually in the past years after several rounds of legal proceedings in court.

Well after the agreement was signed members of the SCC started realizing that the project may not be financially viable. After visiting several European high-end hospitals the council realized that the projected cost of the hospital was much higher than for similar ventures in many other European countries. While the price per square meter for similar ventures in Denmark and Norway were approximately 20,000–30,000 SEK (approximately US$ 2500–3500) the price at New Karolinska was estimated to be 46,000 SEK (US$ 5,000)

(Ennart and Mellgren, 2016, p. 138–139). As a result of these concerns, in 2012, McKinsey was commissioned to investigate the high costs related to the project. Curiously, McKinsey recommended that at least a quarter of planned investments in other public hospitals be postponed to accommodate the high public costs incurred for the Karolinska hospital. This would mean not addressing the urgent need for more beds in these hospitals. (Ennart and Mellgren, 2016, p. 140).

Crisis in hospital care in Sweden and the new Karolinska Sweden is a high income country, which has over the years, invested in building a strong welfare system. Yet it is in the midst of a crisis in hospital-based care, involving shortages of hospital beds and staff and overflowing emergency rooms. Sweden ranks third from the bottom among OECD countries and ranks at the bottom among all countries in the EU as regards availability of hospital beds per 1000 inhabitants (OECD, 2017). When beds are physically available, utilization is low due to shortages of staff, especially of nurses. Shortage of nurses is related to low wages and low increments in wages, and tough working conditions. As a result waiting times can be very long for patients seeking care. Though financial resources are available, issues linked to low wages for staff and their working conditions are not prioritized, while funds are diverted to consulting firms and expensive contractors. The new Karolinska does not address this growing crisis and in fact the number of beds planned for the new hospital is less than in the existing hospital.[7]

Furthermore the new hospital, conceived as a speciality care centre, would mainly cater to patients requiring critical care or those with rare disorders. This means that a bulk of patients in need of care, including the elderly, will not be able to access care from the new hospital. The elderly, who form the bulk of patients in Sweden's emergency rooms and hospitals, will not to be treated at the new Karolinska but at other hospitals in Stockholm which are already overcrowded. At the same time, the expansion of staff, beds and medical equipment at hospitals that treat patients, not welcome at the 'new world-class hospital', is lagging behind. These hospitals are not expected to reach full capacity until years after the new Karolinska hospital is commissioned. The additional cost incurred in expanding capacity in other hospitals is estimated to cost the SCC an additional 33 billion SEK (aproximately US$ 3.5 billion).[8]

Consultants, conflict of interest and profit-hungry contractors So if money spent in building the 'new' Karolinska is not going to increase the number of hospital beds available for patients in need, where is it going? In addition to money spent in hiring expensive contractors, large amounts of money are being spent to hire management consultancy firms. SCC paid 1.2 billion SEK (approximately US$ 140 million) to consultants between 2012–2014, who billed SCC at the rate of 2300 SEK per hour (approximately US$ 250)

(Ennart and Mellgren, 2016, p. 57; Westin, 2015). Boston Consulting Group (BCG) has been central in the implementation of a new management model called 'value based solutions' at the new Karolinska. For this BCG was paid 618,270 SEK (approximately 70,000 US$) per week. Interestingly McKinsey had bid for the same contract at a quoted rate of 406,100 SEK (approx. US$ 45,000) per week (Westin, 2015). Perhaps it is not a coincidence that the current program director of Karolinska hospital is a past employee of BCG (Ennart and Mellgren, 2016, p. 58). The journal Vårdfokus estimates that the sum Karolinska overpaid to consultancy firms, over and above the allocated budget between 2012–2014 is approximately 186 million SEK (approximately US$ 20 million USD) – which corresponds to the wage bill of 400 full-time nurses for a year (Westin, 2015).

Another consultancy company in bed with the SCC is Pricewaterhouse-Coopers (PwC). PwC has been one of the major promoters of PPPs since the mid-1990s and its consultant, Paul De Rita, was the leader of the expert group who conducted a 'neutral' investigation into the financing model chosen by the SCC for the New Karolinska (Ennart and Mellgren, 2016, p. 242). It is thus not surprising that he endorsed the PPP-model as being best suited best to run the Karolinska hospital project. PwC has also assisted Swedish Hospital Partners (SHP) to set itself up in the tax haven of Luxembourg (Ennart and Mellgren, 2016, p. 181). (For a detailed discussion on the role of management consultancy firms in the health sector, see Chapter D3.)

Karolinska is not an isolated example The PPP model has been extensively used in the UK to build and manage hospitals. An example is the Barts Health Trust in London which consists of St Bartholomew Hospital and Royal London Hospital. Since its reconstruction in 2010 the hospital is owned by Skanska and Innisfree and consultancy for the contract was provided by PwC. There are several similarities with the new Karolinska hospital.

How has the Barts Health tTust been performing? In 2015 the trust incurred a loss of 1.8 billion SEK (approximately US$ 200,000,000). It was, as a consequence, forced to reduce the number of employees by 10 per cent. Two-hundred beds were not functional due to lack of staff and the trust failed to deliver promised services in several areas. Surveys show that only one third of the employees would recommend someone to work at Barts Health Trust, the third lowest number of all hospitals in the UK. All employees had been forced to sign contracts that prevented them from making statements about the situation at the hospital. Due to its dire economic situation, Barts Health Trust had been put under the administration of the British health authorities[9].

The contracts of several other PPP-hospitals in the UK have been terminated by the government. The compensation paid by the government to terminate the contracts was huge but the costs would have been even greater (for decades to come) if the government had not terminated the contracts. (BBC News,

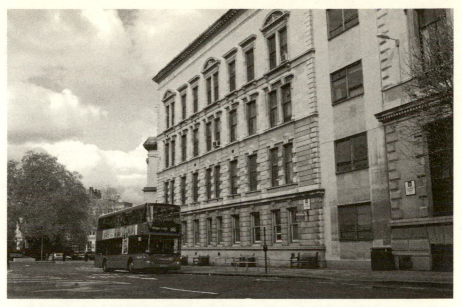

Image B5.1 St Bartholomew's Hospital in London, which was privatised (https://commons. wikimedia.org/wiki/Attributions: St_Bartholomew%27s_Hospital0260.JPG#/media/ File:St_Bartholomew%27s_Hospital0260.JPG by MaryG90; License: CC BY-SA 3.0, https:// creativecommons.org/licenses/by-sa/3.0/)

2012). An analysis of the first six PPP-hospitals in Scotland showed that the cost of financing the hospitals is on average double of what it would have been through the traditional route.

While the criticism of the PPP-model and public mistrust grew in the UK, in the early 2000s, the model became an important 'export product'. The British government cooperated closely with several lobby organizations with the aim of facilitating the entry of British investment funds, consultants and construction companies into new markets in low- and middle-income countries (Holden, 2009). Globally, lobbying for PPPs in the hospital business has been successful and these are being promoted through the International Monetary Fund, World Bank and EU. One example is in Lesotho where half the country's health budget goes towards funding a large PPP venture in the capital city (Oxfam, 2014).

The new Karolinska anno 2017 So how much has the new Karolinska actually cost the SCC and the taxpayers in Stockholm? This is not an easy question to answer. In 2002 the predicted cost of the building was 5.3 billion SEK (approximately US$ 600 million) (Ennart and Mellgren, 2016, p. 152). At the time of the signing of the agreement it was revealed that the total cost had increased to 14.1 billion SEK (approximately US$ 1.6 billion). Just a few days later the project manager admitted that the actual cost would be

22 billion SEK (approximately US$ 2.5 billion).[10] This did not include the cost of maintenance (of which SHP has a monopoly) or the interest on loans. The ruling political party in the SCC claims that the bill for constructing and building the hospital and its maintenance until 2040 will be 52 billion SEK (approximately US$ 6 billion) while former member of the SCC claims that the bill will end up at 69 billion SEK (approximately US$ 8 billion) due to high interest rates and the fact that not all costs are included in the final bill (Ennart and Mellgren, 2016, p. 29).

Actually no one knows the final price tag, not even the SCC's own accountants who, after an investigation into the finances of the new Karolinska project, concluded that the SCC has very little control over future costs. What cannot, however, be denied is the enormous cost incurred by the people of Stockholm who will be financing the venture till 2040, as per the agreement. In 2015 approximately 59 per cent of the Swedish population was for a ban against profit-making within welfare.[11] On the other hand Skanska and Innisfree will, in all likelihood, sell their shares at a premium.

As Innisfree is a venture capital company, one can assume that a considerable sum of taxpayers' money will end up in tax havens. Between 2007 and 2012 private for-profit providers services bought by county councils Sweden increased by over 50 per cent (Dahlgren, 2014). The Swedish economist Göran Dahlgren investigated, in 2014, the experience of profit-driven healthcare reforms in Sweden and concluded that private for-profit healthcare services resulted in reduced efficiency and unequal access to healthcare services while putting additional strain and draining public healthcare resources (Dahlgren, 2014). One can only hope that some lesson will be learnt and that the new Karolinska is both the first and last PPP venture of its kind in the Swedish welfare state.

Notes

1 Most of the material in this chapter is collected from the extensive in-depth investigations done by the Swedish journalists Henrik Ennart och Fredrik Mellgren and presented in the book 'Sjukt Hus' published by Ordfront förlag (Ordfront publisher) in 2016. We acknowledge the generous offer by the authors to use the material and share a short version of the story of New Karolinska with an English speaking audience.

2 Web page: https://sweden.se/society/health-care-in-sweden/. Last updated May 2016. Last accessed 2017-04-03.

3 Web page: About Karolinska, Karolinska University Hospital. Editor: Paulina Lundberg. Last updated 2016-12-06. Last accessed 2017-04-03 http://www.karolinska. se/en/karolinska-university-hospital/about-karolinska/

4 NKS-rapport 1 – Beskrivning av OPS-upphandling, Stockholms läns landsting, Published 2010-05-01. Last accessed 2017-04-03 http://www.nyakarolinskasolna.se/globalassets/nks-rapport-1---beskrivning-av-ops-upphandling.pdf

5 ibid

6 Nya Karolinska Solna – Informations promemoria OPS-upphandling Oktober 2008, Stockholms läns landsting http://www.nyakarolinskasolna.se/contentassets/c60bc21996b44131a67f0c3c1434a89c/moi-tryckoriginal.pdf

7 NKS-rapport- mål och verksamhetsinriktning, NKS-förvaltningen vid

Stockholms läns landsting. Mars 2011. LS 1103-0541. http://www.nyakarolinskasolna.se/conte ntassets/3210ca994ce74d1498ce3d96a8bd93a5/ nks_rapport-mars-2011.pdf

8 Tjänsteutlåtande 2013-04-15 Karolinska universitetssjukhusets uppdrag, verksamhetsinnehåll och kapacitet, samt fastighetsutnyttjande vid Karolinska Solna, LS 1304-0528 http://www.nyakarolinskasolna. se/globalassets/dokument/ls-1304-0528-verksamhetsinnehall-nks-tjut.pdf;

and: Tjänsteutlåtande 2013-02-17 landstingsstyrelsens arbetsutskott, LS 1302-0194, LS1202-0263 Tilläggsavtal http://www.sll.se/Global/Politik/ Politiska-organ/Landstingsstyrelsen/ Arbetsutskottet/2013/2013-02-19/punkt-3-tillaggsavtal.pdf

9 Barts Health NHS Trust, Annual report 2014/2014 https://www. healthwatchtowerhamlets.co.uk/wp-content/ uploads/2015/07/150911-Barts-Annual-Report-FINAL-Online-version.pdf

10 Protokoll Landstingsstyrelsens FoUU-utskott 2009-02-03. Last accessed 2017-04-03. http://www.nyakarolinskasolna.se/globalassets/ politiska-beslut/ls_fouu_2009_02_03.pdf

11 SOM-institutet Svenska trender 1986–2015 s. 49.

References

BBC News 2012, 'Seven NHS trusts to get access to £1,5bn bailout fund' BBC News 2012-02-03 http://www.bbc.com/news/health-16874630

Bordeleau C 2014, 'The emergence and Diffusion of Public Private Partnership in Canada, the United Kingdom and the United States of America (thesis) School of Public Policy and Administration, Charleton University Ottawa, Ontario, Canada, 2014.

Dahlgren G 2014, ´Why public health services? Experiences from profit-driven health care reforms in Sweden´, International Journal of Health Services, Volume 44, Number 3, 2014, Pages 507–524.

Ennart H and Mellgren F 2016, Sjukt Hus. Globala miljardsvindlerier – från Lesotho till nya Karolinska, Stockholm, Ordfront, 2016

Holden C 2009, 'Exporting public-private partnership in healthcare: export strategy and policy transfer', 2009, Policy studies Vol 30 (3), page 313-332 http://www.tandfonline. com/doi/full/10.1080/01442870902863885?s croll=top&needAccess=true

OECD, 2017, Hospital beds (indicator). doi: 10.1787/0191328e-en (Accessed on 18 June 2017)

Oxfam 2014, 'A dangerous diversion – Will the IFC flagship health PPP bankrupt Lesotho's Ministry of Health?' Oxfam, CPA 2014-04-07. https://www.oxfam.org/sites/ www.oxfam.org/files/file_attachments/ bn-dangerous-diversion-lesotho-health-ppp-070414-en_o.pdf

Westin J 2015, `Konsulternas överdrag motsvarar 400 sjuksköterskor`Vårdfokus 2015-06-1 https://www.vardfokus.se/ webbnyheter/2015/juni/konsulternas-overdrag-motsvarar-400-sjukskoterskor/

B6 | ACCESS TO HEALTHCARE OF MIGRANTS IN THE EU

Introduction

Over the last decades, issues related to migration have emerged as a funda-mental and defining factor in European societies. As a consequence, migrants' access to healthcare has also become a pressing social and political issue with multiple implications – ranging from human rights, individual and collective well-being, to public budgets. Moreover, migrants' health is a crucial deter-minant of social cohesion, as illness and marginalization are part of a vicious circle that hinders integration (Ingleby et al., 2005).

The response in Europe has been far from uniform. The direct remit of the European Union (EU) on matters related to health is limited. Apart from a role in matters of public security, the EU only has an 'advisory' role on health issues (limited to raising concern and encouraging countries to take action). It does not have the authority to prescribe actions which are binding on all EU members or harmonize policies and measures on health.[1] EU member states are free to design the way their health systems are funded and the coverage they provide. Thus, identifying common patterns regarding migrants' access to healthcare is not an easy task. However, the following general trends are worth noting:

1. *Migrants are among the most disadvantaged population groups in Europe.* Ac-cording to a report by the Organisation for Economic Cooperation and Development (OECD) and the European Commission, "Immigrants are twice as likely [as the] native-born to live in households which fall within the poorest income decile and below the national poverty threshold" (OECD/ EU, 2015, p. 161). This is linked to multiple factors: their economic back-ground and pre-migration conditions, restrictive access to the labour market, exploitation, lack of efficient integration policies and lack of representation in political and social structures.

2. *Several studies have shown that seeking healthcare is not a major motivation for most migrants to come to Europe* (Médecins du Monde, 2014, p. 19; 2015, p. 25; 2016a, p. 17). In fact, the use of healthcare facilities by migrants is significantly lower than by local populations (Sarría-Santamera et al., 2016).

3. *The European Commission encourages member states to articulate inclusive healthcare systems.* In its advisory capacity, the European Commission has issued several communications raising concerns over the special vulnerability of migrants regarding health inequalities (Commission of the European

Communities 2009, p. 8) and called for EU countries to ensure universal access to healthcare (European Commission 2016, p. 12).

4. *National legislations group migrants into various categories, providing different sets of access rights.* Students, workers from third-party countries, asylum seekers and undocumented migrants are categories typically identified in many European countries, with different and varying levels of access associated with each of them. Most countries grant full access rights to migrants who have acquired permanent residence. At the other end of the spectrum, access for undocumented migrants is usually restrictive.

5. *The recent increase in the arrival of refugees has added a new challenge: an unprecedented flow of people in transit with health needs significantly different from those of settled migrants* (Médecins du Monde 2016a, p. 45). Europe's response to this situation has been far from ideal; it has turned a blind eye on widespread human suffering, a case in point being the EU-Turkey Agreement (Box B6.1).

6. *Legal implementation tends to be deficient, exacerbating migrants' exclusion from healthcare.* Migrants themselves are more often than not unaware of their entitlements, even as desk personnel and health professionals in the healthcare system ignore the applicable law. As a consequence, even if they are eligible, fewer migrants attempt to access the healthcare system and many are wrongfully denied their rights. This circumstance tends to be exacerbated by migrants moving from one country to another.

7. *Despite the different national regulations, European countries remain bound by international human rights commitments.* One of the most notable is the International Covenant on Economic, Social and Cultural Rights (ESCR), which recognizes in its Article 12 "the right of everyone to the enjoyment of the highest attainable standard of physical and mental health". This has been interpreted by the ESCR Committee to entail the obligation to "respect the right to health by, *inter alia*, refraining from denying or limiting equal access for all persons, including prisoners or detainees, minorities, asylum seekers and illegal immigrants, to preventive, curative and palliative health service" (UN Economic, Social and Cultural Rights Committee 2000, para. 34).

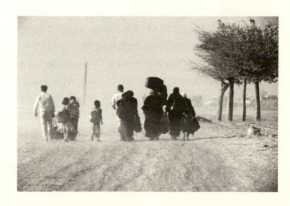

Image B6.1 Refugees from Syria
(Cem Terzi)

Box B6.1: It is not a 'refugee crisis'

The situation of refugees in Turkey

Since April 2011 approximately 7 million Syrians were forced to migrate because of the civil war, which intensified after the intervention of several countries. Of this number almost 4 million fled to Turkey. This is not a 'refugee crisis', but a humanitarian, political, historical and economic crisis.

The recently published UN report Global Trends – Forced Displacement in 2015 (UNHCR 2015) finds that the number of forcibly displaced people has reached its highest number ever: 65.3 million (1 out of 122 people in the world). Unfortunately, the EU has not kept its promise to relocate 22,000 people from the UN camps to Europe, and until the end of 2015 only 600 of these were relocated. In 2015, developed countries admitted a total of only 107,100 refugees for resettlement. In contrast, developing regions (mostly Turkey, Pakistan, Lebanon, Iran, Ethiopia and Jordan) hosted 86 per cent of the world's refugees (ibid.). Closing the borders to the refugees and signing an agreement for returning them back to Turkey means ignoring the problem and bearing no responsibility.

The EU-Turkey Readmission Agreement is akin to an act of official human trafficking. Since its implementation, 1,487 people have been transferred to Turkey from Greece in one year and, as of March 2017, 3,565 refugees have been resettled from Turkey into the EU. These numbers fall far below the stipulated relocation limit of 72,000 refugees from Turkey to Europe. Moreover, in comparison to the more than 3 million Syrians in Turkey, setting the limit of uptake into Europe to such a low number is clearly inadequate.

So-called illegal (economic) migrants are being sent back, under the assumption that we do not have any special obligations towards migrants as we do towards refugees. However, today concepts like refugee, migrants, economic migrants, irregular/undocumented workers, exiled or asylum seekers, and the differentiation between forced migration and economic migration, have lost their relevance. For instance, those who are stateless; those who have lost their houses and jobs and do not have a future in their homelands; those who are marginalized under the economic, political and cultural pressures enforced by neoliberal policies and have to leave their homes are not considered refugees by the UN.

Turkey has nearly 4 million refugees, of which 3.5 million are Syrians (official numbers are less than this as the official figures include only registered people). Only 10 per cent of the Syrian refugees live in 25 refugee camps close to the border with Syria, while the rest are scattered in other parts of Turkey (Figure B6.1). They struggle to live by begging,

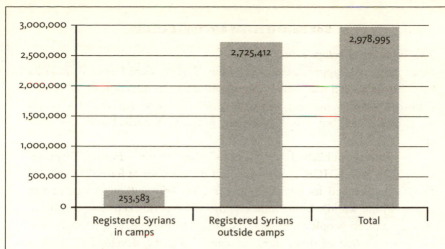

Figure B6.1 Syrians under temporary protection staying in and outside of accommodation centers

Source: Directorate General for Migration Management (2017).

Note: Numbers as at 13 April 2017; these are the official numbers and are generally less than the actual numbers as they include only registered people.

through temporary jobs of a precarious nature and employment in the informal sector, or by getting social aid, which for 'non-camp residents' is very limited.

Conditions of living

Turkey refuses to grant legal refugee status to refugees from outside Europe, thereby depriving them of the rights and benefits they are entitled to. Syrians living in Turkey are considered to be 'guests' with temporary protection status. Of the Syrian refugee population, 75 per cent are women and children (87 per cent of refugee women have no employment); 55 per cent are less than 18 years of age; 42 per cent are between 18 and 59; 3 per cent are over 60 (Directorate General for Migration Management 2017). There are nearly 1 million school-aged children, but only 14 per cent of primary school-aged children outside the refugee camps are enrolled in school in Turkey. Moreover, 150,000 Syrians have given birth in Turkey and their children have no citizenship – either Syrian or Turkish.

Without a work permit Syrian migrant workers in Turkey (uninsured and undocumented) survive by doing dangerous and heavy physical work. They earn far below the minimum wage, and have no recourse to justice in the case of wage disputes or accidents at work.

As on July 2016, only 5,500 Syrian refugees have been granted an official work permit. This means that a million people are either jobless or work illegally. This has led to the rise of a new ethnic underclass in

Turkey. Since parents have difficulty in finding jobs and are underpaid, children tend to work to support the household. Among Syrian refugees child labour is a prominent problem, while a 'lost generation' takes shape.

Access to health

The health conditions of Syrian refugees in Turkey are adversely affected due to lack of adequate housing and food. There are also problems in accessing health services, as most Syrian refugees have temporary identity documents (IDs) that cover only emergency medical problems. Preventive healthcare, especially for children and women, is not available for most people. Except for a few public health centres, routine follow-up for infants and pregnant women is not offered. Thousands of children have not been vaccinated or have received incomplete vaccination.

Since most refugees are forced to keep changing locations to find a job, they cannot register with a family physician and access primary healthcare. They also find it very difficult to reach secondary and tertiary care facilities due to lack of documentation, the complex organization of the Turkish healthcare system, lack of information about the health system, and language barriers.

A need for a change

As a middle-income country Turkey cannot cope with 4 million refugees. European countries and others, especially those that are militarily active in the region, should take responsibility for the refugees. The ploy of keeping refugees away from Europe by providing political benefits and financial aid to countries such as Turkey should be ended. Legal and safe passage should be ensured to those who want to go to Europe. Anti-immigrant border policies that cause deaths and human rights exploitation should be stopped.

(Substantial material for this box has been sourced from The 'Association of Bridging Peoples'. See: http://www.halklarinkoprusu.org/en/)

Migrants' health in times of crisis

The vulnerability of migrants has been aggravated by the economic crisis affecting Europe since 2008. Higher unemployment rates and precarious conditions of employment have pushed many migrants even further to the margins of the system. Poor living conditions are worsening migrants' health, counteracting the initial 'healthy immigrant effect' -- the better health status of newly arrived migrants, as compared to that of the national population due to the fact that sick persons are less likely to migrate/flee (Ingleby 2009,

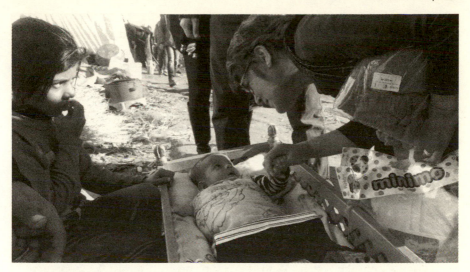

Image B6.2 Volunteer physicians examine children at a refugee camp (Cem Terzi)

p. 11). Xenophobia has also been on the rise: recession and absence of opportunities have made national populations more prone to hate discourses that use migrants as a scapegoat for the country's problems (Médecins du Monde, 2013, pp. 28–29).

In such contexts, the states' responsibility to protect and promote the right to health for all is of paramount importance. However, as austerity has become the new dogma in response to the economic crisis, constraints on public budgets have translated into reduced investments in healthcare. For example, the obligation contained in the Stability and Growth Pact (SGP)[2] to reduce public deficit has been used by the Spanish government to defend its policy of social sector cutbacks, particularly in the field of healthcare.[3] Highly indebted countries, such as Greece, Ireland, Portugal, etc. have received EU loans conditional to strict structural adjustment policies. In certain cases, as in Portugal, such requirements include concrete demands to reform the healthcare system (Eurofound, 2014, p. 7).

Regressive social measures, when unavoidable, should always refrain from targeting the most disadvantaged sectors of the population. Unfortunately, this has not been the case in several European countries with regards to migrants' access to healthcare. While some countries, such as Luxembourg, have been traditionally closed to undocumented migrants (undocumented migrants are not entitled to free healthcare), in recent years we have seen an increase in the number of countries following this approach (Médecins du Monde, 2016b, pp. 85–86).

Spain (Médecins du Monde, 2014, pp. 31–32) and the UK (Médecins du Monde, 2015, pp. 8–9), once home to the most inclusive national healthcare systems in Europe, have now adopted national legislations excluding

Box B6.2 Migrants' access to healthcare in Spain

A major turning point for the Spanish healthcare system was 20 April 2012. Until that date, the National healthcare system (NHS) in Spain was seen as a model in Europe due its inclusive nature which granted access to the care to all citizens and residents, whether authorized or not. While this system was far from perfect, since administrative barriers prevented some migrants from receiving assistance, it did provide some level of secure access to care for migrants. In 2012 the government imposed, without any parliamentary or popular debate, the Royal Decree Law (RDL) 16/2012. The RDL altered the principle of universality by linking the right to access to contribution to the social security system. The requirement of residence (to access care) was replaced by an insurance/benefit scheme which removed around 900,000 undocumented migrants from the system. With the enforcement of the RDL, assistance for undocumented migrants was available only for emergencies; pregnancy, childbirth and post-partum; minors; applicants for international protection; and victims of human trafficking (REDER, 2015, pp. 11–15).

Due to the high level of decentralization of the Spanish NHS, and in the absence of adequate and sufficient information, the RDL was applied in an arbitrary manner by hospitals and healthcare centres. As a consequence, denial of assistance even in cases allowed by the RDL (pregnant women and minors, for example) and the invoicing of emergency services that should have been free of charge became common. (REDER, 2015, pp. 18–20).

This outrageous exclusion from healthcare was contested by civil society. Médecins du Monde, Amnesty International, the Spanish Society of Family and Community Medicine, social movements such as Yo Sí Sanidad Universal and other platforms for the defence of public health, as well as healthcare professionals (who refused to implement the RDL and continued assisting all patients) denounced the grave breach of human rights that was being perpetrated, and demanded that the RDL be repealed. This mobilization in turn triggered the creation of a national network – REDER (Network for Denouncing and Resisting the Royal Decree-Law 16/2012) – of more than 300 social organizations and professional associations, which has been actively advocating for the adoption of a new legislation to ensure a universal system for every person living in Spain, regardless of her/his administrative status.

As a result of the mobilization, some regional governments did not implement the RDL while most political parties signed a declaration committing to repeal the RDL should they be in government (Medicos Del Mundo, 2015). Following the regional elections of May 2015, several new regional governments adopted measures to provide some sort of access to healthcare to undocumented migrants (REDER, 2016). Nonetheless, as regional governments lack the competence to undo national legislation, these measures are inadequate. Meanwhile the source of the problem remains: a structural reform of the system where the human right to health has been stripped of its very nature to make its enjoyment dependent on economic criteria rather than ethics (REDER, 2017).

undocumented migrants from healthcare (Box B6.2). Both governments have argued in favour of this policy, alleging that their respective healthcare systems are on the verge of collapse as a result of migrants' 'abuse' of social services. In Spain, this justification uses the term 'healthcare tourism' in a misleading way, by intentionally mixing two very different phenomena. On one hand, wealthy Europeans travel to Spain to receive medical treatment; and, on the other, undocumented workers from non-EU countries using healthcare resources to a significantly lower degree than the native population. The UK has passed the Immigration Act 2014, according to which even children of undocumented migrants and pregnant women are to be charged for healthcare and maternity care, in what constitutes a clear breach of minimum obligations under human rights law (Justfair, 2015, pp. 118–19). There is no evidence that these policies result in any significant financial savings for public budgets. Clearly undocumented migrants are being blamed to divert attention of the public from unpopular social sector cutbacks.

While regulations openly discriminating against migrants are easy to identify, less obvious provisions often produce similar effects. In the Netherlands, for example, the government has elevated drastically the minimum amount a patient has to pay for healthcare in order to be entitled to a reimbursement (Médecins du Monde, 2015, p. 8). This decision disproportionately affects the poorest sectors of the population, including most migrants.

Fortunately, not all countries affected by the economic crisis have resorted to restricting migrants' right to health. Italy (Médecins du Monde, 2016b, pp. 170–73) and Portugal (Eurofound, 2014, p. 23) have maintained, at least on paper, an inclusive healthcare system that allows access to undocumented migrants (Box B6.3). France has been promoting access to health services by increasing the income ceiling for the *Aide Complementaire de Santé*, which supports healthcare for the poor, and for the *Aide Medicale d'Etat*, which supports undocumented migrants (Médecins du Monde, 2016b, pp. 38–44). Even Greece, undergoing the consequence of both the economic crisis and the high inflow of refugees, has introduced a reform to open its public healthcare system to the most disadvantaged groups, although this does not cover all undocumented migrants (ibid., pp. 64–66). However, even in countries

Box B6.3: Migrants' access to healthcare in Italy

Health policy for migrants in Italy has, from its very origin, been shaped by an engaged civil society. This has given the country one of the most progressive and inclusive legislations on access to healthcare for foreigners, compared to other European countries (Marceca, 2017). Article 32 of the Italian Constitutional Charter, 1848, grants the right to health to all 'individuals', de-linking it from citizenship. However, in spite of this, migrants face difficulties in accessing care.

Civil society has played a role in drafting the two health articles in the 1998 Immigration Law, which are still in force today and grant full rights to immigrants who can enrol in the NHS. This includes immigrants and their families who have a work permit as well as asylum seekers and refugees. Undocumented migrants can access emergency care for free, but are also entitled to second- and third-level care for health needs that are 'urgent or essential'. This includes all interventions that, if not done or postponed, may cause harm to their health. Migrants from other countries of the EU, who hold the European Health Insurance Card, have access to some level of care, while those who regularly work in Italy can enrol in the NHS. However, those who have lost their job, or their legal residency, have to cover the full cost of care through the NHS.

The interpretation of the immigration law has been highly uneven in the country, creating situations of unjustifiable inequalities between regions and between urban and rural areas. An interregional effort has attempted to promote a harmonized document, aimed at offering binding guidelines for shaping health policies at the local level. Despite being signed by all the regional governors in December 2012, the interregional agreement is not being implemented in large measure.

While the right to access exists on paper, enforcement is weak. Since in the Italian NHS, family doctors are the entry point in the system, and undocumented migrants do not have access to family doctors, alternate primary healthcare facilities need to be in place. Often voluntary doctors' organizations and NGOs fill this gap between health needs and health services. Another requirement involves ensuring that access is economically sustainable. Despite the national law providing for user-fee exemption for the most deprived, in many regions this is not applied to migrants who are not registered with the NHS. Finally, there are other requirements: training health professionals in 'soft technologies', such as relational, intercultural and linguistic skills, and the overall organization of the health service, which is too often informed by rationality and efficiency and not centred around effectively responding to health needs, particularly of the most disadvantaged.

Given this situation, there are inequalities in access to healthcare and in health outcomes between native and migrant populations (Barsanti and Nuti, 2013; Tognetti, 2015). Several studies have shown that migrants underuse primary care and hospital services and overuse emergency services. This has much to do with immigrants' awareness of their rights and the means of exercising them; health workers' knowledge of these rights and procedure related to them; and resources within the health system for granting these rights. Studies have also shown that immigrants' access to services is conditioned by various factors: organizational, cognitive and bureaucratic. Clearly it is not enough to offer health services and make them claimable, one needs to promote and actively inform people (and workers) if such resources are to become truly accessible.

where the law allows access to healthcare for undocumented migrants, actual implementation is flawed and migrants continue to face exclusion from the healthcare system.

Barriers and challenges for migrants seeking healthcare

Regardless of the differences in national legislations, migrants face some common barriers and challenges, preventing them from accessing the healthcare system.

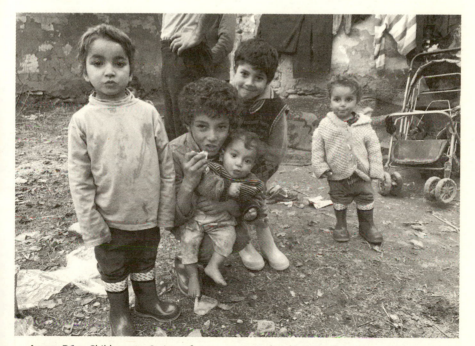

Image B6.3 Children at a Syrian refugee camp in Turkey (Cem Terzi)

Lack of information and fear of being reported Absence of adequate information regarding the functioning of the healthcare system and available entitlements constitutes the first obstacle. Confronted with a different reality than the one in their country of origin and often lacking a social network in the country of destination to ease them into the system, migrants usually ignore the most basic processes in seeking healthcare (Médecins du Monde, 2014, p. 27; 2015, p. 34; 2016a, p. 27).

Moreover, legal ambiguities and insufficient state action to ensure that health workers know and apply correctly the law leads to arbitrary interpretations, resulting in denial of access (International Organization for Migration, 2016, p. 18; Médecins du Monde, 2014, p. 28; 2015, p. 35; 2016a, p. 30). This has the effect of reinforcing migrants' perception of lack of right of access, and as a consequence they desist from demanding assistance even if needed (Médecins du Monde, 2016a, p. 29).

Undocumented migrants may also refrain from seeking health services out of fear of being reported to the police (Médecins du Monde, 2015, p. 36; 2016a, p. 30). This fear is justified as legislation in a majority of European countries explicitly requires health workers to notify the authorities whenever they assist an irregular immigrant. (International Organization for Migration, 2016, p. 19).

Administrative barriers Lack of information is made worse by complex administrative processes, tedious and difficult to understand. Moreover, the fact that identity documents are usually required is often an impediment in accessing care (Médecins du Monde, 2014, p. 27; 2015, p. 34; 2016a, p. 27). The issue is particularly complicated for undocumented migrants, especially in countries (for example, Belgium, France and Spain) where they are eligible for certain entitlements. Proof, in the form of an identity card, cannot always be presented by people who have recently migrated from distant places and might have lost all or most of their material possessions in the course of an extremely traumatizing process. Another obstacle is posed by the necessity to provide a proof of residence, as undocumented migrants often lack a rent contract or are simply homeless (Médecins du Monde, 2016b, pp. 17, 41–43).

Financial barriers Most European countries have some sort of a co-payment scheme where the cost of medical attention is partly borne by the patients. As is obvious, paying for social services has a greater impact on the most disadvantaged and impoverished sectors of the population, including most migrants. While some countries such as France and Belgium have exceptions for the poorest, not everyone can qualify to benefit from these mechanisms (Médecins du Monde, 2016b, pp. 14–18, 37–43). Undocumented migrants are the worst affected when co-payments become necessary. This is particularly so in Germany (Box B6.4) where, in order to get refunded for non-emergency

Box B6.4: Migrants' access to healthcare in Germany

In Germany, healthcare is organized through an insurance-based healthcare system. As in most European countries, access to healthcare for immigrants depends on their legal status. International migrants with work or study permits are usually insured and can access healthcare free of cost like most Germans.

However, migrants from some countries of the EU face major barriers to healthcare as health insurance in these countries is often insufficient or invalid despite the theoretical existence of a European Health Insurance Card. Migrants from the southern and eastern European countries make up a major proportion of migrants seeking help from the many support organizations that assist in accessing healthcare in Germany (Medibuero, 2016).

Asylum seekers are entitled to access healthcare for acute or painful medical conditions and everything that is indispensable to maintaining health, leaving the comprehensiveness of care to the interpretation of the local government or doctor (Fluechtlingsrat Berlin e. V, 2016; Medizinische Flüchtlingshilfe Göttingen e. V, 2016). In practice, access to healthcare varies substantially in scope and quality between German federal states, ranging from electronic health insurance cards for asylum seekers with nearly equal access to care as for Germans to paper-based referral cards that are hard to get and entitle one to care only for acute or painful diseases (ibid.). Changes in asylum legislation in 2014 and 2015 have failed to address the lack of clarity in defining access to care for asylum seekers and missed the opportunity to establish a uniform regulation for comprehensive access to care (Medizinische Flüchtlingshilfe Göttingen e. V, 2016). The restrictive interpretation of laws by healthcare personnel has resulted in asylum seekers being denied care because of the refusal to provide or accept paper-based referral cards. Many asylum seekers have suffered severe medical consequences, including death (Fluechtlingsrat Berlin e. V, 2016). As healthcare services remain insufficient, many people have volunteered to support asylum seekers in their struggle to access healthcare. While voluntary help is necessary to address the immediate need of asylum seekers, it remains impossible to guarantee rights, including access to healthcare, on the basis of volunteer work. (Medibuero, 2016).

Undocumented migrants are entitled to emergency care; however, accessing such care may result in deportation as state institutions are, with some exceptions, obliged to report undocumented migrants to migration authorities. These exceptions are however largely unknown to healthcare institutions, and undocumented migrants continue to risk deportation when they officially access healthcare in case of emergency. Although many NGOs, anti-racist initiatives and individuals are volunteering to improve healthcare and organize medical appointments within the networks of volunteer doctors and hospitals, healthcare remains inadequate.

care costs, migrants need to apply to the social welfare office, which is obliged to report the matter to the authorities (ibid., p. 56).

Language barriers Communication is a basic requirement while seeking health-care. Yet, as Médecins du Monde (2016a, p. 27) has shown, a significant number of migrants all across Europe require translation services, which are not always available.

Xenophobia and discrimination Racism in healthcare services is a barrier that migrants have to face, intermittently or all the time, across Europe (Médecins du Monde, 2014, p. 28; 2015, p. 36; 2016a, p. 30). While at the moment, the number of cases remains relatively low, there is serious concern that they may escalate in the near future as xenophobic extreme right-wing parties are gaining more support within several EU countries.

Conclusion

In 2017, the EU celebrates 60 years since its establishment by the Treaties of Rome. We should not forget, however, that the EU is primarily 'a common market', and that economic, not social, priorities have been guiding the shaping of the EU from its inception until today. Also, in 60 years the EU has not been able to inform, design and implement progressive health and social policies, or to protect the most vulnerable sectors of society and promote their rights.

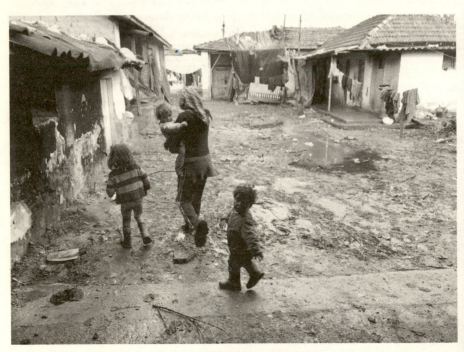

Image B6.4 Living conditions ata refugee camp (Cem Terzi)

In 1907, the pathologist and founder of social medicine Rudolf Virchow wrote "How sad it is that thousands have to die in misery, so a few hundred may live well". Over a century later, the situation seems similar, with inequalities still on the rise as reflected also in health indicators. If what should be 'our' institutions are not acting in the interests of people and in the direction of equality, we should join forces and advocate more to radically change them, challenging with the power of the many the interests of a few.

Notes

1 While this is the theory, we shall later discuss how this legal framework has been bent in the context of the economic crisis, enabling the troika (the EU Commission, the European Central Bank and the International Monetary Fund) to impose health budget constraints on certain EU member states.

2 The SGP is the mechanism established by the EU to control member states' budget deficits and limit public debt. According to the SGP, budget deficit cannot exceed 3 per cent GDP while public debt should be maintained under 60 per cent GDP. States which incur deficits in a breach of these terms could be subjected to sanctions. See European Commission (n.d.).

3 The Stability And Growth Pact is an agreement involving the countries of the European Union (EU) and use the Euro as currency. The SGP, enacted in 1997, was created to establish rules to ensure that all involved countries help maintain the value of the euro by enforcing fiscal responsibility.

References

Barsanti, S & Nuti, S 2013, *Migrant health in Italy: the right and access to health care as an opportunity for integration and inclusion*, working paper no. 04/2013, Istituto di Management Scuola Superiore Sant'Anna di Pisa, http://www.idm.sssup.it/wp/201304.pdf

Commission of the European Communities 2009, *Communication from the Commission to the European Parliament, the Council, the European Economic and Social Committee and the Committee of the Regions—solidarity in health: reducing health inequalities in the EU*, COM (2009) 567 final, Brussels.

Directorate General for Migration Management 2017, *Temporary protection*, http://www.goc.gov.tr/icerik3/temporary-protection_915_1024_4748

Eurofound 2014, *Access to health care in times of crisis*, Publications Office of the European Union, Luxembourg.

European Commission 2016, *Communication from the Commission to the European Parliament, the Council, the European Central Bank, the European Economic and Social Committee, the Committee of the Regions and the European Investment Bank—annual growth survey 2017*, COM (2016) 725 final, Brussels.

European Commission n.d., *Stability and growth pact*, http://ec.europa.eu/economy_finance/economic_governance/sgp/index_en.htm

Fluechtlingsrat Berlin e. V 2016, *Dokumentation Menschrechtsverletzungen durch Mangelmedizin nach AsylbLG*, Berlin, http://www.fluechtlingsinfo-berlin.de/fr/asylblg/Classen_AsylbLG_Gesundheit_08Juni2016.pdf

Ingleby, D 2009, *European research on migration and health*, International Organization for Migration background paper, University of Utrecht.

Ingleby, D, Chimienti, M, Ormond, M & De Freitas, C 2005, 'The role of health in integration', in Fonseca, M L and Malheiros, J (eds), *Social integration and mobility: education, housing and health*, IMISCOE Cluster B5 State of the art report, Estudos para o Planeamento Regional e Urbano no. 67, Centro de Estudos Geográficos, Lisbon, pp. 88–119.

International Organization for Migration 2016, *Recommendations on access to health services for migrants in an irregular situation: an expert consensus,*

International Organization for Migration (IOM) Regional Office Brussels, Migration Health Division, Brussels.

Justfair 2015, *Implementation of the international covenant on economic, social and cultural rights in the United Kingdom of Great Britain and Northern Ireland. Parallel report. Submission to the Committee on Economic, Social and Cultural Rights*, http://tbinternet.ohchr.org/Treaties/CESCR/Shared%20Documents/GBR/INT_CESCR_ICO_GBR_21702_E.pdf

Marceca, M 2017,'Migration and health from a public health perspective', in Muenstermann, I (ed.), *People's movements in the 21st century – risks, challenges and benefits.* https://www.intechopen.com/books/people-s-movements-in-the-21st-century-risks-challenges-and-benefits/migration-and-health-from-a-public-health-perspective.

Médecins du Monde 2013, *Access to healthcare in Europe in times of crisis and rising xenophobia: an overview of the situation of people excluded from healthcare systems*, https://www.medicosdelmundo.org/index.php/mod.documentos/mem.descargar/fichero.documentos_MdM_Report_access_healthcare_times_crisis_and_rising_xenophobia_edcfd8a3%232E%23pdf

Médecins du Monde 2014, *Access to healthcare for the most vulnerable in a Europe in social crisis: focus on pregnant women and children*, http://www.epim.info/wp-content/uploads/2014/05/mdm-access-to-healthcare-europe-2014.pdf

Médecins du Monde 2015, *Access to healthcare for people facing multiple health vulnerabilities – obstacles in access to care for children and pregnant women in Europe*, http://mdmgreece.gr/app/uploads/2015/05/MdM-Intl-Obs-2015-report-EN.pdf

Médecins du Monde 2016a,*Access to healthcare for people facing multiple vulnerabilities in health in 31 cities in 12 countries*, International Network 2016 Observatory report, https://mdmeuroblog.files.wordpress.com/2016/11/observatory-report2016_en-mdm-international.pdf

Médecins du Monde 2016b, *Legal report on access to healthcare in 17 countries*, https://mdmeuroblog.files.wordpress.com/2016/11/mdm-2016-legal-report-on-access-to-healthcare-in-17-countries-15112016.pdf

Medibuero 2016, *Netzwerk für das Recht auf Gesundheitsversorgung aller Migrant*innen: 20 Jahre Medibuero*, Netzwerk, Berlin.

Medicos Del Mundo 2015, *Los principales líderes políticos de la oposición dicen 'sí' a la Sanidad Universal*, https://www.medicosdelmundo.org/index.php/mod.conts/mem.detalle_cn/relmenu.111/id.4256>

Medizinische Flüchtlingshilfe Göttingen e. V 2016, *Gesundheit fuer Gefluechtete*, Göttingen, http://gesundheit-gefluechtete.info/

OECD/EU 2015, *Indicators of immigrant integration 2015: settling in*, OECD Publishing, Paris http://dx.doi.org/10.1787/9789264234024-en

REDER 2015, *Anatomy of the healthcare reform: the universality of exclusion*, Network for Denouncing and Resisting the Royal Decree-Law 16/2012, Madrid.

REDER2016, *Un aniversario sin nada que celebrar*, Network for Denouncing and Resisting the Royal Decree-Law 16/2012, Madrid.

REDER 2017, *Five myths for five years of health exclusion*, Network for Denouncing and Resisting the Royal Decree-Law 16/2012, Madrid.

Sarría-Santamera, A, Hijas-Gómez, AI, Carmona, R & Gimeno-Feliú, L A 2016, A systematic review of the use of health services by immigrants and native populations, *Public Health Reviews*, vol. 37, no. 28, DOI 10.1186/s40985-016-0042-3.

Tognetti, M 2015,'Health inequalities: access to services by immigrants in Italy', *Open Journal of Social Sciences*, vol. 3, pp. 8–15, http://file.scirp.org/pdf/JSS_2015032714224331.pdf

UN Economic, Social and Cultural Rights Committee 2000, *General observation no. 14 – the right to the highest attainable standard of health*, UN Doc. E/C 12/2000/4, August, para. 34.

UNHCR 2015, *Global trends: forced displacement in 2015*, http://www.unhcr.org/statistics/unhcrstats/576408cd7/unhcr-global-trends-2015.html

Introduction: global context of 'informal' employment in the health sector

In the past decades public provisioning of healthcare has declined dramatically (see Chapter B1). Within the public health sector, the retreat of the state from the provision of healthcare has been accompanied by reforms in the internal management and organization of public institutions and systems along the lines of the new public management (NPM) strategy. The main characteristic of the NPM strategy is "the attempt [to introduce] within the public services, which are not yet private, the motivation in accordance with the performances and the disciplines specific to the market" (Moore, Stewart and Haddock, 1994, p. 13). Such reform seek to introduce private-sector practices in the management, organization and labour dynamics of the public sector, thus creating 'internal markets' within public institutions, facilities and systems (Vabø, 2009). A common feature in countries that have adopted the NPM is the pressure they face as a result of dwindling public budgets (Mascarenhas, 1993, pp. 319–28). With a prime focus on reduction of the wage bill various practices are resorted to including: fixed-term work, temporary work, contractual work through manpower agencies, and dependent self-employment (where workers are contracted as individuals and payment is linked to productivity).

Even in times of slowing economic growth, as during the global financial crisis of 2008–2009, employment in the health and other social sectors has maintained a steady growth.[1] However, there is a growing trend towards use of non-standard forms of employment to replace permanent public health service employment (ILO, 2017, p. 21). This directly impacts the wages of health workers and, over the first decade of this century, the remuneration of health workers has decreased in relation to total health expenditure globally (ibid., p. 23).[2] (See Table B7.1)

While the trend towards informalization (see Box B7.1 regarding informal employment) of work is relatively new in high-income countries (HICs) and related to the financial crisis of 2008–2009 and the austerity measures that followed, it is a much older phenomenon in LMICs, linked to introduction of neoliberal policies and Structural Adjustment Programmes (SAPs) in the 1980s and 1990s (People's Health Movement, Medact and TWN, 2014b, 2014).

Financial constraints in the health system contribute to low motivation of health workers, difficulties in retention of the workforce and outward migration.

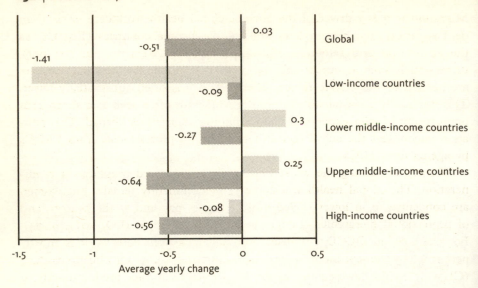

Average yearly change

Average yearly change in remuneration of salaried workers as per cent of GDP

Average yearly change in remuneration of salaried workers as per cent of total health expenditure

Table B7.1: Yearly change of health workers' remuneration of total health expenditure and GDP by country income level, 2000–10 (percentage)

Source: ILO: World Social Protection Report 2014–15: Building economic recovery, inclusive development and social justice (Geneva, 2014)

Box B7.1: What is informal employment?

The International Labour Organization defines this as:

"…employees are considered to have informal jobs if their employment relationship is, in law or in practice, not subject to national labour legislation, income taxation, social protection or entitlement to certain employment benefits (advance notice of dismissal, severance pay, paid annual or sick leave, etc.) for reasons such as: nondeclaration of the jobs or the employees; casual jobs or jobs of a limited short duration; jobs with hours of work or wages below a specified threshold (e.g. for social security contributions); employment by unincorporated enterprises or by persons in households; jobs where the employee's place of work is outside the premises of the employer's enterprise (e.g. outworkers without employment contract); or jobs, for which labour regulations are not applied, not enforced, or not complied with for any other reason.

Source: Hussmanns, R 2003, 'Statistical definition of informal employment: Guidelines endorsed by the Seventeenth International Conference of Labour Statisticians' (2003) Bureau of Statistics, International Labour Office, Geneva

Migration is a key driver of the current global health workforce crisis (Van de Pas, 2013). Further, in low- and middle-income countries (LMICs) as the absorption and retention of health workers (especially, but not only, professionals such as nurses and technicians) in public facilities fall, workers are pushed to the private sector, where the pay is often substantially lower. This financially unsustainable option for workers is often seen as a short-term opportunity to gain experience before finding alternatives abroad. This situation encourages the active recruitment of health professionals from LMICs by agents from HICs.

Women are among the worst impacted by downward pressure on remuneration. The global health workforce is predominantly female, but women are concentrated in lower skilled jobs, with less pay and at the bottom end of professional hierarchies (Langer et al., 2015, cited in ILO, 2017, p. 24). For example, in OECD countries, low-skill long-term care work is mostly performed by women; and in several Asian countries, community health workers (CHWs), on the lowest rung in the healthcare chain, are predominantly, if not exclusively, women. As they work within their communities and provide care that women have traditionally performed without pay, CHWs are rarely remunerated on par with the legal wage and usually work under highly informal employment conditions.

In many LMICs, especially in Africa and South Asia, the 'informal' sector dominates the economy and employment opportunities. Employment conditions are characterized by poverty wages and wage theft, employment insecurity, and abusive and undignified working conditions. Workers often accept substandard employment terms and work conditions in the expectation that in the near future this will give them access to a 'government job', that is, secure and dignified employment with a real wage.

Insecurity of tenure in the case of informal employment makes it more difficult for workers to join or form unions. Without the right to unionize and engage in collective bargaining, health workers remain vulnerable to exploitation by their employers. Ultimately this also means that public health is undermined, as informalization has a negative impact on health workers' ability to perform their duties, the organization of work within an institution and the relationship between workers and patients (Thresia, 2016). This chapter examines working conditions of two categories of health workers in South Asia: workers in public hospitals and community health workers. The case studies documented are based on primary fieldwork and research by Public Services International (PSI).

Informalization of hospital workers in South Asia: case studies

The three case studies that follow document the trends of informalization in public hospitals in Delhi, Kathmandu and Colombo.

Delhi Informal employment conditions have existed, to a limited extent, in public hospitals in Delhi prior to the introduction of neoliberal reforms in India in 1991. Since the early 1990s, reduced government expenditure on healthcare and the policy of providing a greater role for the private sector, mostly through public–private partnerships, has led to a push for contracting out non-clinical services and the use of fixed-duration contracts for unskilled workers, such as sweepers, washermen/washerwomen, kitchen staff, drivers, security personnel.[3] Professional staff were affected by these labour reforms in the early 2000s, starting with facilities run by the state government of Delhi.[4] For example, nurses were hired by hospitals on short-term contracts as a temporary measure on the pretext that it took too long to fill regular posts. However, this practice has now become the norm. After a legal struggle, nurses on fixed-duration contracts in state hospitals started receiving wages equal to those of nurses in permanent posts. However, this parity does not extend to other working conditions and benefits. The hiring of nurses on fixed-term contracts began four to five years ago in hospitals under the central Ministry of Health and Family Welfare (MoHFW) (Basu, forthcoming). MoHFW-run facilities have not followed the court order on pay parity between contractual and permanent workers.

In the early 2000s, a ban on hiring was adopted for Group C and D employees (the two 'lowest rungs' of workers in the government system). In the case of technical staff, the ban was revised to enable the filling of a third of the vacancies. This was challenged by the workers, who claimed it was impossible to decide which technical post was more important and thus qualify for permanent recruitment. In 2005, the ban on hiring was lifted for Group C workers, though hiring on fixed-term contracts continued (ibid.).

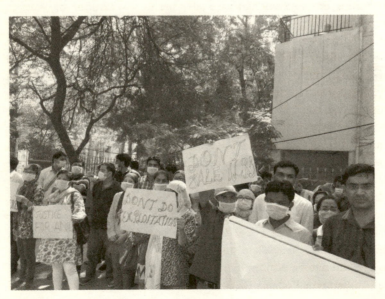

Image B7.1
Health workers demanding better service conditions at a hospital in New Delhi, India (Santosh Mahindrakar)

As hiring on fixed-duration contracts increased for professional staff (mainly nurses), even direct hiring of 'non-medical' staff was stopped and outsourced to contractors. This has led to a deskilling of workers.[5] For instance, out of a total of 150 posts for *ayahs* (helpers) in the prestigious MoHFW facility, the 1,000 bedded Ram Manohar Lohia Hospital, only 25 are permanent. In Lala Ram Swarup (LRS) Institute of Tuberculosis & Respiratory Diseases, an autonomous institute under the MoHFW, out of the 500 Group C and D workforce, 200 are employed through contractors.[6] Workers employed through contractors are subjected to a number of labour law violations, including low pay, absence of social security, and absence of paid and maternity leave and pension.[7]

Typically, the contractor enters into an agreement with the hospital management, which specifies the number of workers required. The agreement is generally for the duration of one year after which it is either renewed or a new contractor is hired. Workers are supervised by a hospital supervisor as well as by one hired by the contractor. The hospital supervisor has the final say on the work assigned and the quality of work; however, the supervisor hired by the contractor micro-manages the workers, who directly report to her/him.[8] Supervisors are not interested in, nor capable of, dealing with occupational health issues of workers who risk exposure to infections and chemicals. The contractor receives the wages from the hospital management and passes it on to the supervisor who then pays each worker. In the process, the worker is at risk of wage theft, i.e. the risk that the entire amount due is not actually passed on to the worker.

Reduction in public funding has also resulted in an increase in the number of public–private partnerships for provision of healthcare services. Consequently, a large number of employees have had to shift from being public-sector employees to becoming employees of private enterprises. Conditions of work in the private sector are worse than in the public sector. Outsourcing of services that are considered non-essential, such as laundry, has been a regular practice in public hospitals. Outsourced services have now expanded after the Delhi government passed orders to all public facilities to outsource security and cleaning services.[9] More recently, the trend has extended to clinical services such as laboratory and radiological diagnostics. In some public facilities, dialysis units have been outsourced to a private company (PHRN et al., 2017). Increased outsourcing of services by public hospitals is accompanied by a rapid rise in the number of private companies that offer these services.

Kathmandu In Nepal, most tertiary hospitals are concentrated in Kathmandu. In Kathmandu the situation regarding non-formal employment in public hospitals is similar to what has been described regarding Delhi, except that an even larger proportion of workers fall in the non-formal category.

The change in the nature of employment commenced with the adoption of the Structural Adjustment Policies (SAPs) in 1986. The reforms were justified as necessary to reduce costs and improve efficiency (Dixit 2014). Reduced funding from the government and the promotion of 'decentralization policies', whereby hospitals have to generate parts of their budgets, resulted in hospitals seeking new avenues for income generation. This has led to the mushrooming of autonomous public facilities. This changes the ethos of the institution, and "[H]ospitals become more concerned with reducing the costs of service delivery than with delivering improved quality of care" (Basu, 2016).

In Nepal nurses have been hired on fixed-term contracts for decades. Nurses in general are paid disproportionately less than doctors and they are usually hired on fixed-term contracts of six months. Recently many nurses are being hired on three-month contracts, which are not renewed.[10] In the aftermath of the earthquake of April 2015 nurses were hired without written contracts.

For non-professional staff, 'contract work' is the norm. They face similar conditions as in Delhi: wage theft, denial of paid maternity leave and pension, multiple supervisors and insecurity of tenure. Workers report that they are often asked to change their location of work by the contractor, based on the changing demand from different hospitals. This creates difficulties in the case of occupational hazards or accidents at work as workers and their families are not sure which agency would process their claims.[11]

As well as a highly challenging situation created by insecurity of tenure, public-sector health workers' trade unions also face legal hurdles. Workers need to show a permanent contract with a government institution (which they do not have), in order to register with the Labour Department in Nepal. Under the Health Service Act, if a public-sector health worker does not register, they do not get an identity number, without which they cannot get membership in a union. This prevents the formal membership of unregistered health workers in unions and union representatives see this as a bid to weaken unions.[12]

Colombo Of the three countries studied, Sri Lanka's health system is the least privatized. While Sri Lanka too has adopted reforms to facilitate the entry of private enterprises in provisioning of health services, these reforms are primarily in the form of public subsidies to private enterprises – incentives to purchase land for private hospital construction, loans for expansion of private facilities, duty free imports of biomedical equipment and permission for professionals in the public sector to work part-time in private facilities (Kumar, 2015).

Unlike in Delhi and Kathmandu, in Colombo the norm regarding employment of the medical workforce (such as nurses and technicians) in the public sector is permanent employment with standard wages and benefits.

While there are some levels of informal employment among unskilled and non-medical workforce, the scale is limited. Contractual hiring through man-power agencies is common for security services, and for workers in cleaning and laundry departments. However, the conditions of work and benefits for fixed-duration workers are better than for their counterparts in India and

Nepal. They are generally provided with medical insurance and paid leave, and their salaries are comparable to those in permanent employment (Basu, 2016).

A common form of informal employment of medical staff is the hiring of retired nurses on fixed-duration contracts for a period of a year or two. While nurses were initially remunerated at the level of their last drawn salary, in order to reduce costs the policy was later changed to remuneration equivalent to the starting salary in the corresponding occupation. This has reduced interest in rejoining among retired nurses. In the case of posts remaining vacant, there is anecdotal evidence of existing staff taking on extra work for which they receive additional payment.[13] This trend is also seen in the case of ward attendants, where the proportion of posts kept vacant is typically high. While this is generally seen as an opportunity to augment income, in the long run the practice can negatively impact quality of care (ILO, 2017, p. 32).

Overall trends In all three countries studied, informal employment relations first cover unskilled workers, who are not directly in touch with patients, and whose work is often seen as not core to the work of the hospital, such as laundry, security and kitchen staff. As informalization spreads, ward attendants and cleaning staff are also affected. It often takes some time before technicians and laboratory staff is affected, and nurses are affected at the end of the chain.[14] Thus the level of skill plays an important role in shaping the terms of employment across the workforce.

Different categories of workers face varying degrees of deterioration of their employment conditions. Employees with fixed-duration contracts, who work directly under the management of the hospital, have relatively better terms of employment and working conditions than those who are supervised by contractors or manpower agencies.

informalization is less prominent where penetration of the private sector in the health system is low. While direct causalities are difficult to establish, it would appear that informalization of the health workforce, weakening of public healthcare institutions and the expansion of the role of the private sector are interlinked in multiple and complex ways.

Community Health Workers

The WHO characterizes Community Health Workers (CHWs) as follows: "Community health workers should be members of the communities where they work, should be selected by the communities, should be answerable to the communities for their activities, should be supported by the health system but not necessarily a part of its organization, and have shorter training than professional workers." (WHO, 2007)

Though a precise classification is difficult due to the wide variation in the profiles of CHWs (Table B7.1), this definition is understood to include both a generic community-based workforce, as well as a more specialized community-

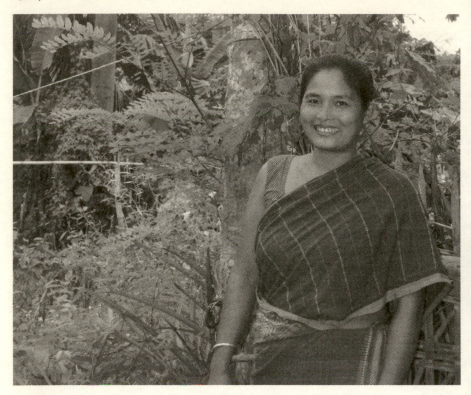

Image B7.2 A community health worker in Tripura, India (Sulakshana Nandi)

based workforce, and to exclude auxiliary or mid-level health cadres that are generally facility-based (Haines et al., 2007).

In the 1970s and 1980s, CHWs were a key component of comprehensive primary healthcare.[15] However, by the early 1990s, the enthusiasm for CHWs had diminished with many national CHW programmes having been abandoned (ibid.). The shortage of professional health workers in the mid-2000s and the move to delegate tasks (task-shifting) earlier performed by them to less trained health workers, such as CHWs, created renewed interest in CHW programmes (WHO, 2007).

There are two different perspectives on the role of CHWs. One that they are community based health advocates and agents of social change, and second, that they are an extension of the formal healthcare system. While early programmes emphasized the role of CHWs as community advocates, today's programmes emphasize their technical and community healthcare function; thus, essentially, treating them as extensions of the formal healthcare system (ibid.).

There is evidence of positive impacts of CHW programmes on health outcomes, such as a substantial reduction in child mortality (UNICEF, 2004). However, strengthening of public health systems remain necessary to maintain and build on the health gains brought about by these programmes (Haines et al., 2007). Yet, in most LMICs public healthcare systems are fragile and under-funded, and the extensive deployment of CHWs goes hand in hand with their inadequate remuneration.

While the question as to whether CHWs should be volunteers or paid in some form remains controversial, 'satisfactory remuneration' (through material and/or financial incentives) has been identified as a factor that motivates individual CHWs, and, conversely, inconsistent and/or inequitable remuneration has been identified as a disincentive (WHO, 2007).

The following three case studies examine CHW programmes in Pakistan, India and Nepal, and discuss, respectively: the process of regularization of CHWs in Pakistan and key factors of attrition; the context in which the Nepal CHW programme has sustained on volunteerism; and the unifying demand in India for the recognition of CHWs as health workers. Table B7.1 provides details about the CHW programmes in the three countries.

TABLE B7.1: CHW Programme profile in South Asian countries

	Pakistan	India	Nepal
Workforce	Lady Health Workers (LHW)	Accredited Social Health Activist (ASHA)	Female Community Health Volunteer (FCHV)
Year of commencement of programme	1994	2005	1998
Total workforce	125,000	939,000	53,000
Population per CHW	175 Households (1,000-1,200 people)	200 households (approx. 1,000 people)	125 households (approx. 600 people)
Main tasks	Maternal, neonatal and child health, family planning, health promotion, immunization	Family planning, institutional delivery, child health, health education	Safe motherhood, child health, family planning, immunization
Training	3 months + 3 months in field	23 days	18 days
Remuneration (annual)	US$ 1650	US$ 180 + incentives	US$ 75

Source: Compiled from descriptions of the respective programs

Lady health workers in Pakistan The Lady Health Workers (LHWs) Programme (officially the National Programme for Family Planning and Primary Health Care, FP & PHC) was created in 1994 with the aim to improve the health of communities by providing maternal, neonatal and child health, and family planning services, by integrating existing vertical health promotion programmes.

The programme has expanded over the years from an initial deployment of 30,000 LHWs to more than 125,000 LHWs. After a 15-month basic training, a LHW is responsible for the basic health needs of between 1,000 to 1,200 people, roughly 175 households. Despite visible impacts such as immunization coverage and coverage by skilled birth attendants, there are wide disparities in the reach of the programme between and within provinces. Sindh and Punjab are significantly better served than Khyber Paktunkhwa (KP) and Balochistan, where security is issues for LHWs. Urban areas are better covered than rural areas, where delivery of health services in general is limited.

The programme has been substantially scaled up in the past decades. From a coverage of 50–60 per cent of the population in rural areas and urban slums in 2006 (Haines et al., 2007), it expanded to cover 85 per cent of the households in 2009 (Perry, 2017). Since then, the workforce has increased by more than a third, from about 91,000 to 125,000 today. A major portion of the funds for the programme come from government revenues, with an estimated 11 per cent covered by external donors (Perry, 2017).

The programme is a major employer of women in the non-agricultural sector in rural areas. LHWs hail from economically vulnerable households and poverty is one of the factors responsible for women seeking a job as a LHW (Khan, 2011). According to a recent survey, in the province of Sindh, the income of LHWs represents 69 per cent of their household income (Muhammad, 2017). It has also been documented that in many cases LHWs are the first women in their families, communities and villages to acquire education up to the matriculation level (10 years of schooling) and to have a paid government job (Inam, 2017).

Yet, their recognition as employees of the state with remuneration on government scales only came after a long and bitter struggle. Formed in 2010, the All Pakistan Lady Health Workers Association (APLHWA) emerged as the national platform to fight for the rights of LHWs (Diwan, 2013). The PLHWA's campaigns (including sit-ins, road blocks, rallies and national strikes) led to a gradual increase in the remuneration of LHWs and the granting of employment benefits. The struggle culminated in the recognition of LHWs as government employees through an order of the Supreme Court of Pakistan in March 2013. The Supreme Court took the view that LHWs are state employees and the court instructed the federal government to formalize their services and grant them legal wage-based remuneration and other labour rights such as holiday pay and pension.[16]

Wages are not paid regularly and LHWs have to agitate for the wages to be released – often earnings for several months remain pending. A recent survey (Muhammed, 2017) found that irregular wage payments mean that LHWs have to borrow from shopkeepers for food (including rice, wheat, pulses and vegetables) as well as to cover utility bills, medical expenses and children's education.[17]

The recognition of LHWs as paid workers in the public sphere contributes to overcoming the gendered division of public and private spaces. However, it also makes them possible targets of regressive pushbacks, verbal abuse and violence by the communities they serve (Inam, 2017). This is in addition to the attacks on them by religious extremists, as was seen especially during the polio campaign.[18] The formal recognition of an employer–employee relationship places a greater responsibility on the state, especially in the current challenging work environment.

Accredited social health activists in India In India the National Rural Health Mission (NRHM) aimed to improve health outcomes in rural areas. To do so, the NRHM, in 2005, created a large pool of community health workers called Accredited Social Health Activists or ASHAs.[19] Initially deployed in rural areas, according to the revised guidelines of the National Health Mission (2013), state governments can deploy ASHAs in urban areas as well. ASHAs receive 23 days of training. As of September 2016, over 939,000 ASHAs had been deployed across the country (Ministry of Health and Family Welfare, 2017).

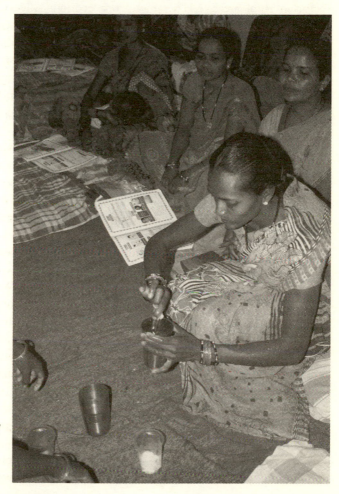

Image B7.3 A community health worker training women to make oral rehydration solution (Sulakshana Nandi)

Specific tasks of ASHAs, as well as their remuneration, are decided by the state governments. Their remuneration is based on task-based incentives and ASHAs have to report to the health post once a week. At the end of the month the tasks completed by ASHAs are reviewed and the remuneration is calculated accordingly.

Studies have shown that the incentivized system of payment has resulted in low remuneration for a large amount of work and delayed payments (Bhatia, 2014; Som, 2016, pp. 26–42). In addition, ASHAs have irregular work hours requiring them to work at odd hours, for instance when they have to accompany pregnant women for institutional deliveries. The irregular work hours coupled with irregular remuneration puts them under great strain. Further, ASHAs are not recognized as government employees. This has implications for the employment conditions of ASHAs. There is no provision for paid leave, including maternity leave, allowances for washing of uniforms, or compensation for occupational risks encountered.

Across different states in India, ASHAs have organized themselves and are agitating for better working conditions and remuneration and for their formal recognition as health workers. In the wake of the nationally coordinated movement of ASHAs demanding a minimum fixed wage in addition to existing incentives, in December 2013 a fixed monthly honorarium of Rs 1,000 (roughly US$ 15, equivalent to less than 10 per cent of the government notified minimum wage for full-time unskilled workers) was announced for ASHAs. Some state governments have announced honorariums above this level. For instance, as 2015, while ASHAs in West Bengal receive an honorarium of Rs 1,800, those in Kerala received only Rs 1,000 (Anonymous, 2015). While the fixed monthly honorariumis an important gain, it remains grossly inadequate. Along with other social service workers in a similar situation, ASHAs across 23 states went on a strike in January 2017 to demand recognition as workers, minimum wages, pension and other social security benefits (Anonymous, 2017).

The government (federal as well as state governments) argues that the flexible system of payment for ASHAs and their non-recognition as health workers is related to the fact that they are not workers but women who have 'volunteered' their services for the betterment of their community.[20] However, it is important to note that ASHAs do not receive adequate institutional support to be able to play the role of 'agents of change'. The tasks listed linked with their remuneration are specific to healthcare extension services and ASHAs are often burdened with additional tasks (such as conducting census related activities). Most ASHAs spend almost as much (or in some cases similar) time as full-time workers in accomplishing the tasks assigned to her. Thus, their possible role as 'agents of change' mostly falls between the cracks and is dependent on individual interest in playing such a role against all odds.

The size and spread of the mobilization of ASHAs demanding their rights as workers is a sign of widespread discontent that cannot be brushed aside.

Arguably, the decision of the government with regard to the demand of ASHAs to be recognized as workers in the health sector will have consequences for the long-term sustainability of this workforce.

Female community health volunteers in Nepal Nepal's Female Community Health Volunteer (FCHV) programme was started in 1988–1989 with the aim to promote safe motherhood, child health, family planning and immunization. FCHVs also treat cases of lower respiratory tract infections and refer more complicated cases to health institutions. There are more than 54,000 FCHVs working all over Nepal, except in urban municipalities. Currently, one FCHV is in charge of around 125 households (around 600 people).

FCHVs undergo an 18-day basic training course on key elements of primary healthcare. While an estimated 70 per cent of FCHVs are illiterate (Schwarz et al., 2014), imparting of basic education is not part of the training. After completion of training FCHVs are provided with a certificate from the Ministry of Health, and a medicine kit consisting of supplies such as ORS packets, vitamin A capsules, iron tablets and so on.

FCHVs have to report to the local health post once a month. They are provided with an identity card and a register with 30 to 40 indicators to be filled in, such as maternal, infant and child deaths and details of vertical programmes implemented in their areas. Yet, FCHVs work with minimal financial support. They are provided NPR 7,000 (US$ 60) a year for their uniform, about NPR 1600 (US$ 15) during the immunization campaigns, and a stipend for refreshments during the training period. In addition, the Ministry of Health and Population (2010) has established a FCHV fund in each village for the setting up of income-generating activities.

Despite the fact that FCHVs are delivering regular and vital public services, the FCHV programme was conceptualized as a short-term exercise, and it is not integrated into the regular budget of the MoH. As at 2013, the costs of the FCHV programme were fully financed by donor agencies, such as the US Agency for International Development and the United Nations Children's Fund (Perry, 2017, p. 69).

In Nepal, FCHVs have an unusual profile. Most of them come from families that have another regular source of income, a trend that is stronger in the hills and less seen in the plains.[21] A 2003 study (UNICEF, 2004) showed that poorer, lower-caste and tribal women were mostly excluded from the selection process. FCHVs themselves recognize that a woman from a poor family would not be able to become a FCHV as her family would not be able to 'afford it'. This gives an indication as to why it has been possible to run this programme which is based largely on voluntary work. However, some FCHVs have expressed concerns that, with the changes in the economy, it is becoming increasingly difficult to absorb all the costs involved in their work.[22]

The Nepal Health Sector Programme for 2010–2015 (NHSP2) has scaled up the services provided by FCHVs. However, the policy does not provide for an increase in the incentives for FCHVs. The expectation that FCHVs will provide more services without any additional support or remuneration might, in the long term, compromise the retention and recruitment of these workers (Pratap, 2012).

FCHVs have organized themselves into trade unions and associations during the last decade and are demanding better working conditions and an increase in their remuneration. While the current attrition rates are very low – 4 per cent according to some estimates – working conditions are emerging as a disincentive to FCHV recruitment and motivation (USAID, 2016).

Currently the relationship of FCHVs with the community is crafted on the understanding that the former provide voluntary services. Any change in the nature of this relationship has to be dealt with carefully to maintain the current high level of acceptance that FCHVs have in the community.

Conclusion

Community Health Workers contribute greatly to the health outcomes of rural and poor communities in South Asia. While their role has been recognized and their work valued in different ways, remuneration is inadequate. It can be argued that the underpaid (or unpaid) work of CHWs in the health system amounts to a hidden subsidy towards society at large.

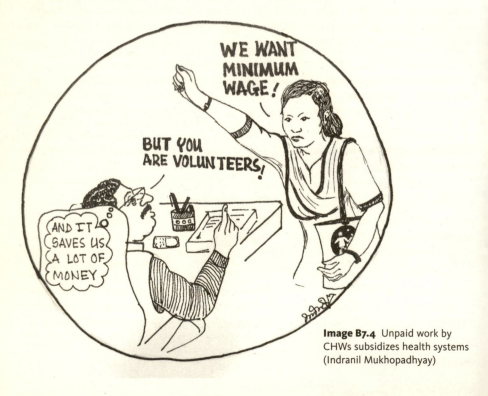

Image B7.4 Unpaid work by CHWs subsidizes health systems (Indranil Mukhopadhyay)

This seems to fit the pattern where, with the increase in the proportion of women in the workforce or in an occupation, wages often decline (ILO, 2017, p. 24). However, CHWs have successfully organized themselves and managed to steadily increase their remuneration. For the public health community, ensuring that adequate service provision is maintained is paramount. Only through engagement of the larger public health community with the demands of organized CHWs can both decent work and quality services be effectively realized.

Notes

1 Though there was a deceleration of employment growth in 2013, this was probably related to the impact of austerity measures in high-income countries (ILO, 2017, p. 13).

2 High-income countries and upper-middle-income countries accounted for most of the decrease of remuneration as a share of total expenditure, while salaries of health workers as a proportion of GDP decreased in low-income countries (ibid., p. 23).

3 The classification of government employees under the Central Civil Services (Classification, Control & Appeal) Rules, 1965 categorizes employees based on their salary level, where A is the highest pay scale and D the lowest. The groups are based on salary level and not occupation. See Representatives of Hospital Employees Union (HEU), interview.

4 The National Capital Territory (NCT) of Delhi has more than fifty public hospitals. This includes four hospitals under the Municipal Corporation of Delhi (municipal level); close to forty hospitals under the Government of the NCT of Delhi (state level), including autonomous bodies; four hospitals under the Ministry of Health and Family Welfare under the central government (MoHFW); as well as six hospitals under other central government ministries; and the All India Institute of Medical Sciences (under the central government).

5 Representatives of HEU and the All India Health Employees and Workers' Confederation (AIHEWC), interviews

6 Ibid.

7 Ibid.

8 Ibid.

9 Representatives of AIHEWC, interview.

10 Representative of the Nursing Union of Nepal, interview.

11 Representative of Health Professionals Organization of Nepal (HEPON), interview.

12 Ibid.

13 Representative of the Confederation of Public Service Independent Trade Union (COPSITU) (2017), interview, 26 April.

14 In the case of doctors, the process is slightly different because a mid-level or senior consultant, though on an informal contract, does not face the same level of vulnerability and can leverage the advantages of this 'flexible' employment condition.

15 The Alma-Ata Declaration defined comprehensive community healthcare as including, at least: i) education concerning prevailing health problems and the methods of preventing and controlling them; ii) promotion of food supply and proper nutrition; iii) an adequate supply of safe water and basic sanitation; iv) maternal and child healthcare, including family planning; v) immunization against the major infectious diseases; vi) prevention and control of locally endemic diseases; vii) appropriate treatment of common diseases and injuries; and viii) provision of essential drugs (WHO, 1978).

16 In an earlier order, in November 2012, the Supreme Court had increased the remuneration of LHWs to the prevalent minimum wage of PKR 7,000 at that time, or EUR 60.

17 The study finds that though 83 per cent of the children in LHWs' families go to school, the major reason for children not going to school is erratic income, and that 87 per cent of the children not going to school are girls.

18 See, for instance, *The Guardian*, 2017.

19 For more details on the programme, see People's Health Movement, Medact and TWN, 2014c.

20 The NRHM Mission Document (2005–2012) explicitly states that the ASHA "[W]ill be an honorary volunteer, receiving performance-based compensation for promoting universal immunization, referral and escort services for RCH [Reproductive Child Health], construction of household toilets, and other healthcare delivery programmes."

21 Nepal's territory is divided into three geographical regions that have specific characteristics and social dynamics, the terai (plains), the hills and the Himalayas (mountains). There is anecdotal evidence that in the terai, FCHVs are from a lower-caste community of traditional birth attendants.

22 Focus group discussion, 8 March 2017.

References

Anonymous 2015, 'Accredited social health activists workers to go on strike from today'http://www.thehansindia.com/posts/index/Telangana/2015-09-02/ASHA-workers-to-go-on-strike-from-today/173947

Anonymous 2017, 'CITU congratulates scheme workers for successful all India strike', *Peoples Democracy*, vol. 41, no. 26, http://peoplesdemocracy.in/2017/0129_pd/citu-congratulates-scheme-workers-successful-all-india-strike

Basu, A2016, *Non-standard work in the healthcare sector in South Asia – informalisation of work: a regional overview*, Public Services International, Faridabad.

Basu, A R *Report on the emerging patterns of informal employment in the public health sector and associated trade union struggles: a study of New Delhi*, Public Services International (forthcoming).

Bhatia, K 2014, 'Performance-based incentives of the ASHA scheme: stakeholders' perspectives', *Economic and Political Weekly*, vol. 49,no. 22.

Diwan, M 2013, 'The nation's caregivers: work experiences, professional identities and gender politics of Pakistan's lady health workers', Master of Arts thesis, Queens University, Canada.

Dixit, H 2014, *Nepal's quest for health*, Educational Publishing House, Kathmandu.

Frenk, J 2015, 'Women and health: the key for

sustainable development', *The Lancet*, vol. 386, pp. 1165–210.

Haines, A, Sanders, D, Lehmann, U, et al. 2007, 'Achieving child survival goals: Potential contribution of community health workers', *The Lancet*, vol. 369, pp. 2121–31.

ILO 2017, *Improving employment and working conditions in health services*, report for discussion at the Tripartite Meeting on Improving Employment and Working Conditions in Health Services, International Labour Organization, Geneva.

Inam, M 2017, *Sexual harassment of lady health workers at office and field*, Workers Education and Research Organization, Public Services International, Karachi.

Khan, A 2011, 'Lady health workers and social change in Pakistan', *Economic and Political Weekly*, vol. 46,no. 30.

Kumar, R 2015,*Preserving 'free health' under Sri Lanka's privatisation policy* http://www.sundaytimes.lk/150208/business-times/preserving-free-healthunder-sri-lankas-privatisation-policy-134353.html

Mascarenhas, R C 1993, 'Building an enterprise culture in the public sector: reforms in Australia, New Zealand and Great Britain', *Public Administration Review*, vol. 53, no. 4, pp. 319–28.

Ministry of Health and Family Welfare 2017, *Supporting mechanism for ASHA*, viewed 2 May 2017, http://nhm.gov.in/communitisation/asha/asha-support-mechanism/supporting-mechanism.htm.

Ministry of Health and Population 2010, *Annual Report 2009–10*, Government of Nepal, Kathmandu.

Moore, M, Stewart, S & Haddock, A 1994, *Institution-building as a development assistance method: a review of literature and ideas*, report to the Swedish International Development Authority, Stockholm.

Muhammad, Q 2017, *Impact of delayed wages on lady health workers in Sindh: an exploratory survey*, Workers Education and Research Organization, Public Services International, Karachi.

People's Health Movement, Medact & TWN 2014a, 'The current discourse on Universal Health Coverage (UHC)', *Global Health Watch 4*, New Delhi.

People's Health Movement, Medact & TWN

2014b, 'The health crisis of neoliberal globalisation', *Global Health Watch 4*, New Delhi.

People's Health Movement, Medact & TWN 2014c, 'The revival of community health workers in national health systems', *Global Health Watch 4*, New Delhi.

Perry, H, Zulliger, R, Scott, K, Javadi, D, Gergen, J, Shelley, K, Crigler, L, Aitken, I, Arwal, S H, Afdhila, N, Worku, Y, Rohde, J, Chowdhury, Z & Strodel, R 2017, *Case studies of large-scale community health worker programs: examples from Afghanistan, Bangladesh, Brazil, Ethiopia, Niger, India, Indonesia, Iran, Nepal, Pakistan, Rwanda, Zambia, and Zimbabwe*, USAID and Maternal and Child Health Integrated Program (MCHIP),Washington, DC.

Pratap, N 2012, *Technical consultation on the role of communitybased providers in improving maternal and neonatal health*, Community Health Workers Meeting, Amsterdam.

Public Health Resource Network, Jan Swasthya Abhiyan & Oxfam India 2017, *Public private partnerships in healthcare: outsourcing of haemodialysis services in Delhi: a case study*, New Delhi.

Schwarz, D, Sharma, R, Bashyal, C, Schwarz, R, Baruwal, A, Karelas, G, Basnet, B, Khadka, N, Brady, J, Silver, Z, Mukherjee, J, Andrews, J & Maru, D S 2014, 'Strengthening Nepal's female community health volunteer network: a qualitative study of experiences at two years', *BMC Health Services Research*, vol. 14, no. 473.

Som, M 2016, 'Volunteerism to incentivisation: changing priorities of mitanins work in Chhattisgarh', *Indian Journal of Gender Studies*, vol. 23, no. 1, pp. 26–42.

The Guardian 2017, 'Pakistan polio vaccinator's murder by militants raises health workers' fears', 25 March, https://www.theguardian.com/society/2014/mar/25/pakistan-polio-vaccinators-murder-militants-salma-farooqi

Thresia, C U 2016, *Non-standard work and quality of healthcare services*, Public Services International, Faridabad.

UNICEF 2004, *What works for children in South Asia: community health workers*, UNICEF Regional Office for South Asia, Kathmandu.

USAID 2007, *An analytical report on national survey of female community health volunteers of Nepal*, Kathmandu.

USAID 2016, *Female community health volunteers in Nepal: what we know and steps going forward*, PowerPoint slides.

Vabø, M 2009, *New public management the neoliberal way of governance*, working paper no. 4, viewed 7 May 2014, <thjodmalastofnun.hi.is/sites/thjodmalastofnun.hi.is/files/skrar/working_paper_4-2009.pdf>.

Van de Pas, R 2013, *Human resources for health—a bottleneck for primary health care?*, Get Involved in Global Health. Conference 50 years Medicus Mundi" Primary Health Care and Cooperation: a Utopia? 7-6-2013

WHO 1978, *Declaration of Alma Ata, International Conference on Primary Health Care*, Alma Ata, 6–12 September, World Health Organization.

WHO 2007, *Community health workers: what do we know about them?* Policy brief, World Health Organization, Geneva.

Workers Solidarity 2000, *Critical condition: a report on workers in Delhi's private hospitals*, Workers Solidarity, Delhi.

BEYOND HEALTHCARE

C1 | CLIMATE CHANGE, ENVIRONMENTAL DEGRADATION AND HEALTH: CONFRONTING THE REALITIES[1]

Introduction

Worldwide, environmental conditions have changed more rapidly in the past half-century than at any other time in human history (McNeill, 2000). The almost unfathomable magnitude of human-induced environmental degradation since the Industrial Revolution, and the attendant impact on climatic conditions, has led scientists to characterize the post-1800 period as a new geologic era: the Anthropocene (Waters et al., 2016).

Most prominently, based on the work of more than 2,000 scientists in the 195-member-country UN Intergovernmental Panel on Climate Change (IPCC), there is overwhelming scientific consensus that climate change is taking place and that human activities – shaped by the forces propelling the global economy – are driving it. Importantly, climate change aggravates and is aggravated by many other forms of environmental degradation – that is, the depletion and contamination of the earth's air, water and land. These all, in turn, have an array of health consequences.

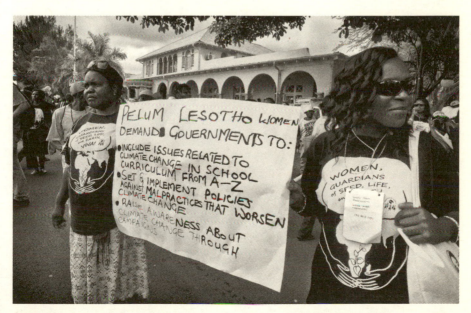

Image C1.1 Women in Lesotho advocating for climate literacy (Louis Reynolds)

Despite this broad consensus, and a shared understanding that climate change requires concerted global action – since its drivers and effects transcend borders and are shared globally (even as those bearing the brunt of climate change consequences are in low- and middle-income countries (LMICs)) –the global response has been timid and late in coming. This chapter reviews the underlying forces of climate change within the broader crisis of environmental degradation, and the consequent effects on human health and health inequities. We discuss what kinds of overall approaches are warranted and explore a range of promising, albeit insufficient, global, national and local responses and environmental justice movements. We also examine how the task of addressing the ongoing environmental degradation and dealing with the refusal by some governments to even acknowledge the existence of climate change, let alone act to mitigate it, will require creative and persistent forms of organization and mobilization.

Underlying forces (and consequences) of environmental degradation

While the effects of environmental contamination and resource depletion are typically experienced locally, the underlying drivers are global in nature – tied to market-based, consumption-driven, growth- and profit-oriented economies and their unsustainable industries, which affect the environmental landscape in a myriad of ways transcending geopolitical boundaries. Ultimately, global capitalism drives this destructive path (Foster, Clark and York, 2011). Under capitalism's contemporary phase of neoliberal globalization, the distance between consumption and the consequences of production is lengthened, masking how they are inextricably linked: people purchasing 'low-cost' clothing or electronics in, for example, Barcelona or Baltimore may not participate in, witness or even contemplate the environmental and human consequences of production in Bangkok or Bangalore. Moreover, in a global market economy, production costs rarely reflect social and environmental costs, from air pollution and chemical waste produced by garment factories to water and soil contamination from coltan mining, not to mention extreme labour exploitation.

Since contaminating and depleting natural resources do not directly affect profits, there is no inherent reason for businesses to refrain from production that harms the environment (or to make efforts to minimize these harms), notwithstanding the ubiquitous slick 'corporate social responsibility' campaigns that claim otherwise. Indeed, industrial production, mining, energy extraction and agribusiness are the prime generators of environmental degradation whenever they are not checked by effective government regulation.

Perhaps most illustrative, since the Second World War more than 85,000 new industrial chemicals have been produced and released into the environment with minimal testing or government oversight. This includes several thousand substances manufactured in vast quantities: 450 metric tons or more annually (Domínguez-Cortinas et al., 2013, pp. 351–57). Even when the harmful health and environmental effects are known and chemicals are regulated in high-income countries (HICs), as with benzene, they may still be exported, used and produced in LMICs with few regulations (Sellers 2014, pp. 38–71). The case of lead is telling in this context. Its toxicity was recognized as early as the 1890s, but it took nearly a century for mounting scientific evidence and activism to translate into its wide-ranging ban in gasoline and paints (Markowitz and Rosner, 2014).

Toxic waste is also an ever-present by-product of industrial production. Over 200 million people worldwide are directly exposed to dangerous waste toxins, and millions more are indirectly exposed (Blacksmith Institute and Green Cross Switzerland, 2014). Another key perpetrator of environmental contamination is the military–industrial complex, involving the production, testing, storage and detonation of both nuclear and conventional weapons, with the US and Russian military bases and munitions factories, especially, responsible for a toxic stew of dangerous chemicals linked to elevated cancer rates and reduced life expectancy among nearby populations (Blacksmith Institute and Green Cross Switzerland, 2013; Westing, 2008).

Resistance to landfills and industrial waste in Western Europe and North America has led HICs to enact stricter regulations against toxic dumping. But the practice continues illegally, especially through the annual export of at least 8.5 million tons of toxic waste to LMICs, where the largest hazardous dumpsites in the world are located (UNEP, 2011). Electronic waste (e-waste) – including consumer electronics such as computers, mobile phones and household appliances – increasingly ends up in Chinese, Indian and African landfills (UNEP, 2015). The world's largest e-waste dumpsite in Agbogbloshie (in Accra, Ghana) affects some 40,000–250,000 people living and working in proximity to lead, mercury and other metals that contaminate the air and soil (Blacksmith Institute and Green Cross Switzerland, 2013).

In the lucrative agribusiness sector, massive pesticide application and wasteful irrigation practices cause major soil and groundwater contamination and resource depletion. A whopping 70 per cent of the world's water is utilized by agriculture, mostly agribusiness (WWAP, 2014). Large-scale commercial farming is also associated with occupational safety and health concerns; farmer exposure to pesticides without adequate protection results in up to 5 million poisonings and 250,000 fatalities each year (Marrs and Karalliedde, 2012; Orozco et al., 2009, pp. 255–68), on top of the untold exposure of workers and local populations, such as communities in proximity to floriculture operations in Ecuador, to harmful toxins (Breilh, 2012).

The mining sector, meanwhile, remains one of the world's most profitable – and destructive – industries (see Chapter C5). Mining, whether of gold, uranium, cobalt, coal, other metals, rocks or minerals, invariably has devastating environmental consequences: stripped terrain and forests; mudslides; seepage of heavy metals, acids and other toxic by-products into soil and watersheds; and the release of particulate matter and greenhouse gases that damage the ecological resources of nearby communities.

The energy sector is at the crux of any critical discussion on climate change and environmental degradation. Non-renewable fossil fuels – namely, oil, natural gas and coal – have extensive negative environmental effects through their extraction, refining and distribution. For example, every part of the oil extraction process, even before combustion, is hazardous to health due to spills, leaks, collision-related fires and the burning of 'excess' methane and other gases at oil wells, rigs and refineries – processes that also release carbon emissions into the air, contributing to pollution and climate change (Union of Concerned Scientists, 2015). Similarly, the emissions of 'cleaner fuels' such as natural gas remain associated with asthma, chronic bronchitis, cancers and blood disorders (Davoudi et al., 2013, pp. 7–19).

Further exacerbating carbon emissions and contamination is the conversion of raw bitumen from tar sands into crude oil – a process employed in Alberta, Canada. Communities near strip-mining, drilling and processing facilities are exposed to hazardous chemicals used in the conversion process, which are linked to elevated cancer rates downstream. These chemicals accumulate in the food chain, posing a particular threat to nearby indigenous communities who rely on hunting and fishing for their livelihoods (National Resources Defense Council, 2014). Unconventional gas and oil drilling through hydraulic fracturing (fracking), too, uses harsh chemicals, with massive water and air contamination potential (Saunders et al., 2016, pp.1–57).

And so, the forces driving the global economy shape and are shaped by the self-perpetuating cycle of human activities (extraction, production and consumption), in turn generating climate change and other forms of environmental degradation, all with detrimental health effects.

Leading environmental and health problems

The major health problems resulting from environmental degradation include air pollution and the overuse, misuse and contamination of water, land and forests in an intertwining of natural resource (ab)use with market-driven features of the built environment, jeopardizing the spaces and places where people work, play and live. According to a recent estimate, environmental factors – polluted air, built environment hazards, agricultural practices, occupational hazards, radiation, climate change, chemical exposures and inadequate water and sanitation – were associated with 12.6 million deaths (23 per cent of deaths worldwide) in 2012 (Prüss-Ustün et al., 2016).

Air pollution Air pollution is one of the most prevalent environmental problems, linked to industrial contamination, power plants, building heating and cooling, household fuel use and transport (including aircraft) exhaust. The combustion processes that generate air pollution also contribute to climate change (Field et al., 2014).

Outdoor air pollution was an underlying factor in some 3.7 million premature deaths in 2012, nearly 90 per cent of them in LMICs (WHO, 2014a). Almost all city dwellers worldwide breathe unsafe air rife with particulate matter (PM), a mixture of fine solid particles, including dirt, dust, mould and, especially, aerosols formed from by-products of combustion: for example, sulphur dioxide and nitrogen oxides (WHO EURO, 2013). The health consequences of PM inhalation include lung cancer, cardiopulmonary diseases, and the aggravation of asthma and chronic obstructive pulmonary disease.

The problem is worse in many LMICs due to generally fewer controls on vehicle and industrial emissions; unregulated burning of household fuels and garbage; limited renewable energy source-based public transport; and large-scale industrial use of inexpensive high-sulphur fuels, including brown coal, as well as 'slash and burn' approaches to clearing land, such as for palm oil plantations in Indonesia.

India and Pakistan have the cities with the worst air pollution, topped by New Delhi whose 25 million inhabitants, especially children, face spiralling rates of upper and lower respiratory diseases (Mathew et al., 2015, pp. 421–27). India also has the highest mortality rate from respiratory diseases in the world at 155 deaths per 100,000 people (WHO, 2015a), with an estimated 1.3 million excess deaths annually due to air pollution. China, too, has record-breaking air pollution, especially in the most rapidly industrializing and urbanizing regions such as Hebei province. Still, per capita air contaminant emissions remain far higher in HICs, especially from vehicle exhaust (WHO, 2015b).

Indoor air pollution is even more deadly than its outdoor counterpart, responsible for a staggering 4.3 million annual deaths (WHO, 2014b). This is mostly caused by inhalation of biomass fuels (including animal dung, wood and logging waste, crop waste and coal) in poorly ventilated (open) heating and cook-stoves – involving approximately 3 billion people world-wide. Children, women and the elderly are particularly exposed to smoke and gases from cooking due to social roles keeping them indoors for long periods (WHO, 2016).

Waterways The basic human need of freshwater is wracked by intertwining problems of unequal access, scarcity and contamination. One-third of the world's population – predominantly in rural areas and informal settlements of LMICs – faces some level of water shortage or inadequate sanitation facilities (UNICEF and WHO, 2015), with particularly high water stress among displaced persons and refugees. Yet industrial and agribusiness interests capture public water supplies at discounted rates (WWAP, 2015), illustrating how water and sanitation access constitute a political problem of resource allocation rather than a primarily technical one.

To meet daily survival needs, billions of people must rely on contaminated water from rivers, streams, lakes and reservoirs or from rainwater collected in industrial barrels, usually lined with toxic chemicals. Ingestion of contaminated water and compromised hygiene can lead to a variety of bacterial illnesses such as cholera, typhoid and salmonella; skin infections; cryptosporidium infection and other parasitic diseases; and infection by food-borne pathogens. As well, toxins entering water supplies from industrial and agricultural run-off can cause acute poisonings and a variety of cancers.

Water- and sanitation-related diseases kill at least 1.4 million people each year (Forouzanfar et al., 2015, pp. 2287–323). Infants and malnourished young children are the hardest struck, with more than 750,000 dying annually from diarrhoea – 90 per cent attributable to unsafe/inadequate water and sanitation (UNICEF, 2015).

Anthropogenic climate change is also associated with the 'deadly trio' of ocean-related changes with health implications: ocean warming, acidification and deoxygenation (Burkett et al., 2014, pp. 169–94). The ocean absorbs one-third of global carbon dioxide (CO_2) emissions, accelerating acidification; meanwhile, oxygen levels have declined due to warming and everyday sources of contamination, including sewage, and chemical, agricultural and industrial run-off carried out to sea. These effluents create 'dead zones' where fish and other marine life can no longer thrive (Bijma et al., 2013, pp. 495–505), threatening food sovereignty and livelihoods for communities with seafood-based diets, such as northern Canada's Inuit population (Laird, Goncharov and Chan, 2013, pp. 33–40).

Land degradation and deforestation Arable land, which covers less than 10 per cent of the earth's surface, has been grossly overworked for decades. Land degradation – stemming from rising salinity levels due to deforestation and harmful agricultural practices such as overgrazing, poor irrigation, pesticide and fertilizer application, excess water use, over cultivation and mono-crop production – destroys 20,000–50,000 square kilometres of soil annually, with soil erosion rates up to six times higher in LMICs than HICs (Hester, 2012). The effects are dire for the approximately 1.5 billion people whose livelihoods depend upon farming and who are increasingly subject to food shortages, escalating poverty and forced migration (UNEP, 2014).

Large-scale deforestation – some 130 million hectares between 1990 and 2015 – is linked to intensive logging and clear cutting for construction materials, timber harvesting, domestic charcoal fuel, and urban and agricultural expansion (FAO, 2016). Deforestation jeopardizes health: it alters ecosystems' ability to remove pollutants from air and water, increases the spread of malaria, diminishes pollination and pest control, reduces the sources of new medicines and worsens the effects of floods, landslides, tidal waves and hurricanes (Whitmee et al., 2015, pp. 1973– 2028). LMICs are disproportionately affected: Haiti,

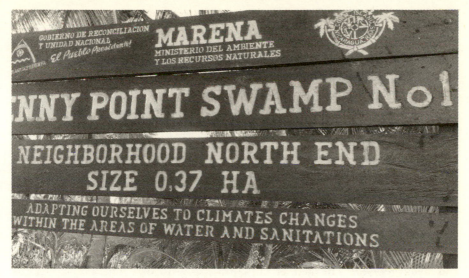

Image C1.2 Climate mitigation in Nicaragua (Mariajose Aguilera)

for example, has lost over 80 per cent of its original forest cover, exacerbating topsoil erosion, shrinkage of arable land and food insecurity (Swarup, 2009).

Climate change The predictions of dramatic environmental changes from climate change seemed improbable only a generation ago, yet today they already constitute lived experience for many (Baer and Singer, 2009). The greatest scientific certainty is around increase of surface and sea temperatures and ocean acidification. Other changes in all likelihood due to climate change are increased heat waves, melting polar ice caps, rising sea levels, heavy precipitation and droughts (Field et al., 2014).

Most directly, climate change is likely to increase the intensity and frequency of extreme heat events: between 1999 and 2010 there was a quadrupling of heat waves in Europe, leading to 70,000 excess deaths in 2003 alone (Christidis et al., 2012, pp. 225–39). In 2015, a heat wave in South Asia saw temperatures soaring to 49°C (120°F), killing approximately 2,500 people in India and 2,000 in Pakistan. Heat-related mortality involves dehydration and heat stroke, and the exacerbation of existing health problems such as heart, lung and kidney disease, and diabetes. Repeated dehydration can also lead to chronic kidney disease (Kjellstrom, Holmer and Lemke, 2009).

Secondary and indirect health consequences of climate change, mediated through environmental and ecosystem changes, stem from temperature and precipitation pattern changes that can be conducive to the proliferation and virulence of food- and water-borne pathogens, including enteric bacteria (for example, cholera) and viruses (Smith et al., 2014). For instance, heavy rainfall causes sewage overflow, allowing faecal waste run-off to contaminate surface water; conversely, low rainfall and drought result in higher concentration of pathogens in the available water (El-Fadel et al., 2012, pp. 15–21).

Other secondary consequences include vector-borne diseases such as malaria, dengue and chikungunya, transmitted by temperature-sensitive arthropods. Even modest warming may enhance mosquito survival and reproduction, while rain and stagnant water create favourable breeding sites. Indirect health effects also extend to food sovereignty and nutrition. Droughts lower agricultural output and cause food shortages and under-nutrition in poor, already food-insecure areas (Smith et al., 2014).

Finally, there are tertiary, more diffuse health effects of climate change, mediated through economic, social and political factors. Heat waves, sea level rise, drought and other phenomena can lead to a whole range of stresses on well-being: livelihood loss, population displacement and social conflict, all affecting physical and mental health (McMichael, 2013, pp. 1335–43). For example, storms and floods have profound effects on people's mental health, leading to depression, anxiety and other forms of psychological distress, as has been documented in the aftermath of cyclones and floods in Bangladesh, which have hit women and the poor especially hard (Nahar et al., 2014). Populations forcibly displaced due to harsh, sudden or escalating environmental changes may experience similar mental health effects, plus under-nutrition, respiratory illness and increased maternal mortality (Smith et al., 2014).

All told, the World Health Organization estimates that climate change will cause an *additional* 250,000 deaths per year between 2030 and 2050 (WHO, 2014c). This is a conservative estimate, accounting only for deaths via direct pathways; the economic and social conflict effects are much greater, considering that there are over 1 billion people worldwide, living on ecologically fragile land (UNDP, 2015).

Spaces and places of inequity and injustice

As well as understanding how climate change-linked phenomena affect health, it is crucial to recognize that across and within countries, those most likely to be affected are impoverished, socially excluded and otherwise vulnerable people. For instance, during heat waves, the elderly, infants and young children are particularly susceptible to harm because their bodies are less adept at thermo-regulating. People living alone, outdoor workers, indoor workers in buildings lacking cooling mechanisms, and persons with chronic conditions, mental health problems and disabilities are also vulnerable during extreme heat events. Poverty worsens these conditions by limiting access to resources that mitigate heat stress; those from the lower socioeconomic groups die at higher rates during heat waves (Basu, 2015).

Virtually all health problems linked to environmental degradation are experienced most acutely by historically oppressed groups, such as African Americans in the USA. The concept of environmental racism, popularized in the 1980s amid resistance to the siting of toxic landfills in predominantly African American communities in the US South, drew attention to the racialized dimension of environmental injustice (Bullard et al., 2008, pp. 371–411). Indigenous peoples are especially exposed to the injustices of environmental degradation. Due to the connection of indigenous livelihoods to the natural resources of their traditional lands, and to historic and ongoing political, economic and cultural oppression, many indigenous populations directly experience the consequences of environmental destruction (Ford, 2012, pp.1260–66). As highlighted by 'Idle No More', many indigenous groups are also at the forefront of resistance to abuses (Klein, 2014).

Environment and health inequities persist within both LMICs and HICs, but there is a difference between the two in the injustice experienced. It is a misconception that population size or growth per se drives these issues. Instead, even as ever-intensifying production, extraction and consumption patterns that lead to environmental degradation and climate change are deeply shaped by transnational corporations (TNCs) and HIC policies and population demands, those bearing the most deleterious effects are disproportionately located in LMICs. These include African countries and many small islands especially vulnerable to and burdened by the costs of climate change mitigation and adaptation efforts. Likewise, toxic waste largely generated in/by HICs is systematically exported to LMICs, together with the outsourcing of hazardous industries and jobs (Clapp and Dauvergne, 2011). Meanwhile, the TNCs reap the profits of exporting to LMICs hazardous products, such as certain pesticides, banned in HICs.

Though workers and consumers necessarily participate in the nexus of production and consumption, they do not control these economic activities or the global arrangements that sustain them, and the poorest, wherever located, benefit the least. Within and between countries, the uneven control and use of resources are central to the reproduction of capital, placing both HIC and LMIC elites literally and figuratively in the driver's seat of the economic order and of resource contamination and depletion. In sum, the high costs of environmental degradation and its health consequences are borne by those excluded from power and decision-making, even as the greatest advantages accrue to the more powerful (Brulle and Pellow 2006, pp. 103–24).

What is to be done?

With the massive health implications of fossil fuel energy dependence, large-scale agribusiness, hazardous waste dumping and other features of global capitalism, action is needed at all levels: global, national and local. The phasing out of chlorofluorocarbons (CFCs), a key contributor to ozone layer depletion, through the Montreal Protocol in 1987, stands out as a success in global co-operation for environmental protection, even as attenuating CFC effects is taking far longer than projected. But most other international efforts have struggled to make concrete advances. The challenge of reaching consensus on obligatory greenhouse gas emission reduction targets, for instance, has made the Kyoto Protocol and its successor, the Paris Agreement, diluted, market-oriented and unenforceable responses to climate change.

The Paris Climate Agreement, which entered into force in 2016, is at best insufficient to achieve its central goal of limiting the global rise in temperature to below 2°C above pre-industrial levels. At worst, given that national emissions reduction targets are voluntary, with no penalties for non-compliance, the agreement may be of little use – especially given President Donald Trump's June 2017 announcement that the USA intended to withdraw from the agreement. Trump also made clear that the USA would not fulfill its US$ 3 billion pledge to the Green Climate Fund, which was set up to support climate change mitigation and adaption efforts in low-income and otherwise vulnerable countries. As the second largest current per capita CO_2 emitter, and largest cumulative CO_2 emitter in history, the United States's decision to withdraw from the Paris agreement clearly signals its unwillingness to participate in global efforts on climate change, even as China, India, and multiple European Union countries have reaffirmed their commitments. Still, even if it were fully implemented by all parties, the Paris Agreement provides no panacea – ultimately it sidesteps addressing climate change's economic, social and political drivers.

At the national level, governments can undertake a wider range of policy and regulatory actions to slow some of the driving forces of climate change and environmental degradation by setting regulations, standards (for example, air and water quality) and green taxes; holding corporations accountable (including for their practices overseas); and enabling the development and use of sustainable technologies and energy sources. The 2007 regulation of the European Union (EU) – Registration, Evaluation, Authorization and Restriction of Chemicals (REACH) – is a promising approach: all companies are required to "identify and manage the [health and environmental] risks linked to the substances they manufacture and market in the EU" or face regulatory restrictions (ECHA, 2015).

China, now the world's largest greenhouse gas emitter with the fastest growing industrial sector and major mining and energy extraction interests across the world, has started to address health and environmental consequences, especially as they manifest in dangerous levels of air pollution in its industrial belt. Yet while China has invested in renewable energy, electricity and public transport alternatives, and has closed polluting factories, it continues under a global capitalist drive. Other burgeoning polluters with major industrial, energy extraction and mining interests, such as India, Pakistan, Russia, Nigeria, Indonesia and Brazil, are strangled by moneyed interests at the national level, leaving transformative change to the local level.

Indeed, many of the most progressive advances in environment and public health protection occur at local levels. Municipal initiatives for green/healthy cities show the merits of ecological planning and design for reducing carbon emissions through investment in public transport, bicycling infrastructure, ecological housing and buildings, and urban agriculture – efforts that reduce the carbon footprints of cities and towns. For example, in Curitiba, Brazil, decades of ecological urban planning has produced one of the world's most efficient bus rapid transit systems and an extensive recycling system, while in Amsterdam, the Netherlands, a network of bicycle paths allows a third of all trips to be made by bike. Cuba, meanwhile, has provided a model of organic urban agriculture, enabling it to attenuate food shortages and improve nutrition, ban chemical pesticides, generate sustainable employment and move towards a carbon-neutral economy.

There are also individual – and household – level responses that encourage an array of lifestyle adaptations: using eco-friendly products; recycling and composting; home gardening; using energy efficient appliances; expanding the use of public transport, biking and walking; lowering thermostats in the winter; reducing or eliminating the use of air conditioners; and limiting car use or using fuel-efficient vehicles. Of course, appealing to the individual assumes that people have the time, access and resources, or the education or desire to make these behavioural changes, making these responses far more relevant to middle-to-high-income residents of middle-to-high-income countries than to members of the working class or people in low-resource settings.

Effective as some of these efforts can be, they offer only a first step in transforming the profit-oriented, polluting global political economic order. For example, individual- or household-level solutions do not affect underlying structural determinants, including energy, industrial and military production and waste processes that drive global environmental degradation. And the most forward-looking local policies cannot supersede the effects of pro-TNC industrial production policies and subsidies at the national level.

Moreover, the impact on equity must be assessed for all responses. To illustrate, while technological innovations, such as renewable energy and water desalination, can provide effective solutions at all levels, they do not in and of themselves address the equitable distribution and control of resources needed to attain environmental justice.

By contrast, environmental justice movements and resistance, from local to transnational, often take issues of inequity directly to the sources – confronting agribusiness, energy, mining and other industrial interests. Methods for seeking justice include litigation, divestment campaigns, advocacy and protest.

Farm-worker lawsuits brought by Latin American and US lawyers have been among these effective channels. For example, in 2002, chemical TNCs like Dow, Shell and Dole were ordered to compensate almost 600 Nicaraguan banana workers US$ 490 million. The workers had been sterilized by the hazardous pesticide Nemagon, banned in the late 1970s in the USA but utilized for many more years in US-owned plantations in Latin America, Asia and Africa (Boix and Bohme, 2012, pp. 154–61). Still, while such lawsuits may meaningfully affect policies in legalistic societies, they may be less useful where legal costs and legal systems are inaccessible, and they can drag on for years. For instance, Chevron (then Texaco) engaged in dirty methods to extract oil in Ecuador for nearly 30 years, dumping billions of gallons of toxic waste, including 19 million gallons of oil spilled from a pipeline. Although the company left the area in 1992 and litigation has been ongoing for over 25 years, the community has yet to be compensated for health and environmental damages amid continuing litigation (Kimerling, 2013, pp. 241–94).

In another vein, divestment from fossil fuels, spearheaded by environmental organizations such as 350.org, entails getting rid of stocks, bonds and other investments linked to fossil fuel industries. Echoing divestment campaigns against apartheid South Africa, these largely HIC efforts seek to delegitimize and eventually eliminate major greenhouse gas-emitting industries. As of early 2017, there were over 700 institutions worldwide that had committed to the fossil fuel divestment campaign, totaling over US$ 5.4 trillion (Fossil Free, 2017).

Numerous civil society organizations are mobilizing resources to bear witness to corporate abuses and government neglect, and are advocating for rights and policies that are protective of the environment and health. Among these, La Via Campesina, an international movement of peasants, small- and medium-sized producers, landless people, rural women, youth, indigenous groups and agricultural workers, advocates for food sovereignty, preservation of natural resources, sustainable agriculture, gender equity and fair economic relations. Its efforts are closely tied to land rights activism and the resistance against displacement, which is often a crucial part of environmental struggles globally.

Protest is a powerful form of resistance, while also being potentially dangerous for activists. With mining alone, there have been numerous resistance efforts in recent years, often led by indigenous groups. From Apurimac, Peru, to Papua province, Indonesia, local communities have protested mining operations due to environmental pollution that affects their daily lives. In North Dakota, USA, the nearly year-long protest by the Standing Rock Sioux tribe and allies against the Dakota Access Pipeline cited indigenous treaty rights to land and water, initially persuading a halting of the pipeline plan by the Obama administration, later reversed under Trump.

Elsewhere, years of resistance in El Salvador led in 2017 to a path-breaking nationwide ban on metal mining to protect the nation's fragile water supply from contamination by toxic mining tailings. This illustrates how widespread civil society mobilization can embolden state legislatures to value environmental protection over good standing with TNCs (MiningWatch Canada, 2017).

Whatever the means for pursuing environmental justice, what is needed are paradigms that question the global political economy and provide ecological alternatives. Degrowth is one framework that critiques economic growth as a necessary social objective and capitalism as a system that necessitates and

Image C1.3
Demonstration in Melbourne for measures against climate change (PHM Australia)

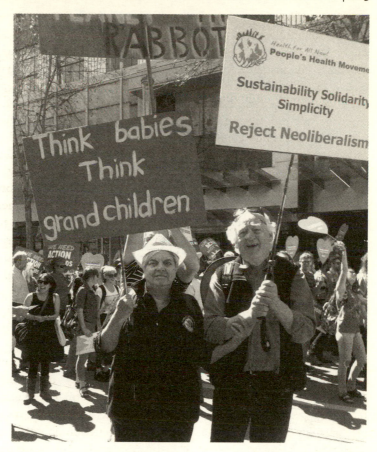

perpetuates growth. It promotes the prospect of a smaller society (in terms of production and consumption) and of re-structuring society away from commodification and toward other functions, such as economies of care and the reclaiming of commons – the shared management and responsibility for resources (Kallis, Demaria and D'Alisa, 2015). 'Buenvivir', a contemporary indigenous development in the Andean region of Latin America, questions conventional assumptions about 'growth' and 'development' and their links to well-being. Instead, buenvivir calls for a new paradigm of 'living well' in harmony with the natural environment and within existing resources.

Still, it is questionable whether concrete measures framed around degrowth or buenvivir go far enough to question capitalism, as seen in countries like Ecuador, which has enshrined buenvivir and the rights of nature in its Constitution but continues to depend on resource extraction as a vehicle for development. Of course, Ecuador per force operates within a global market order: alternative paradigms have the potential to generate lasting change by raising consciousness, shifting values and ultimately pressuring political processes towards the building of societies that favour equity over growth.

Conclusion

Although manifesting distinctly in different locales, environmental degradation and its health consequences are interrelated across the world, transcending place and ultimately affecting everyone (McMichael, 2013, pp. 1335–43). The human population is now at a crucial crossroads. Addressing the myriad environmental challenges and their interconnected health effects is complex and difficult, and will require broad co-operation, creative ideas and intense political struggle.

Alas, the present reality is one of substantial political recalcitrance to transformative change by some of the largest polluters. Among the early measures adopted by the Trump administration are a proposed 30 per cent budget cut to the US Environmental Protection Agency (EPA), relaxing of clean water regulations (Jaffe, 2017, pp.1180–81), reviving of major oil pipeline projects, overturning a moratorium on new coal mining leases and derailing the Obama administration's Clean Power Plan, which sought to implement regulations that would curb greenhouse gas emissions. Outrageously, Trump's choice for head of the EPA, former Oklahoma attorney general Scott Pruitt, has a history of close ties to the fossil fuel industry (Davenport and Lipton, 2017) and has openly questioned the anthropogenic factor in climate change and advocated against (including by partaking in lawsuits) many of the EPA's regulations.

But even those governments that recognize climate change and have publicly committed to the Paris Agreement remain mired in the contradictions of an environmentally degrading, climate change-producing global capitalist system. Canada, for example, having abandoned the Kyoto Protocol, has signed the Paris Agreement, yet continues to provide billions of dollars in government support (tax breaks, subsidies, approvals and lax securities/regulation) to tar sands exploitation, the mining industry and to building two giant pipelines.

Meanwhile, as per the example of El Salvador, smaller countries are taking the most transformative and even desperate measures, given the immediate and current effects of environmental degradation on population well-being. While it is inspiring that a small and vulnerable country has taken such a bold move, it remains shameful that for the principal environmental perpetrators – chiefly TNCs and their government partners – for the most part it is business as usual. If Naomi Klein is correct in arguing that 'this changes everything', political and social movements everywhere will need to participate in their own Leap Manifesto: a call for a new buenvivir-type ethic of a society based not on profits but on caring for one another and the earth (The Leap Manifesto, 2015).

Note

1 This chapter draws heavily from Birn, Pillay and Holtz (2017, Ch. 10).

References

Baer, H A & Singer, M 2009, *Global warming and the political ecology of health: emerging crises and systemic solutions*, Left Coast Press, Walnut Creek.

Basu, R 2015, 'Disorders related to heat waves', in Levy, B & Patz, J (eds), *Climate change and public health*, Oxford University Press, New York.

Bijma, J, Pörtner, H, Yesson, C & Rogers, A D 2013, 'Climate change and the oceans – what does the future hold?' *Marine Pollution Bulletin*, vol. 74, no. 2, pp. 495–505.

Birn, A E, Pillay, Y & Holtz, T H 2017, *Textbook of global health*, 4th edn, Oxford University Press, Oxford.

Blacksmith Institute & Green Cross Switzerland, 2013, *The world's worst 2013: the top ten toxic threats – cleanup, progress, and ongoing challenges*, Blacksmith Institute, New York.

Blacksmith Institute & Green Cross Switzerland 2014, *Top ten countries turning the corner on toxic pollution 2014*, Blacksmith Institute, New York.

Boix, V & Bohme, S R 2012, 'Secrecy and justice in the ongoing saga of DBCP litigation', *International Journal of Occupational and Environmental Health*, vol. 18, no. 2, pp. 154–61.

Breilh, J 2012, 'Coping with environmental and health impacts in a floricultural region of Ecuador', in Charron, D F (ed), *Ecohealth research in practice: innovative applications of an ecosystem approach to health*, International Development Research Centre, Ottawa.

Brulle, R J & Pellow, D N 2006, 'Environmental justice: Human health and environmental inequalities', *Annual Review of Public Health*, vol. 27, pp. 103–24.

Bullard, R D, Mohai, P, Saha, R & Wright, B 2008, 'Toxic wastes and race at twenty: Why race still matters after all of these years', *Environmental Law*, vol. 38, pp. 371–411.

Burkett, V R, Suarez, A G, Bindi, M, Conde, C, Mukerji, R, Prather, M J, St. Clair, A L & Yohe, G W 2014, 'Point of departure', in Field, C B, Barros, V R, Dokken, D J, Mach, K J, Mastrandrea, M D, Bilir, T E, Chatterjee, M, Ebi, K L, Estrada, Y O, Genova, R C, Girma, B, Kissel, E S, Levy, A N, MacCracken, S, Mastrandrea, P R & White, LL (eds), *Climate change 2014: impacts, adaptation, and vulnerability. Part A: global and sectoral aspects*, contribution of Working Group II to the Fifth Assessment Report of the Intergovernmental Panel on Climate Change, Cambridge University Press, Cambridge and New York, pp. 169–94.

Christidis, N, Stott, P A, Jones, G S, Shiogama, H, Nozawa, T & Luterbacher, J 2012, 'Human activity and anomalously warm seasons in Europe', *International Journal of Climatology*, vol. 32, no. 2, pp. 225–39.

Clapp, J & Dauvergne, P 2011, *Paths to a green world: the political economy of the global environment*, 2nd edn, MIT Press, Cambridge.

Davenport, C & Lipton, E 2017, 'The Pruitt emails: E.P.A. chief was arm in arm with industry', *The New York Times*, 22 February.

Davoudi, M, Rahimpour, M R, Jokar, S M, Nikbakht, F & Abbasfard, H 2013, 'The major sources of gas flaring and air contamination in the natural gas processing plants: A case study', *Journal of Natural Gas Science and Engineering*, vol. 13, pp. 7–19.

Domínguez-Cortinas, G, Díaz-Barriga, F, Martínez-Salinas, R I, Cossío, P & Pérez-Maldonado, I N 2013, 'Exposure to chemical mixtures in Mexican children: high-risk scenarios', *Environmental Science and Pollution Research International*, vol.20, no. 1, pp. 351–57.

ECHA [European Chemicals Agency] 2015, *Understanding REACH*, viewed 11 April 2017, http:// echa.europa.eu/ web/ guest/ regulations/ reach/ understanding-reach.

El-Fadel, M, Ghanimeh, S, Maroun, R & Alameddine, I 2012, 'Climate change and temperature rise: implications on food- and water-borne diseases', *Science of the Total Environment*, vol. 437, pp. 15–21.

FAO 2016, *State of the world's forests 2016, forests and agriculture: land-use challenges and opportunities*, FAO, Rome.

Field, C B, Barros, V R, Dokken, D J, Mach, K J, Mastrandrea, M D, Bilir, T E, Chatterjee, M, Ebi, K L, Estrada, Y O, Genova, R C, Girma, B, Kissel, E S, Levy, A N, MacCracken, S, Mastrandrea, P R & White, L L (eds) 2014, *Climate change 2014: impacts, adaptation, and vulnerability. Part A: global and sectoral aspects*, contribution of Working

Group II to the Fifth Assessment Report of the Intergovernmental Panel on Climate Change, Cambridge University Press, Cambridge and New York.

Ford, J D 2012, 'Indigenous health and climate change', *American Journal of Public Health*, vol. 102, no. 7, pp.1260–66.

Forouzanfar, M H, Alexander, L, Anderson, H R, Bachman, V F, Biryukov, S, Brauer, M, Burnett, R, Casey, D, Coates, M M, Cohen, A & Delwiche, K 2015,'Global, regional, and national comparative risk assessment of 79 behavioural, environmental and occupational, and metabolic risks or clusters of risks in 188 countries, 1990–2013: a systematic analysis for the Global Burden of Disease Study 2013',*TheLancet,*vol. 386, no. 10010, pp. 2287–323.

Fossil Free 2017,*Divestment commitments*, viewed 11 April 2017, https://gofossilfree. org/commitments/.

Foster, JB, Clark, B & York, R 2011, *Theecological rift: capitalism's war on the earth*, Monthly Review Press, New York.

Hester, RE 2012, *Soils and food security*, The Royal Society of Chemistry, London.

Jaffe, S 2017, 'US health and science advocates gear up for battle over EPA', *The Lancet*, vol. 389, no. 10075, pp.1180–81.

Kallis, G, Demaria, F & D'Alisa, G 2015, 'Introduction: degrowth', in D'Alisa, G, Demaria, F &Kallis, G (eds), *Degrowth: a vocabulary for a new era*, Routledge, New York and London.

Kimerling, J 2013, 'Lessons from the Chevron Ecuador litigation: the proposed intervenors' perspective', *Stanford Journal of Complex Litigation*, vol. 1, no. 2, pp. 241–94.

Kjellstrom, T, Holmer, I & Lemke, B 2009, 'Workplace heat stress, health and productivity – an increasing challenge for low- and middle-income countries during climate change', *Global Health Action*, vol. 2, no. 1.

Klein, N 2014,*Thischanges everything: capitalism vs the climate*, Simon and Schuster, New York.

Laird, B D, Goncharov, A B & Chan, H M 2013,'Body burden of metals and persistent organic pollutants among Inuit in the Canadian Arctic', *Environment International*, vol. 59, pp. 33–40.

Markowitz, G & Rosner, D 2014, *Lead wars: the politics of science and the fate of America's children*, University of California Press, Berkeley.

Marrs, T C & Karalliedde, L 2012,'The toxicology of pesticides', in Baker, D, Karalliedde, L, Murray, V, Maynard, R & Parkinson, NHT (eds), *Essentials of toxicology for health protection: a handbook for field professionals*, 2nd edn, Oxford University Press, Oxford.

Mathew, J, Goyal, R, Taneja, K K & Arora, N 2015,'Air pollution and respiratory health of school children in industrial, commercial and residential areas of Delhi', *Air Quality, Atmosphere & Health*, vol. 8, no. 4, pp. 421–27.

McMichael, A J 2013,'Global health: globalization, climate change, and human health', *The New England Journal of Medicine*, vol. 368, no. 14, pp. 1335–43.

McNeill, J R 2000, *Something new under the sun: an environmental history of the twentieth-century world (the global century series)*, WW Norton & Company, New York.

MiningWatch Canada 2017, *Salvadoran legislature votes for water over gold, becoming first nation to ban metals mining worldwide*, viewed 11 April 2017,http://us4.campaign-archive2.com/?u=c89185f430617e4dc1a02762 e&id=95a0c16eb0&e=987d9afab0.

Nahar, N, Blomstedt, Y, Wu, B, Kandarina, I, Trisnantoro, L & Kinsman, J 2014, 'Increasing the provision of mental health care for vulnerable, disaster-affected people in Bangladesh', *BMC Public Health*, vol. 14, no. 708.

National Resources Defense Council 2014,*Tar sands crude oil: health effects of a dirty and destructive fuel*, National Resources Defense Council, New York.

Orozco, F A, Cole, DC, Forbes, G, Kroschel, J, Wanigaratne, S & Arica, D 2009,'Monitoring adherence to the International Code of Conduct: highly hazardous pesticides in central Andean agriculture and farmers' rights to health', *International Journal of Occupational and Environmental Health*, vol. 15, pp. 255–68.

Prüss-Ustün, A, Wolf, J, Corvalán, C, Bos, R & Neira, M 2016, *Preventing disease through healthy environments: a global assessment of the burden of disease from environmental risks*, WHO, Geneva.

Saunders, P J, McCoy, D, Goldstein, R, Saunders, A T & Munroe, A 2016,'A review of the public health impacts of unconventional natural gas development', *Environmental Geochemistry and Health*, 5 December, pp.1–57.

Sellers, C 2014,'From poison to carcinogen: towards a global history of concerns about benzene', *Global Environment*, vol. 7, no. 1, pp. 38–71.

Smith, K R, Woodward, A, Campbell-Lendrum, D, Chadee, D, Honda, Y, Liu, Q, Olwoch, J, Revich, B & Sauerborn, R 2014,'Human health: Impacts, adaptation, and co-benefits', in Field, C B, Barros, V R, Dokken, D J, Mach, K J, Mastrandrea, M D, Bilir, T E, Chatterjee, M, Ebi, K L, Estrada, Y O, Genova, R C, Girma, B, Kissel, E S, Levy, A N, MacCracken, S, Mastrandrea, P R & White, L L (eds), *Climate change 2014: impacts, adaptation, and vulnerability. Part A: global and sectoral aspects*, contribution of Working Group II to the Fifth Assessment Report of the Intergovernmental Panel on Climate Change, Cambridge University Press, Cambridge and New York.

Swarup, A 2009, *Haiti: 'a gathering storm' – climate change and poverty*, Oxfam International, Port-au-Prince.

The Leap Manifesto 2015, *The Leap Manifesto:a call for Canada based on caring for the earth and one another*, viewed 11 April 2017, https://leapmanifesto.org/en/resources/

UNDP 2015,*Human Development Report 2015: work for human development*, UNDP, New York.

UNEP 2011, *Waste: investing in energy and resource efficiency*, UNEP, Nairobi.

UNEP 2014, *Assessing global land use: balancing consumption with sustainable supply*, UNEP, Nairobi.

UNEP 2015, *Waste crime – waste risks gaps in meeting the global waste challenge: a rapid response assessment*,UNEP, Nairobi.

UNICEF 2015, *Committing to child survival: a promise renewed. Progress report 2015*, UNICEF, New York.

UNICEF & WHO 2015, *Progress on sanitation and drinking water – 2015 update and MDG assessment*, WHO, Geneva.

Union of Concerned Scientists 2015,*All about oil*, viewed11 April 2017, http://www. ucsusa.org/clean-vehicles/all-about-oil#. WO1PU6IjXIU

Waters, C N, Zalasiewicz, J, Summerhayes, C, Barnosky, A D, Poirier, C, Gałuszka, A, Cearreta, A, Edgeworth, M, Ellis, E C, Ellis, M & Jeandel, C 2016, 'The Anthropocene is functionally and stratigraphically distinct from the Holocene', *Science*, vol. 351, no. 6269.

Westing, A 2008,'The impact of war on the environment', in Levy, B S & Sidel, V W (eds), *War and public health*, Oxford University Press, Oxford.

Whitmee, S, Haines, A, Beyrer, C, Boltz, F, Capon, A G, De Souza Dias, B F, Ezeh, A, Frumkin, H, Gong, P, Head, P, Horton, R, Mace, G M, Marten, R, Myers, S S, Nishtar, S Osofsky, S A, Pattanayak, S K, Pongsiri, M J, Romanelli, C, Soucat, A, Vega, J & Yach, D 2015, 'Safeguarding human health in the Anthropocene epoch: report of The Rockefeller Foundation-Lancet Commission on planetary health', *The Lancet*, vol. 386, pp. 1973– 2028.

WHO 2014a, *Burden of disease from ambient air pollution for 2012*, WHO, Geneva.

WHO 2014b, *Burden of disease from household air pollution for 2012*, WHO, Geneva.

WHO 2014c, *Quantitative risk assessment of the effects of climate change on selected causes of death, 2030s and 2050s*, WHO, Geneva.

WHO 2015a,*Global health observatory data repository*, viewed 24March 2015, http:// apps.who.int/gho/data/?theme=main

WHO 2015b, *Reducing global health risks through mitigation of short-lived climate pollutants. Scoping report for policymakers*,WHO, Geneva.

WHO 2016, *Burning opportunity: clean household energy for health, sustainable development, and wellbeing of women and children*,WHO, Geneva.

WHO EURO 2013, *Healtheffects of particulate matter: policy implications for countries in Eastern Europe, Caucasus and Central Asia*,WHO EURO, Copenhagen.

WWAP [United Nations World Water Assessment Programme] 2014,*The United Nations world water development report 2014: water and energy*, UNESCO, Paris.

WWAP 2015,*The United Nations world water development report 2015: water for a sustainable world*, UNESCO, Paris.

Historically, women's ability to make choices and exercise autonomy in matters of sexuality and reproduction have been conditioned and constrained by social (caste, class, gender, race religion, ethnicity, sexuality), economic and political structures, responding to a model that prescribes normative behavior, and disallowing behavior which deviates from this. Women's health is, for example, persistently relegated to 'maternal health' and 'family planning', especially for married women. Women's identities as 'reproductive beings' has been the basis for their domestication, relegating them to the private sphere of family. Reproduction, however, is in itself a site of coercion and social inequality, regulated by 'hetero-normativity' and social hierarchies. Further, non-normative gender and sexual expressions (e.g., same-sex sexual expressions) are largely marginalized and continue to remain invisible despite recognized violations of health and human rights.

Any conversation, therefore, on reproductive and sexual health and rights (SRHR), must employ the lens of intersectionality, whereby multiple tropes of identity and social locations are factored into analyses and policy perspectives. An intersectional approach to SRHR is necessary to understand and address inequities that impact autonomy, personhood, dignity, health and human rights. These are indelibly linked with the political economy of health and its intersections with the deep-rooted, multiple and structural discriminations. The abdication of its role in the provision of services by the State with the simultaneous promotion of privatization and corporatization has adversely impacted access, for a large number of people, to healthcare as well as other determinants necessary for their health. Inequalities within and across countries continue to grow, stoked by global policies that deny social, economic and political justice. This is further challenged by the rise in religious and political fundamentalisms that, in many parts of the globe, consolidate patriarchy, challenging democratic aspirations and institutions world-over. Following long struggles, the hard won rights to bodily integrity and autonomy, freedom from violence, access to safe abortion and to other reproductive and sexual health information and care stand threatened.

The Sustainable Development Goals (SDGs)[1], like their predecessor the Millennium Development Goals (MDGs), aim to transform global realities and inequalities. Specifically, goals [5] and [3] target the achievement of gender equality and empowerment of all women and girls and ensure healthy lives and promote well-being for all at all ages, respectively. Cross-cutting both SDG 3 and 5 is the issue of SRHR (arrow, 2016). While the SDGs' call to 'leave no one behind' is significant, neither are the targets and indicators exhaustive, nor do they present a transformative potential (Hickel, 2015). (See Chapter A1.)

The following sections of the chapter illustrate a few pertinent debates, issues that are marginal in the public health discourse as well as in policies that build upon the preceding arguments vis-à-vis identities, intersectionality and inequity, in the context of SRHR.

Queering the right to health and healthcare

Discrimination on the basis of non-normative sexuality and gender identities is deeply entrenched and an area of grave concern. The public healthcare system has historically been at the centre of fostering such discrimination and violations of the health and human rights of those with marginalized sexualities and gender identities. With laws that criminalize homosexuality in many countries across the world, access to healthcare remains a particularly important challenge. The International Lesbian, Gay, Bisexual, Trans and Intersex Association (ILGA) in its 12th edition of 'State Sponsored Homophobia – A World Survey of Sexual Orientation Laws: Criminalisation, Protection and Recognition' has identified 72 countries where there is some form of criminalization, including 13 where homosexual acts can be punished with the death penalty (Carrol and Mendos, 2017). Among these 72 countries, most are located in the Global South. Thus the vulnerabilities of queer people regarding their right to health and healthcare are compounded due to their location as well as their identity.

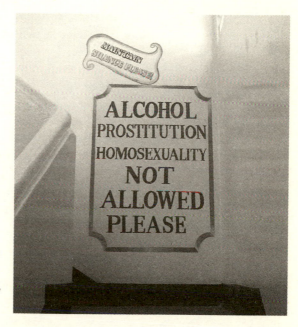

Image C2.1 House rules in a guest house in Malindi, Kenya (By Nicor - Own work; License: CC BY-SA 3.0, https://commons.wikimedia.org/w/index.php?curid=8077400)

According to a Report of the United Nations High Commissioner for Human Rights titled 'Discriminatory laws and practices and acts of violence against individuals based on their sexual orientation and gender identity' (United Nations, 2011) "The criminalization of homosexuality may deter individuals from seeking health services for fear of revealing criminal conduct, and results in services, national health plans and policies not reflecting the specific needs of LGBT persons…In countries where no criminal sanctions exist, homophobic, sexist and transphobic practices and attitudes on the part of health-care institutions and personnel may nonetheless deter LGBT persons from seeking services" (paragraphs 55 and 56).

The recognition of gender identities beyond the male and female binary, has however, witnessed some progress. During 2012–15 many countries accorded legal recognition to the identity of transgender people. For example, in Argentina in 2012 and in Denmark in 2014, self-identification became the sole criteria for legal recognition and change of name in identity documents for transgender people. In both countries, sex reassignment surgery or certification of any other medical or psychological intervention is not mandatory to obtain such recognition. Argentina includes the provision of surgical intervention and hormonal therapy as a right for those who desire to have them, in public, private as well as trade-union run services in the country as part of the

---

Box C2.1: Right to health of queer communities in India

In the context of India, for example, the Section 377 of the Indian Penal Code (IPC) that criminalizes 'sex against the order of the nature' is used to target and violate the rights of the queer community, including to healthcare. In 2009, a two-judge bench of the Delhi High Court recognized that section 377 obstructs people's right to health by hindering the outreach of public health measures for HIV/AIDS prevention. However, the Supreme Court of India's ruling in 2013 reaffirming the provisions of Section 377, while hearing an appeal against the Delhi High Court judgement of 2009 dealt a blow to human rights and health rights especially for the queer community in India[2]. The reference by the Supreme Court in its 2013 judgement to the queer community as a "miniscule minority" was a stark reflection of the prevalent attitudes as well as obfuscation of the right to sexual autonomy and non-discriminatory access to healthcare. While the struggle continues with curative petitions against the judgement being admitted by the Supreme Court towards determining the constitutional validity of the Section 377 (Rajagopal, 2016), 'queering' of the public health discourse, policy and programmes must remain central to the health movement and other campaigns.

'Compulsory Medical Plan' for citizens[3]. Denmark, represents an exception in Europe, where in 34 countries legal recognition by way of change of name and change of sex assigned at birth is linked with certification of some form of medical intervention (Ansari 2017). In India, in 2014, the Supreme Court of India accorded recognition to transgender and intersex people as the 'other' gender, upholding their right to self-identification and recognizing their fundamental rights guaranteed under the constitution as full citizens[4]. However, the implementation of this judgment through the Transgender Persons (Protection of Rights) Bill, 2016, and multiple state-level policies have met with criticism as they have placed disproportionate emphasis on medical diagnosis, proof of sex-reassignment surgeries and a plethora of 'evidences' that go against the very essence of self-identification as a trans-person. Iran too promotes the 'medicalization' of gender identity for transgender people. This has made it easier to access sex reassignment and transition related healthcare since 1987. However, an emphasis on medical intervention designates transgender identities as pathologies – as though it is a disorder in need of rectification (ibid.). Further, these measures stop short of facilitating access to social security measures including access to comprehensive healthcare by people who have been historically marginalized and been largely invisible in society.

Moreover, fundamentalisms – religious or otherwise – pose a great danger to the life and liberty of homosexual and transgender persons. In April 2016, two prominent gay rights activists of Bangladesh Xulhaz Mannan and Mahbub Tonoy were brutally murdered in Dhaka by religious fundamentalists. According to a compilation by the 'Trans Murder Monitoring Project', there were 2,343 reported killings of trans and gender-diverse people in 69 countries worldwide between 2008–2016. The report reveals: "Throughout all six world regions, the highest absolute numbers have been found in countries with strong trans movements and civil society organisations that carry out forms of professional monitoring: Brazil (938), Mexico (290), Colombia (115), Venezuela (111), and Honduras (89) in Central and South America; the United States (160) in North America; Turkey (44) and Italy (32) in Europe; and India (62), the Philippines (43) and Pakistan (39) in Asia (Transgender Europe (TGEU) 2017)."

Sex workers' health: an agenda for public health

For women in sex work, their identity as a 'sex worker' prevails over all else; ignoring their experiences as women affected by gender, norms related to sexuality, and their social locations. These, as well as stigmatization, as a consequence of criminalization and social control impact varied aspects of their lives, including their access to healthcare, housing, etc. (Pai et al., 2014). Stigma also reduces sex workers' access to institutions of law and order, justice in situations of violence. For sex workers, violence is rampant in intimate relationships, in their work as well as through interface with representatives of institutions of health, law, justice (ibid.). Stigma and consequent self-imposed invisibility increases the risk of violence, and creates obstacles for public health interventions to reach them.

Moreover, sex workers have been historically targeted in a very instrumentalist manner – as 'vectors' of HIV, as high risk groups who need access to drugs or treatment so as to curb the spread of the disease among the 'general population' (Crago, 2015). Reports of sex workers being tested for HIV without their consent and the public disclosure of the results have repeatedly violated accepted standards of confidentiality and consent, while severely hindering their access to quality health services (SAMA, 2017). Such response to the HIV/AIDS pandemic also acted as one of the major catalyst for sex workers to organize themselves to advocate for rights against such targeting and to be seen as rights bearing individuals who are entitled to health as a human right. According to a *Lancet* paper, "sex workers' health programmes, including interventions focusing on safer sex, should be for the promotion of health of sex workers and not just a way to slow down the dissemination of HIV" (Wolffers and Beelen, 2003).

However, quality healthcare to address sex workers own health needs – access to safe abortion, access to pre- and post-natal care, healthcare in cases of sexual or domestic violence, counselling to deal with violence and stigma and other mental health issues – is virtually absent[5]. Sex workers are highly vulnerable to physical and mental health issues but have minimal access to medical and psychosocial care. Sex workers who access healthcare in public hospitals, are frequently denied treatment or find themselves at the receiving end of abuse and discrimination, and receive treatment of poor quality.

Sex work is frequently conflated with trafficking and is responsible for the rights of sex workers being severely compromised. While a proportion of sex workers are 'trafficked', a higher number enter sex work of their own volition. Poverty, caste and gender inequality are often underlying motivations for their entering sex work, but their decision is not without agency. In some countries, this leads to criminalization of sex workers and enforces invisibility. While trafficking – understood as illegal confinement, coercion, bonded labour and deception – are definitely a problem, most countries have laws to address these generally, as well as particularly in the realm of labour laws. Therefore, if sex workers enjoy the rights of workers, issues linked to their conditions at the workplace can also be addressed by existing laws against violation of labour rights. Sex workers have often argued for their recognition as workers and effective implementation of existing laws, instead of anti-trafficking laws that violate their rights. "Repressive policies toward prostitution and prostitutes and/or repressive, restrictive policies towards migration per se under the denominator of anti-trafficking policy, actually *preclude* an effective, adequate policy against those abuses that anti-trafficking policies should be designed to address (i.e. the abuse and violence in relation to the process of recruitment and in relation to working conditions in prostitution). Anti-trafficking policies mostly address the wrong phenomena" (Vanwesenbeeck, 2011).

Laws and policies must distinguish between sex work and trafficking, measures to address trafficking in persons must not interfere with the human rights of sex workers, and the model of raids, 'rescue' and rehabilitation for sex workers must be abolished. Decriminalization of sex work and measures to safeguard health and occupational safety must be instituted. In order to establish a rights-based approach to sex work, participation of sex workers must be ensured in the design, implementation and monitoring of policies and laws (Sama, 2017). The Government must take steps to provide a full range of non-stigmatizing and confidential health services that is relevant to their needs.

Whither the *right* to safe abortion?

Women's rights over their own bodies and their reproductive autonomy are often rendered secondary, pitted against the conceptualization of the foetus as a 'person' which bears the 'right to life'. Access to safe abortion is a hugely contested issue globally with complete bans in some states. Abortion, under any circumstance, is banned in 11 African countries[6], 7 Latin American and Caribbean countries[7] and 3 Asian countries[8]. One of the major incidents that rekindled global debates on abortion was the death of Savita Halappanavar, a woman of Indian origin in Ireland in 2012. She died of septicemia that resulted from denial of medical care following a miscarriage.

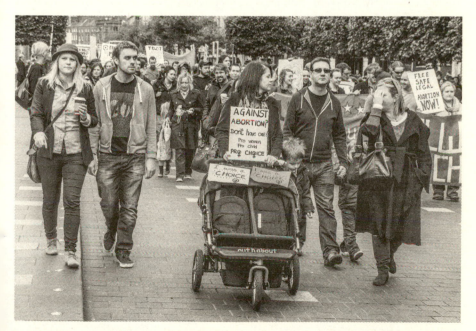

Image C2.2 March for Choice in Dublin (William Murphy; License: CC BY-SA 2.0, https://creativecommons.org/licenses/by-sa/2.0/)

Though updated statistics are not available, according to 2008 data of the World Health Organization (WHO), "In developed regions, it is estimated that 30 women die for every 100 000 unsafe abortions. That number rises to 220 deaths per 100 000 unsafe abortions in developing regions and 520 deaths per 100 000 unsafe abortions in sub-Saharan Africa. Mortality from unsafe abortion disproportionately affects women in Africa. While the continent accounts for 29% of all unsafe abortions, it sees 62% of unsafe abortion-related deaths[9]".

The recent reinstating of the 'Global Gag' Rule in 2017 by the current US President, Donald Trump, has only sparked further debate on the issue of abortion (see Box C2.2). The most recent version of the gag rule has been imposed on all US federal funding on global health, including family planning and also funding that comes as 'foreign aid'. It affects sexual and reproductive rights globally and also threatens access to safe abortion services and pushes women to pursue unsafe abortions that put their health and lives at risk (Redden, 2017). Moreover, the 'Global Gag' Rule affects not just access to safe abortion, but also sexual and reproductive health and rights, including programmes against HIV/AIDS, Zika, etc. (ibid.).

In Brazil, the spread of the Zika virus and rising cases of children born with microcephaly has given impetus to women's rights campaigns that are demanding an expansion of very restrictive abortion laws. Brazil criminalizes abortion and permits them only in case of a pregnancy resulting from rape, necessity to save a mother's life and anencephaly in the foetus (Carless, 2016).

In 2016, thousands of women in Poland took to the streets to protest against a proposal to ban abortions in the country by the conservative government in the country. In response, the government dropped the proposal, yet refused to liberalize existing laws to facilitate greater access – which was a demand of the protesters (Borys, 2016). The law in Poland permits abortion only for pregnancy following rape and in case of danger to the mother's life. More recently in June 2017, women in Poland have hit the streets yet again,

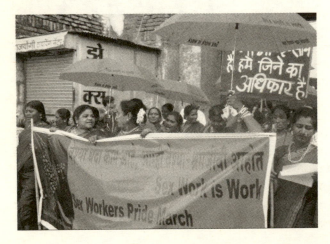

Image C2.3 International Sex Workers Day, 2012, Sex Workers Pride March (National Network of Sex Workers, India)

Box C2.2: What is the 'Global Gag' Rule?

The controversial 'Global Gag' Rule (also known as the Mexico City Policy) prohibits international family planning organizations receiving US aid from providing information, counselling, or referrals related to abortion – even if using their own non-US funding and even if the practices are legal in their own countries.

When reinstated as a matter of law, the GGR has terrible consequences for women and their families. While it was in effect between 2001 and 2009, the policy forced clinics to cut back on a range of critical health services that have nothing to do with abortion, such as family planning, obstetric care, HIV testing and malaria treatment.

A Stanford University study also suggested that the policy may be linked to a dramatic rise in induced abortions in Africa, including in Ghana, Guinea and Mozambique. These countries, which experienced the greatest cuts in US support for health organizations under the policy, saw the number of induced abortions double between 2001 and 2008, along with a decline in contraceptive use. Reduced access to contraceptives resulting from funding cuts may have led women to substitute abortion for contraception, according to the study, which is the first quantitative effort to examine the policy's impacts.

The GGR was first adopted in 1984 by President Ronald Reagan but has since been removed and reinstated several times. President Obama rescinded the policy when he took office in January 2009. President Donald J. Trump reinstated the 'Global Gag' Rule in 2017.

Source: Reproduced from Engender Health n.d. 'Raise Your Voice: Raise Your Voice: End the Global Gag Rule!' http://www.engenderhealth.org/media/info/globalgagrule-video.php?gclid=CjwKEAjwqIfLBRCk6vH_rJq7yDoSJACG-18frScL5ER78knJ9AzYXa_yvq95mkFvfTw3wXRzuxVTQMRoCBw3w_wcB

---

to protest against the government's directive to ban over the counter sale of emergency contraceptives. Such a move curtails women's SRHR and allows greater control for medical practitioners (Lampen, 2017).

Towards a conclusion

The chapter suggests approaches to analysing and building the public health discourse and policies related to sexual and reproductive health and rights, which currently fall outside the normative framework. Illustrating three areas – right to health of queer people, sex workers' access to healthcare and access to safe abortion – the chapter focuses on key issues and concerns that are largely marginal in the SRHR discourse. There is a need to chart the

Box C2.3: Abortion laws in India

In India, the law on abortion – the Medical Termination of Pregnancy Act 1971 (amendments in 2002) does not recognize women's absolute right to abortion but allows access to abortion under certain circumstances like pregnancy following rape, contraceptive failure, in case of foetal abnormalities and if a woman is experiencing physical or mental trauma. The Act recognizes termination of pregnancy till 20 weeks, beyond which, courts have the jurisdiction to decide based on the opinion of a duly constituted medical board that weighs the merits of each case. However, even when such boards rule in favour of the woman's plea to be allowed to abort, no legal precedent is set for medical boards to be constituted without the courts' intervention in subsequent cases. Such a stipulation restricts an adult woman's desire for terminating a pregnancy till a medical board determines that there is a danger to her physical and/or mental health in each case (Nadimpally and Banerjee, 2016). Amendments to the MTP Act are under consideration to increase the gestation limit from the present 20 weeks to 24 weeks for special categories of women. In addition, the amendment proposes to do away with the gestational limit for seeking abortions on grounds of foetal abnormality that is incompatible with life (PTI, 2017). An extremely progressive judgment in September 2016 by the Bombay High Court held that, "Pregnancy has profound effects on a woman's health and life. Thus, how she wants to deal with this pregnancy must be a decision she alone can make. Let us not lose sight of the basic right of women: the right to decide what to do with their bodies, including whether or not to get pregnant and stay pregnant" (Arvind, 2016).

Two issues that pose substantive barriers to access to abortion is criminalization of consensual sexual activity below 18 years and its conflation with gender biased selection. Mandatory reporting by healthcare providers under The Protection of Children from Sexual Offences (POCSO) Act 2012 severely curtails access to safe abortion for young girls. The positioning of sex selection versus access to abortion is not only misplaced, it immensely harms women's physical and emotional health whereby they are either forced to continue unintended pregnancies or have little choice but to access abortion in unsafe conditions. Further, the range of technologies, including pre-conception technologies for gender biased selection, continues to thrive and expand.

future trajectory of activism around SRHR afresh. For too long, even major sections of health civil society movements, have been complicit in reducing the discourse on SRHR to one about maternal health and reproduction.

Rather than fragmented voices across the spectrum, there is a need to forge alliances and solidarities to resist retrograde steps that threaten human and sexual and reproductive health and rights. Mobilizations for development of 'shadow' reports by civil society under international instruments like the Universal Periodic Reviews (UPR) and reporting to the Committee under the 'Convention for Elimination of All Forms of Discrimination Against Women' (CEDAW) can be harnessed. Countries that have not signed/ratified some of the international treaties that accord protections and entitlements regarding SRHR must become sites of strategic mobilizations. The Women's March in the USA in January 2017 is an illustration of one such mobilization. People's collective resistances against inequalities and oppressions located at the intersections of hetero-patriarchal structures, neoliberal globalized markets, and other fundamentalisms, must be transformed to ensure that 'leaving no one behind' does not remain an empty slogan.

Notes

1 Under the 2030 Agenda for Development, in 2015 all member states of the United Nations agreed upon working towards achieving Sustainable Development Goals (SDGs). The 17 sustainable development goals (SDGs) are broken down into 169 specific targets that each country has committed to try and achieve voluntary basis over the next 15 years.

2 See: Supreme Court appeals case: Suresh Kumar Koushal and another ... versus NAZ Foundation and others CIVIL APPEAL NO.10972 OF 2013 http://judis.nic.in/supremecourt/imgs1.aspx?filename=41070

3 See: http://tgeu.org/argentina-gender-identity-law/

4 See: NALSA (National Legal Services Authority) Versus Union of India and others, WRIT PETITION (CIVIL) NO.400 OF 2012 http://supremecourtofindia.nic.in/outtoday/wc40012.pdf

5 See: Right to Health and Health Care 21. UPR report SANGRAM http://www.sexualrightsinitiative.com/wp-content/uploads/India-UPR-13-CREA.pdf

6 See: Abortion in Africa, Incidence and Trends https://www.guttmacher.org/fact-sheet/facts-abortion-africa

7 See: Abortion in Latin America And the Caribbean https://www.guttmacher.org/sites/default/files/factsheet/ib_aww-latin-america.pdf

8 See: Abortion in Asia https://www.guttmacher.org/sites/default/files/factsheet/ib_aww-asia.pdf

9 See: Factsheet by WHO, June 2017 http://www.who.int/mediacentre/factsheets/fs388/en/

References

Ansari A 2017, Transgender rights: These countries are ahead of the US, CNN, February 23, 2017 http://edition.cnn.com/2017/02/23/health/transgender-laws-around-the-world/index.html

arrow 2016, Recommendations to governments to firmly integrate gender equality and SRHR into the national SDG plans in the Global South regions "ensuring that no one is left behind" http://arrow.org.my/wp content/uploads/2016/07/Call-to-action-HLPF-2016.pdf

Arvind A 2016, 'Women should be allowed to end pregnancy even when there is no risk: Bombay HC' Hindustan times, Sep 21 2016 http://www.hindustantimes.com/mumbai-news/let-women-abort-foetus-irrespective-of-reason-bombay-hc/story-2tlic6kvwPvl7J7q8WfcDI.html

Borys C 2016, 'Poland's Massive Abortion Protest Shows That Citizens Are Frustrated With The Country's Rightward Surge' Huffpost Oct 12, 2016 http://www. huffingtonpost.com/entry/poland-abortion-protest_us_57fced3ae4b068ecb5e1af88

Carless W 2016, 'The Zika virus has reignited Brazil's abortion debate' Global Post, Public Radio International (PRI) January 28, 2016 https://www.pri.org/stories/2016-01-28/zika-virus-has-reignited-brazil-s-abortion-debate-0

Carrol A and Mendos L R 2017, 'State Sponsored Homophobia, A World Survey of Sexual Orientation Laws, Criminalization, Protection and Recognition, 12th Edition, May 2017, p. 193, ilga.org http://ilga.org/downloads/2017/ILGA_State_Sponsored_Homophobia_2017_WEB.pdf

Crago A L 2008, 'Our Lives Matte: Sex Workers Unite for Health and Rights' Open Society Institute, Public Health program, New York, 2008 https://www.opensocietyfoundations.org/sites/default/files/Our%2520Lives%2520Matter%2520%2520Sex%2520Workers%2520Unite%2520for%2520Health%2520and%2520Rights.pdf

Hickel J 2015, The Problem with Saving the World, Jacobin, 08.08.2015 https://www.jacobinmag.com/2015/08/global-poverty-climate-change-sdgs/

Lampen C 2017 'Poland makes emergency contraception a prescription-only drug — even for rape survivors', Mic Network Inc, June 26, 2017 https://mic.com/articles/180798/poland-makes-emergency-contraception-a-prescription-only-drug-even-for-rape-survivors#.yp2r9qlob

Nadimpally S and Banerjee S 2016, 'Why Do Women Need a Medical Board to Sign-Off on Abortion?' The Wire, 16/08/2016 https://thewire.in/59330/why-do-women-need-a-medical-board-to-sign-off-on-abortion/

Pai A, Seshu M, Gupte M, VAMP, 2014. 'Status of women in sex work in India' 2014 http://tbinternet.ohchr.org/Treaties/CEDAW/Shared%20Documents/Ind/INT_CEDAW_NGO_Ind_17395_E.pdf

Press Trust of India (PTI) 2017 Amendment to MTP Act proposed before Cabinet: Govt,

Indian Express, March 24 2017 http://indianexpress.com/article/india/j-p-nadda-amendment-to-mtp-act-proposed-before-cabinet-govt-4584104/ Accessed on 3 April 2017.

Rajagopal K 2016, 'Five-judge Constitution Bench to take a call on Section 377', The Hindu, 2 February http://www.thehindu.com/news/national/Five-judge-Constitution-Bench-to-take-a-call-on-Section-377/article14056992.ece

Redden M 2017, 'Global gag rule' reinstated by Trump, curbing NGO abortion services abroad' The Guardian, January 2017 https://www.theguardian.com/world/2017/jan/23/trump-abortion-gag-rule-international-ngo-funding

Sama 2017, Unpublished draft

Transgender Europe (TGEU) 2017 'Trans Day of Visibility 2017 Press Release' 30th March 2017 http://transrespect.org/en/tdov-2017-tmm-update/

United Nations 2011, 'Discriminatory laws and practices and acts of violence against individuals based on their sexual orientation and gender identity' Report of the United Nations High Commissioner for Human Rights, Annual report of the United Nations High Commissioner for Human Rights and reports of the Office of the High Commissioner and the Secretary-General, 17th November 2011 http://www.ohchr.org/documents/issues/discrimination/a.hrc.19.41_english.pdf

Vanwesenbeeck E 2011, 'Sex Workers' Rights and Health The Case of The Netherlands', in book: Global Perspectives on Prostitution and Sex Trafficking (Europe, Latin America, North America, and Global)., Landham, M D: Lexington Books, Dalla R L, Baker L M, DeFrain J, Williamson C (Eds), pp. 3–25, 2011 https://www.researchgate.net/publication/289533336_Sex_Workers%27_Rights_and_Health_The_Case_of_The_Netherlands

Wolffers I and Beelen N 2003, 'Public health and the human rights of sex workers', The Lancet, vol. 361, 7 June.

C3 | HEALTH REFORMS IN CHILE: LACK OF PROGRESS IN WOMEN'S SEXUAL AND REPRODUCTIVE HEALTH AND RIGHTS[1]

Introduction

The global recognition of the importance of universalism in health has been acknowledged with the commitment, enshrined in the Sustainable Development Goals (SDGs), to ensuring universal access to sexual and reproductive healthcare services by 2030. Calls for universal access to healthcare to address inequalities in health are not new. The Platform for Action emerging from the 1994 International Conference on Population and Development (ICPD) called for universal access to healthcare services, including, specifically, reproductive health services (Principle 8). Yet despite these global commitments and assertions only limited progress has been made towards meeting this objective and many women across the world are still systematically denied access to these services.

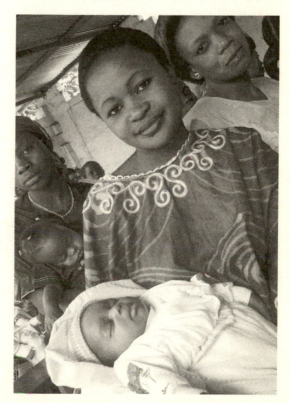

Image C3.1 Health systems often see women as just 'reproducers' (third world health aid)

This has particularly been the case for women in Latin America, where, it has been argued, reproductive health systems are among the largest contributors to gender inequality in the world (UNDP, 2010). Moreover, gender differences in the access to and use of services are not sufficiently factored into debates around universalism (WHO, 2010). Yet universal access goes beyond mere coverage of services. Structural inequalities by gender, as well as by class, race and ethnicity, can reinforce barriers to access and must be accounted for in any discussion of universalism.

The case of Chile can offer some insights into the factors limiting universalism in sexual and reproductive health and rights (SRHR).[1] Chile presents an interesting case study given its status as a middle-income country and its well-developed public and private health sectors. Around 70 per cent of the population is covered by the public system, and in recent years considerable progress has been made towards universal healthcare coverage (Bitrán, 2013). The shift towards universalism began in the early 2000s and studies have suggested that significant improvements have been made towards improving health inequalities (Frenz et al., 2014, pp. 717–31). A central element of the reform is the Plan of Universal Access with Explicit Guarantees, or Plan AUGE as it is commonly known in Chile, which legally guarantees equal rights to both public- and private-sector beneficiaries in terms of accessing timely, affordable and quality healthcare services for 80 prioritized health problems.

Nevertheless, despite the progress towards universal healthcare, there continue to be significant structural constraints within the health system, which remains highly stratified across the public and private systems and continues to prioritize high-income users. Critics have argued that the need to meet the AUGE guarantees has led to a neglect of other health concerns, that overall access continues to be shaped by gender, ethnicity and age, and that the adequacy and quality of care, particularly among low-income users, is a matter of concern (Aguilera et al., 2014). These inequalities are particularly manifested in women's sexual and reproductive health and rights, where there has been a significant lack of progress towards securing better health indicators and outcomes, particularly in the field of SRHR.[2] It is also worth noting that successive Chilean governments have passed extensive legislation advancing gender equality and, indeed, the current president, Michelle Bachelet, has arguably promoted feminist agendas. Yet despite apparent progress in 'pro-gender' policies, particularly in the area of social policy, only limited changes have resulted on the ground. Recently, there has been a push to move the agenda further and there are ongoing discussions in Parliament to approve the de-criminalization of abortion in restricted cases. As Table C3.1 illustrates, there are still a number of significant gaps in women's SRHR health outcomes, which need addressing.

Concerns have been expressed over the lack of progress in a number of areas of women's SRHR in Chile, including the following (CEDAW, 2012):

TABLE C3.1: Some key indicators of women's SRHR in Chile

Indicator	Prevalence
Contraceptive use (2006)a	64.2% (Americas: 73.6%)
Births by caesarean section (2010)b	37.0% (Americas: 35.6%)
Legal situation re. abortion	Completely criminalized (bill to allow therapeutic abortion in three cases presented in January 2015)
Number of abortions per annumc	60,000 to 70,000
Maternal mortality rate (per 100 000 live births)d *	22
Estimated deaths per 100,000 (2008) – cervix uteri cancere	4.8
Estimated deaths per 100,000 (2008) – breast cancerf	7.3
Estimated deaths per 100,000 population (2008) – ovarian cancerg	0.3
Rate of teenage pregnancy (% of 15–19-year-olds who are mothers)h	12.3

Sources: a. WHO (2016); b. Ibid. c. See CEDAW (2012); d. UNICEF (2017); e. WHO (2017); f. Ibid.; g. Ibid.; h. United Nations (2017)

Note: * Regional average 77 per 100,000 live births.

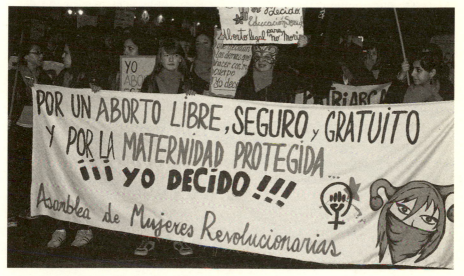

Image C3.2 Pro-choice March in Chile, 25 July 2013 (AshokaJegroo / The Santiago Times; License: CC BY 2.0, https://creativecommons.org/licenses/by/2.0/)

- criminalization of all forms of abortion, and the lack of progress on securing safe
- abortions for women
- high number of teenage pregnancies
- high rates of school dropout and expulsion of teenage mothers
- lack of access to contraception.

This creates a highly contradictory situation in a middle-income country such as Chile where, on the one hand, people have access to highly developed health systems but at the same time experience a significant deficit in terms of personal and health rights. Access to SRHR is clearly shaped by class: for example, economic resources guarantee access to safer abortion in private clinics and with the use of the medication Misoprostol. Moreover, 48 per cent of teenage mothers live below the poverty line, with many coming from the poorest rural communities (CEDAW, 2012).

How do we therefore explain the lack of progress with respect to SRHR in Chile, despite the fact that overall health indicators are good and Chile is a middle-income country? The rest of the chapter focuses on three inter-related factors.

The marginalization of SRHR in health reform debates

The role of power relations in policymaking is often overlooked, yet an idea of the nature of power relationships is critical to understanding the ways in which SRHR issues have been neglected in policy debates. Political scientists have shown how, in order to identify the 'relevant' actors and understand the power structures inherent in health sector institutions, it is helpful to take a historical view. The work of Paul Pierson (1994) has been central to these debates. He has shown how the establishment of welfare states in the Global North created vested interests and 'armies of beneficiaries' that protected it from attack. These historical interests and policies have shaped the politics, including the behaviour of bureaucrats and interest groups, which feed back into contemporary reform processes. These so-called 'policy legacies' help us to identify which actors maintain a vested interest in the health sector and seek to shape reform processes accordingly. Policy legacies can also reveal how particular gender, race and class orders become entrenched within policy processes over time. For example, the historical development of the Chilean health sector shows how men's health needs were prioritized because men were seen as constituting an integral part of the labour force. In contrast, women were seen primarily as mothers whose only role was to give birth and look after young children, and their needs were therefore seen as secondary to those of men. There was no acknowledgement of women having any health issues beyond those directly related to biological reproduction. The replication of this pattern over time has created 'gendered policy legacies', which shed some light on subsequent failures to prioritize women's health needs.

The lack of attention assigned to women's health concerns is further compounded by the marginalization of women within central decision-making arenas in the Chilean legislature. This raises significant questions over the likelihood of SRHR issues being taken up as matters of serious political concern. This was particularly evident when women's groups sought to influence the design of Plan AUGE to ensure, for example, that the inclusion of health conditions reflected women's health priorities alongside men's. In the preliminary phases of the AUGE, 56 health conditions were included but only around one-third specifically addressed questions of gender inequality in health (Vargas and Poblete 2008, pp. 782–92). Moreover, attempts to introduce a more redistributive element to the health system, which would have had important implications for public-sector users (that is, the majority of poor women), were blocked by private insurance companies. This clearly illustrates how particular class and gender interests can be maintained through reform processes.

The role of the Catholic Church and other conservative vested interest groups

The 'policy legacy approach' also underlines the influential role of the Catholic Church in health policymaking. This is particularly evident in the field of women's SRHR where the Church exerts an influence at not only the policymaking stage but also in terms of healthcare delivery, thus impacting health outcomes.

Since the papacy of Karol Józef Wojtyla (1978–2005), the Catholic Church has undergone a conservative shift, and reviews of official papal documents show that it has been increasingly involved in regulating sexuality, reproduction, family structures and gender roles (Casanova 2009, pp. 1–29). Despite there being low popular adherence to the Church in Chile, the Church has successfully maintained a conservative agenda on issues of reproductive rights, precisely because the decreasing attachment of Catholics to the Church has left the latter with the freedom to generate alliances with conservative business and right-wing elites, who are quite empathetic to the Church's moral teachings (Hagopian, 2008, pp. 149–68).

Furthermore, Catholic ideas of women's sexual and reproductive rights in Chile were embedded into the policies and legislation of the military regime in the period 1973–1990, despite the fact that the Church opposed the regime's human rights violation. The influence of Catholicism is also present in the 1980 Constitution; most notably, Jaime Guzmán, a devout Catholic, was one of the commissioners responsible for drafting it. The Constitution set the precedent to criminalize all forms of abortion. Since the return to democracy in 1990, a powerful religious elite has been able to influence policy implementation on sexual education in schools, and access to emergency contraception and abortion. Conservative elites have maintained a close hold over public discussion, and economic elites have stepped in when the government has succeeded in introducing progressive reforms, such as in the case of emergency contraception: conservative mayors stopped access to emergency contraception in their municipalities, based on their own conservative views, even when by law they were mandated to ensure access in all public health establishments. These elites belong to conservative groups within the Church, including Opus Dei, the Legionaries of Christ and the Schoensttadt Movement, and they have successfully penetrated elite educational and health facilities, spiritual groups and community churches. Groups like Opus Dei are not only successful in their reach but also in their hold over members' work and family life, transforming elite members into committed and active advocates with access to resources and power. Even when leftist governments are in place, such as the current Bachelet government in Chile, real progress in SRHR is unlikely as political leaders are either unwilling or unable to accept the potential political fallout that would result from the adoption of a comprehensive and effective SRHR policy.

The role of medical professionals

The 'policy legacies approach' also reveals how the medical profession has been able to maintain its power as a professional body during successive reform periods. Moreover, its inherent gendered nature has meant that the medical profession has failed to prioritize women's own definitions of their health, and it has continued to essentialize women as reproducers. In Chile, the development of the medical profession was closely aligned with nineteenth-century ideals of hegemonic masculinity, and the evidence of this policy legacy is still apparent in the profession across much of the Latin America. Present-day maternal healthcare services are often organized around medical professionals (that is, doctors), rather than 'semi-professionals' (that is, nurses and midwives). This has important implications for decision-making processes with regard to childbirth, where power tends to lie with medical professionals rather than the women themselves (Gamble et al., 2007, pp. 331–40). Moreover, in the context of the privatization of, and 'professionalism' in, healthcare, medical professionals such as obstetricians are becoming increasingly accountable to 'the market' rather than the state (Sandall et al., 2009, pp. 529–53). This is particularly evident in the context of reproductive healthcare services, especially childbirth. In Chile, where the medical profession was one of the main beneficiaries of the public-sector reforms of the 1980s, medical practicioners acquired the possibility of a 'dual practice', that is, a stable public-sector job coupled with private-sector responsibilities and revenue. This has exacerbated inequalities, as private patients in the Chilean system are often given preferential treatment over public-sector patients, particularly in the matter of childbirth (Murray and Elston 2005, pp. 701–21).

Yet it is also necessary to understand how 'gendered policy legacies' shape opportunities for medical professionals to exert power at the policy implementation stage. A recent systematic review highlighted the growth of the microipractice model as an important constraint in implementing health policies (Gilson, Schneider and Orgill 2014, pp. iii51–iii69). Health workers frequently use their own discretion to determine whether or not to offer women family planning services and, moreover, whether or not to restrict women's contraceptive choices. In the case of Chile, private clinics and private university hospitals decide what reproductive and sexual health services to offer, despite national regulations and guidelines. This means that some Catholic health services do not provide access to contraception or voluntary sterilization; there is also anecdotal evidence of medical professionals marking the files of women who are suspected of having undergone an abortion.

While it is important to recognize that discretionary power is not always used to undermine and subvert policy, there is a clear need to understand how power relations shape outcomes so that it is possible to move towards better 'policy ownership' by implementers (Lehmann and Gilson 2013, pp. 358–66). In Chile, health and medical workers maintain power and control over women seeking healthcare services, a situation that has arguably been reinforced in the context of the privatization of health services.

Conclusion

The foregoing discussion on universal access to healthcare has focused attention on the importance of SRHR and its centrality to the wider development process. Yet if governments are serious about their commitment to overcoming inequalities and meeting development goals, it is essential that SRHR issues are fully addressed. The case of Chile clearly demonstrates that even in the context of universal healthcare systems in countries where economic development has occurred and income levels have been raised, women's sexual and reproductive health rights are frequently ignored or even deliberately kept off the political agenda. We therefore advocate the importance of employing a broader approach: governments must not only commit to promoting women's health concerns but must simultaneously address the deeply embedded gendered norms within the society and healthcare system, and in the daily practice of health professionals. If not, policies will fall short at the implementation stage.

Notes

This chapter draws in part on an earlier article by the authors: 'What is hindering progress? The marginalization of women's sexual and reproductive health and rights in Brazil and Chile', *Journal of International and Comparative Social Policy*, vol. 31, 20 Oct. 2015.

Although sexual and reproductive rights have not been explicitly included in the SDGs, we believe that they are an integral part of sexual and reproductive healthcare and must be taken into account.

The definition of SRHR in the ICPD Programme of Action includes family planning; antenatal and postnatal care; prevention of abortion and management of the consequences of abortion; information, education and counselling, as appropriate, on human sexuality and reproductive health and prevention; and prevention of violence against women (UNFPA, 2008).

References

Aguilera, X, Castillo-Laborde, C, Ferrari, MND, Delgado, I & Ibañez, C 2014, 'Monitoring and evaluating progress towards universal health coverage in Chile', *PLoS Medicine*, vol. 11, no. 9, DOI:10.1371/journal.pmed.1001676.

Bitrán, R 2013, 'Explicit health guarantees for Chileans: The AUGE benefits package', UNICO Studies Series 21, The World Bank, Washington DC.

Casanova, J 2009, 'Religion, politics and gender equality: public religions revisited'. In Phillips, A & Casanova, J, *A debate on the public role of religion and its social and gender implications*, United Nations Research Institute for Social Development, Geneva, pp. 1–29.

CEDAW 2012, 'Concluding observations on Chile', 53rd session, U.N. Doc. CEDAW/C/CHL/CO/5–6.

Frenz, P, Delgado, I, Kaufman, J & Harper, S 2014, Achieving effective universal health coverage with equity: evidence from Chile', *Health Policy and Planning*, vol. 29, no. 6, pp. 717–31.

Gamble, J, Creedy, D, McCourt, C, Weaver, J & Beake, S 2007, 'A Critique of the Literature on Women's Request for Cesarean Section', *Birth*, vol. 34, no. 4, pp. 331–40.

Gideon, J & Minte, G A 2015, 'What is hindering progress? The marginalization of women's sexual and reproductive health and rights in Brazil and Chile', *Journal of International and Comparative Social Policy*, vol. 31.

Gilson, L, Schneider, H & Orgill, M 2014, 'Practice and power: a review and interpretive synthesis focused on the exercise of discretionary power in policy implementation by front-line providers and managers', *Health Policy and Planning*, vol. 29, pp. iii51–iii69.

Hagopian, F 2008, 'Latin American Catholicism in an age of religious and political pluralism: a framework for analysis', *Comparative Politics*, vol. 40, no. 2, pp. 149–68.

Lehmann, U & Gilson, L 2013, 'Actor interfaces and practices of power in a community health worker progamme: a South African study of unintended policy outcomes', *Health Policy and Planning*, vol. 28, pp. 358–66.

Murray, S F & Elston, M A 2005, 'The promotion of private health insurance and the implications for the social organization of healthcare: a case study of private-sector obstetric practice in Chile', *Sociology of Health and Illness*, vol. 27, no. 6, pp. 701–21.

Pierson, P 1994, *Dismantling the welfare state? Reagan, Thatcher and the politics of retrenchment*, Cambridge University Press, New York.

Sandall, J, Benoit, C, Wrede, S, Murray, S F, Van Teijlingen, E & Westfall, R 2009, 'Social service professional or market expert? Maternity care relations under neoliberal healthcare reform', *Current Sociology*, vol. 57, no. 4, pp. 529–53.

UNDP 2010, *Regional Human Development report for Latin America and the Caribbean 2010 – acting on the future: breaking the intergenerational transmission of inequality*, United Nations Development Programme, New York.

UNICEF 2017, Maternal mortality fell by almost half between 1990 and 2015 http://data.unicef.org/maternal-health/maternal-mortality

United Nations 2017, Gender Equality Observatory for Latin America and the Caribbean, http://www.cepal.org/oig/ws/getRegionalIndicator.asp?page=02&language=spanish

Vargas, V & Poblete, S 2008, 'Health prioritization: the case of Chile', *Health Affairs*. vol. 27, pp. 782–92.

WHO 2010, *Gender, women and primary health care renewal: a discussion paper*, World Health Organization, Geneva.

WHO 2016, *Global Health Observatory data repository*, http://apps.who.int/gho/data/node.main.REPWOMEN39

WHO 2017, *Health statistics and information systems* http://www.who.int/healthinfo/global_burden_disease/estimates_country/en/

Trade agreements have substantial effects on well-being and livelihoods, including on health. The harmonization of intellectual property protection laws and its consequences for access to medicines are perhaps the most familiar. But the consequences on various social determinants of health – the conditions in which people live, work and die – are probably more important, yet indirect and much harder to assess (McNeill et al., 2017).

In this chapter we look at the possible risks free trade agreements pose to the health of workers. First we give an insight into the changing power relations that have shaped the global trade framework in the last few decades. Before going deeper into the issue of the health of workers, we take a short look at the impact of trade agreements on various aspects of health, such as government revenue, nutrition, and access to medicines and healthcare services. Finally, we look at how trade agreements impact employment and working conditions, and the health of workers.

From WTO to free trade agreements

For almost half of the last century, the General Agreement on Tariffs and Trade (GATT) was the most important international framework shaping the global trade regime. GATT was formed in 1947 with the objective of reducing the barriers to international trade. Therefore, multilateral agreements were negotiated in different 'rounds' to reduce tariff barriers, quantitative restrictions and export subsidies.

Since the end of the Cold War, the ascent of neoliberal globalization has accelerated the expansion of international trade. Trade liberalization was promoted by international institutions as an important economic strategy towards development and poverty reduction. Consequently, the Uruguay Round of the GATT negotiations (1986–1993) gave birth to the World Trade Organization (WTO), which came into being on 1 January 1995. Unlike GATT, which only had a small secretariat, the WTO covers a scope that is much more encompassing. When it was established, GATT had 23 contracting parties and was limited to trade in goods. Today, the WTO has 164 members (who account for over 97 per cent of world trade), and includes trade in goods and services and the protection of intellectual property rights. By contrast, global health governance exhibits little structural coherence, a greater diversity of actors and approaches, and weaker legal obligations on states (Fidler, Drager & Lee 2009, pp. 325–31).

The member countries of the WTO have been negotiating the Doha Development Round since 2001. The name 'development' was added by the rich countries to bring on board the developing countries who were more interested in assessing the existing WTO agreements than engaging in new negotiations. There was also the promise to take into account their concerns. However, the Doha Round is characterized by a ratcheting up of the demand for 'market access' by rich countries – with tariff cuts of up to 55 per cent. Negotiations at the Doha Round have been stuck since the WTO Ministerial meeting at Cancun in 2003 when developing countries refused to commence discussions on the so called 'Singapore Issues' – investment, government procurement and competition.

Since then, the USA and EU have moved to negotiate bilateral treaties with different countries and currently both are pursuing free trade agreements (FTAs) with individual countries and groups of countries. These bilateral agreements do not replace but complement commitments under the WTO and cover a wide range of issues, including investments, trade in services, intellectual property rights, competition policy and government procurement. Often the provisions that were blocked by low- and middle-income countries (LMICs) at the WTO negotiations are now being repackaged in the bilateral FTAs.

A recent study comparing 74 previous agreements, which the Trans–Pacific Partnership (TPP) signatories have signed since 1995, concluded that negotiations can best be thought of as a competition among states to insert their vision for trade cooperation into an important new agreement (Allee and Lugg, 2016). This enhances an often-made point that FTA negotiations between a developing country and a developed country pose additional reasons for concern (Third World Network, 2009):

- FTAs are usually negotiated with little transparency or participation from the public. Civil society involvement during the negotiations is generally very limited or even non-existent. This stands in contrast to the involvement of private lobby groups. For example, 85 per cent of the committee members during the TPP negotiations in the USA consisted of trade advisers of private industry and trade groups (McNamara & Labonté 2016, pp. 1–21).
- Developing countries are usually in a weaker bargaining position due to the lack of capacity of their economies, their weaker political situation and their weaker negotiating resources. These power asymmetries are especially evident in the investor-state dispute settlement (ISDS) provisions. (See Chapter D5.)
- In the WTO, the principle of special and differential treatment (for developing countries) is recognized. Developing countries are, on paper at least, not obliged to open up their markets (or undertake other obligations) to

the same degree as developed countries. Most FTAs, on the other hand, are based on the principle of reciprocity.

- On issues that are the subject of rules in the WTO (for example, intellectual property and services), flexibilities are available to developing countries in interpreting and implementing obligations. However, developed countries attempt to remove these flexibilities for developing countries in the FTAs.

As we can see, existing power imbalances between the global North and the South are reflected in the rules established by trade agreements; they tend to deepen inequalities in multiple ways. (McNeill et al., 2017).

Trade impacts health in several ways1

The FTAs are blueprints for future bilateral and regional trade agreements and include a rewriting of the rules that govern the global economy, promoting corporate interests at the expense of public health priorities. These agreements go further than the traditional trade agreements that concerned themselves only with import and export tariffs, and also influence production rules and standards. Inevitably, their broader scope has more widespread consequences for economies and societies. They are influential in shaping employment, access to technologies, environmental pollution and sustainability, and many other social determinants of health."(McNeill et al., 2016)

FTAs cause a loss of government revenue by the abolition or lowering of tariffs on cross-border trade. As tariffs on cross-border trade represent a significant proportion of government revenues in the poorest countries, this loss limits the capacity of these countries to implement social policies and to make investments in vital sectors such as health and education. For many LMICs, raising public revenues through alternative forms of taxation is not feasible due to their weak formal sectors and the socially regressive nature of consumption taxes. It is projected that middle-income countries are likely, through taxation, to recover only 45–60 per cent of lost revenue (foregone as a result of reduction in tariffs), and low-income countries at best 30 per cent or less (Baunsgaard & Keen, 2005).

Second, and contrary to what is often believed, healthcare in developing countries can be very profitable, so commercial interests are involved. The health sector is one of the fastest growing sectors in the world economy. Consequently, the liberalization of services remains a crucial point in FTAs. Clauses relating to the liberalization of trade in services, including healthcare, encourage commercialization and privatization of health services. The increasing international trade in healthcare services takes different forms: healthcare workers move abroad to work (thus accentuating the health worker crisis in LMICs) , foreign investors invest in hospitals, and insurance companies search for new markets. Moreover, more and more countries try to attract consumers from different countries to promote so-called health tourism (Pollock and

Price, 2003). Opening the health sector to foreign competition through trade agreements lock countries into a situation where privatization of health services becomes irreversible (Legge, Sanders and McCoy, 2009).

Third, high standards of intellectual property rights (IPRs) are now an integral part of FTAs. Provisions in FTAs on IPRs demand stronger protection than those provide in the TRIPS agreement under the WTO. While the TRIPS agreement has been criticized for having a detrimental impact on access to medicines, the so-called 'TRIPS Plus' rules in FTAs are further loaded in favour of transnational pharmaceutical corporations and promote monopolies (Oxfam International, 2009). Access to affordable medicines is compromised, both by limiting the ability of governments to expand coverage and by limiting the ability of poor people to pay for medicines out-of-pocket (WHO, 2006).

Finally, policies that promote trade can lead to alterations in diet and the nutrition status of the population. For example, average tariffs in Central America declined from 45 per cent in 1985 to around 6 per cent in 2000 and food imports, especially of processed foods, more than doubled. This directly influenced the availability and price of processed foods, many of which are energy-dense and high in fats, sugars and salt (Thow and Hawkes, 2009). These trends have been accompanied by rising rates of obesity and chronic diseases, such as cardiovascular disease and cancer. Poor households are most sensitive to changes in food prices are more likely to shift to cheaper processed foods. Trade liberalization also promotes penetration of supermarkets and multinational fast-food outlets, and drives up consumption of alcohol and tobacco (Blouin, Chopra and Van der Hoeven 2009, pp. 502–07).

The rise of precarious employment and its impact on health

Trade also indirectly impacts health through its impact on employment and working conditions. (McNamara and Labonté 2016, pp. 1–21). Labour conditions can affect health of workers, families and communities in a negative way, especially if they are in what is called 'precarious employment'. There is no consensus on the definition of precarious employment, but Benach et al. (Benach et al., 2016, pp. 232–38) surmise that "[P]recarious employment might be considered a multidimensional construct encompassing dimensions such as employment insecurity, individualized bargaining relations between workers and employers, low wages and economic deprivation, limited workplace rights and social protection, and powerlessness to exercise workplace rights." Over the past decade, evidence has accumulated that demonstrates a consistent association between precarious employment and several dimensions of health (Benach et al., 2016, pp. 232–38).

In general, precarious work – such as informal work, temporary work, contract work, child labour and slavery/bonded labour – is associated with poorer health status. Evidence indicates that mortality is significantly higher among temporary workers as compared to permanent workers. Poor mental health outcomes are associated with precarious employment. Workers who perceive work insecurity experience significant adverse effects on their physical and mental health (WHO, 2008).

There are important differences amongst countries, according to the labour standards and social protection policies in place. For example, the relationship between job insecurity and poor health is less in countries with more extensive social security systems, which improve the ability of individuals to cope with stressful events (Bambra, 2011, pp. 746–50). More severe adverse effects on health can be expected in countries with limited social protection (McNamara and Labonté, 2016, pp. 1–21).

On the other hand, redistributive social policies result in better population health outcomes (Wilkinson and Pickett, 2009). While precarious and informal employment is becoming more prevalent, acceptable labour standards and social protection extend only to a proportion of the growing number of workers. The enforcement of labour standards is typically restricted to formal markets, and the availability of social protection is usually restricted to standard, formal employment relationships, and not to different forms of precarious employment relationships (McNamara and Labonté, 2016, pp. 1–21).

Historically, precarious employment was common. Thanks to increased government regulation, better labour standards and social protection policies, precarious employment declined in the developed countries. Currently, precarious employment is again becoming more common in developed countries, and is still widespread in developing countries (Benach and Muntaner, 2007, pp. 276–77). The main causal factors in the rise of precarious employment are the processes of globalization, including trade (McNamara and Labonté, 2016, pp. 1–21).

Since the increase in global market integration in the 1970s, the dominance of neoliberalism has translated into a new model of economic development oriented towards productivity and supply of products to global markets. Institutions and employers wishing to compete in this market argue the need for a flexible and ever-available global workforce (Benach, Muntaner and Santana, 2007; WHO, 2008). Thus a race to the bottom for maintaining competitive prices has been initiated at the expense of workers' rights, leading to a shift away from job or employment security towards 'flexible' employment practices (Scott-Marshall and Tompa 2011, pp. 369–82).

The emergence of a 'new international division of labour' is exemplified by the relocation of labour-intensive production to sites in the developing world, selected on the basis of low wages and minimal social protection for workers (WHO, 2008). An example of this practice is the *maquilas* (manufacturing companies located in *zonas francas* or free trade zones, producing garments for export) in Mexico and Central America. Here working conditions are under constant pressure because of the lethal competition between companies. The North American Free Trade Agreement (NAFTA), enforced in 1994,

Box C4.1: Working women suffer most

Protection and benefits provided are generally poorer for women than men. Women are typically employed in lower paid, less secure and informal occupations. For equivalent work, women worldwide are paid 20–30 per cent less than men (WHO, 2008). When employment and working conditions worsen under the pressure of free FTAs, women are the first to be affected.

In addition, precarious working conditions have a serious impact on workers' social protection. In most countries social security systems are linked to formal employment (International Labour Organization, 2013). Informal workers (the majority of whom are women) do not receive a pension and get no unemployment allowance, no maternity leave or allowance, no replacement income when sick, and no reimbursement of medical expenses. While trade liberalization leads to more informalization and casualization, this has an effect on workers' social protection, hitting women particularly hard.

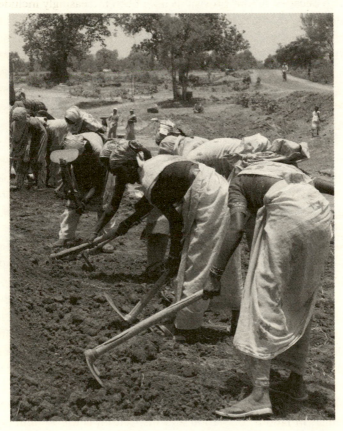

Image C4.1
Working women suffer most (Sulakshana Nandi)

drastically lowered import tariffs among the USA, Canada and Mexico, thus making it more beneficial for American businesses to relocate their production to Mexican *maquiladoras*. It is estimated that the USA and Canada lost up to 750,000 jobs due to NAFTA. Further, 65 per cent of American companies threatened to relocate production away from the USA if they were not allowed to lower wages (Amadeo, 2017).

Precarious employment is particularly prominent in the informal economy, especially in LMICs where employment conditions are unregulated (Benach and Muntaner, 2007, pp. 276–77). Trade liberalization has contributed to an increase in informalization and casualization across the globe (ILO, 2016). At the same time trade liberalization has negative effects on unionization of workers and their bargaining power of employees (ILO, 2013). The disempowerment of workers and their unions has gone hand in hand with the increasing power of large transnational corporations and multilateral institutions and their influence on policies on labour (WHO, 2008).

Labour provisions in free trade agreements: a solution?

Over the past two decades, labour provisions have been increasingly included in free trade agreements, to counterbalance the negative impact of trade liberalization on employment and working conditions and to ensure that labour standards are upheld or improved, rather than put at risk. The ILO defines labour provisions as "any standard that addresses labour relations or minimum working terms or conditions, mechanisms for monitoring or promoting compliance, and/or a framework for cooperation". They are becoming a common tool for promoting labour standards, with over 80 per cent of agreements entering into force since 2013 (International Labour Organization, 2016). But do these provisions really benefit workers, or are they just window dressing? Some observers argue that they will make trade more socially sustainable, others believe such provisions are intended more to limit domestic opposition to new trade and investment agreements than to ensure protection of labour rights (McNamara and Labonté, 2016, pp. 1–21).

In its latest report on this topic, the ILO (2016) concludes that it's hard to make general statements about the effectiveness of labour provisions because labour market outcomes vary according to the context, and depend strongly on governments' and institutions' capacity to implement and monitor labour rights and working conditions. Although the findings are not fully generalizable, several case studies have showed that capacity-building activities, monitoring and involvement of those affected in the framework of labour provisions, were associated with positive institutional and legal changes, and, in some cases, improvements in working conditions.

An example of an FTA with a labour chapter, which has brought about some positive changes in labour legislation and inspection, is the Dominican Republic–Central America FTA (CAFTA–DR) with Honduras.[2] In 2005

Box: C4.2: Work that kills slowly: banana workers in Ecuador

(This section draws on the work of De Ceukelaire and Vervoort (2010).

About 90,000 people work in the banana plantations in Ecuador. Ecuador is the world's leading banana exporting country (30 per cent), mainly producing for the EU market. Through the global supply chain, big companies compete to undercut others, and their buying power allows them to manipulate the market. The prices paid to banana producers by the supermarkets are forced down. And as producer prices are squeezed, production costs, such as labour costs, are forced down. Although Ecuador has signed the ILO conventions on fundamental labour rights — even incorporated them into the national legislation — the level of compliance is inadequate. The systematic violation of environmental, safety and labour standards by many fruit producers is well documented.

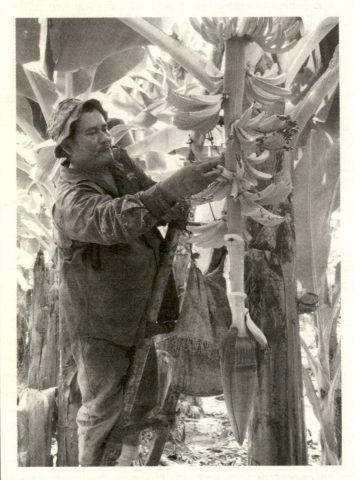

Image C4.2
Banana worker in Ecuador (Julie Steendam)

Workers testify that the work at the plantations is harsh, precarious and underpaid. Most workers are paid under the piece-rate system (payment linked to productivity), and many of them don't get the minimum wage of US$ 366. In most cases, women are paid less for the same work as compared to men. For many workers, the salary isn't sufficient to meet the basic needs of their families, such as healthy nutrition, adequate housing and clothing. Working days of 14 hours aren't an exception, and due to exhaustion there's an increased risk of suffering occupational accidents. In addition, workers generally don't receive the necessary protective clothing, which adds to the risk of their cutting themselves, being bitten by insects or snakes, or being poisoned by agrochemicals. The use of pesticides poses great risks to workers. A recent study (AGU, 2016) comparing workers exposed to pesticides with workers at organic plantations where no chemicals are used, shows that workers in conventional banana production (where extensive use of pesticides is common) suffer significantly more health problems. They suffer from eye and skin irritations (banana workers are often called *losmanchados* or 'the speckled', because of the stains on their skin), fatigue and insomnia. They are also at a six-to eight-times higher risk of developing gastrointestinal symptoms such as nausea, vomiting and diarrhoea. The study also says that workers exposed to pesticides are more likely to develop cancer.

The precarious working conditions have become worse over the years and informal work is increasing. Because of this, workers usually have little or no access to social protection. If they try to organize to change their situation, they may be blacklisted or threatened. Consequently, they are afraid to stand up for their rights, because losing their job means not having any income at all.

Honduras ratified this trade agreement between the USA, Central America and the Dominican Republic. The agreements include an extensive chapter on labour. In 2012, Honduran trade unions, together with the American Federation of Labour, and Congress of Industrial Organizations filed a complaint (Honduras Submission, 2012) stating that several articles of the labour chapter were being violated by the Government of Honduras. Labour inspectors from the US Ministry of Labour went to Honduras for an investigation and found that labour rights were violated in sectors such as the *maquilas* and the agro-industry. In order to comply with its obligations under CAFTA, the Ministry of Labour of Honduras had to agree to an Action Plan. An important step was the approval of a new Labour Inspection Law, more stringent than the previous one. Representatives from trade unions believe this to be an important step forward. However, trade unions warn about the continuing and widespread violation of labour rights in Honduras and significant progress is still to be made.

However, the positive impact of labour provisions is not always a given. As the ILO report (ILO, 2016) states, the impact of these provisions depends crucially on the extent to which they involve different actors, especially those who are adversely affected. A number of these provisions make explicit reference to the involvement of such actors. Nonetheless, the implementation and use of these mechanisms is still very limited in practice. Also, overall transparency is limited, particularly in negotiation processes.

In a prospective analysis of the labour chapter of the TPP, McNamara and Labonté (2016, pp. 1–21) have tried to identify how the TPP can potentially affect health through labour market pathways. Although the TPP has a comprehensive labour chapter, there is little evidence to support the claim that it effectively addresses the negative impact of trade liberalization on labour. Instead, there are several ways in which the TPP might weaken employment relations to the detriment of health. The provisions related to labour standards and rights are unlikely to increase the power of workers and thereby improve employment relations important for health (ibid.). The TPP labour chapter refers to the ILO Declaration on Fundamental Principles and Rights at Work, but in fact that serves merely as a reaffirmation of the membership of countries in the ILO, without providing any incentive or obligation to ratify and implement the eight corresponding Core Conventions of the ILO. A related concern is that reference to the ILO Declaration can result in weak and elastic interpretations of labour rights. The ILO Declaration, unlike the Core Conventions, references broad and undefined fundamental rights. This means that signatory countries may find a potentially divergent and inadequate range of domestic measures to be satisfactory in meeting minimum labour standards. The provisions dealing with the implementation side of the chapter are largely ornamental and seem to offer little in terms of concrete improvements for employment or working conditions. The chapter's stipulations are also found to unevenly distribute power to the detriment of workers, and they establish the priority of trade and market regulation over workers' rights.

A common concern raised is that labour provisions or the so-called Sustainable Development Chapters in trade agreements often lack binding, stringent rules, as regards monitoring and enforcement of the provisions. In a recent study designed to document the specific threats to workers' rights embodied in the Transatlantic Trade and Investment Partnership (TTIP), AnetaTyc (2017, pp. 113–28) finds that the TTIP "implies disregard for workers' rights". Gaps include the lack of mandatory ratification of core labour conventions, the lack of a sanction mechanism in the case of failure of ratification of core conventions by a member of the ILO and the lack of a body that can monitor and assess compliance with commitments connected with the protection of workers' rights.

The future for trade agreements

Supporters of FTAs claim that trade contributes to global economic growth and job creation. But what does this mean, if this growth isn't contributing to improvement of employment and working conditions, better living standards and health for all? Claims that increased trade leads to economic growth and well-being are contradicted by facts. The unacceptably high levels of global inequality, consequence of a failed wealth distribution system, are now recognized as a serious threat by even the International Monetary Fund (IMF), long-time champion of neoliberal policies and structural adjustment (Nunn and White, 2016, pp. 186–231). If employment growth following the implementation of new FTAs is mainly in precarious or informal employment, as the evidence from other trade reforms would suggest, any potential economic and health benefits for workers will be, at best, limited (McNamara and Labonté, 2016, pp. 1–21).

We can conclude that trade agreements result in negative effects on health through various pathways, such as through its negative effect on employment and working conditions. "A flexible workforce may boost economic competitiveness, but brings with it negative effects on the health of workers", concluded the WHO Commission on the Social Determinants of Health (WHO, 2008).

That is why there is an urgent need to think beyond a framework that is bound by the neoliberal recipes of further deregulation, less government control and market liberalization. Adding labour chapters is clearly insufficient since their legal status is often less binding than other provisions directly linked to trade, such as ISDS mechanisms.

Treaties on trade, investment and intellectual property rights often undermine public health. Provisions that are obviously bad for public health, including TRIPS Plus provisions and the liberalization of health services, should never be part of free or any trade agreements. Moreover, developing countries should be compensated for revenue losses arising from lower tariffs by developed countries who demand lowered removal of tariff barriers.

Notes

1 This case draws upon the following sources: AGU (2016), and Oxfam Deutschland (2016)

2 Interview with representatives from Federación de Trabajadores de la AgroIndustria (FESTAGRO), CGT (Central General de Trabajadores) and RSM (Red de Sindicatos de la Maquila).

References

AGU 2016, Investigación epidemiológica sobre los pequeños productores y los trabajadores grícolas en la agricultura convencional y orgánica (banano) en Ecuador, 31 March, https://cumbreagrariaecuador.files. wordpress.com/2017/02/aegu_reporte-pesticidas-bananos_parte1.pdf

Allee, T & Lugg, A 2016,'Who wrote the rules for the Trans-Pacific Partnership?' Research & Politics, vol. 3, no. 3, DOI10.1177/2053168016658919.

Amadeo, K 2017, 'Do NAFTA's 6 pros outweigh its 6 cons?' The Balance, 13 February, https://www.thebalance.com/nafta-pros-and-cons-3970481

Bambra, C 2011, 'Work, worklessness and the political economy of health inequalities', *Journal of Epidemiology & Community Health*, vol. 65, no. 9, pp. 746–50.

Baunsgaard, T & Keen, M 2005, *Tax revenue and (or?) trade liberalization*, IMF working paper, WP/05/112.

Benach, J & Muntaner, C 2007, 'Precarious employment and health: developing a research agenda', *Journal of Epidemiology & Community Health*, vol. 61, pp. 276–77.

Benach, J, Muntaner, C & Santana, V 2007, 'Employment conditions and health inequalities. Final report to the WHO Commission on Social Determinants of Health', Employment Conditions Knowledge Network http://www.who.int/social_determinants/resources/articles/emconet_who_report.pdf

Benach, J, Vives, A, Tarafa, G, Delclos, C & Muntaner, C 2016, 'What should we know about precarious employment and health in 2025? Framing the agenda for the next decade of research', *International Journal of Epidemiology*, vol. 45, no. 1, pp. 232–38.

Blouin, C, Chopra, M & Van der Hoeven, R 2009,'Trade and social determinants of health', *The Lancet*, 7 February, vol. 373, no. 9662, pp. 502–07.

De Ceukelaire, W & Vervoort, K 2010, *The EU's bilateral FTA Negotiations are a threat to the right to health*, Platform for Action on Health and Solidarity – Working Group on North-South Solidarity Issues.

Fidler, D, Drager, N & Lee, K 2009, 'Managing the pursuit of health and wealth: the key challenges', *The Lancet*, 24 January, vol. 373, no. 9660, pp. 325–31.

Honduras Submission 2012, *Public submission to the Office of Trade and Labor Affairs (OTLA) under chapters 16 (Labor) and 20 (Dispute Settlement) of the DR-CAFTA*, 26 March, https://www.dol.gov/ilab/reports/pdf/HondurasSubmission2012.pdf

International Labour Organization 2013, 'Social dimensions of free trade agreements', *Studies on Growth with Equity*, Geneva.

International Labour Organization 2016, 'Assessment of labour provisions in trade and investment agreements', *Studies on Growth with Equity*, Geneva.

Legge, D, Sanders, D & McCoy, D 2009, 'Trade and health: the need for a political economic analysis', *The Lancet*, vol.373, no. 9663.

McNamara, C & Labonté, R 2016, 'Trade, labour markets and health: a prospective policy analysis of the Trans-Pacific Parntership', *International Journal of Health Services*, pp. 1–21.

McNeill, D, Birkbeck, C D, Fukuda-Parr, S, Grover A, Schrecker, T & Stuckler, D 2017, 'Political origins of health inequities: trade and investment agreement', *The Lancet*, vol. 389, no. 10070.

Nunn, A & White, P 2017, 'The IMF and a new global politics of inequality?' *Journal of Australian Political Economy*, vol. 78, pp. 186–231.

Oxfam Deutschland 2016, *Frutasdulces, verdadesamargas*, https://www.oxfam.de/system/files/oxfamalemania_bananoypina_20160531.pdf

Oxfam International 2009, *Trading away access to medicines: how the European Commission's trade agenda has taken a wrong turn* http://www.oxfam.org/en/policy/trading-away-access-medicines

Pollock, A & Price, D 2003,'The public health implications of world trade negotiations on the general agreement on trade in services and public services', *The Lancet*, vol. 362.

Scott-Marshall, H & Tompa, E 2011, 'The health consequences of precarious employment experiences', *Work*, vol. 38, pp. 369–82.

Tyc, A 2017,'Workers' rights and transatlantic trade relations: the TTIP and beyond', *The Economic and Labour Relations Review*, vol. 28, no. 1, pp. 113–28.

Third World Network 2009, *EU EPAs – economic and social development implications: the case of the CARIFORUM-EC economic partnership agreement*, viewed 6 January 2010, http://www.twnside.org.sg/pos.htm

Thow, A & Hawkes, C 2009,'The implications of trade liberalization for diet and health: a case study from Central America', *Globalization and Health*, vol. 5, no. 5. Viewed 10 April 2010. http://www.globalizationandhealth.com/content/5/1/5

Wilkinson, R & Pickett, K 2009, *The spirit level: why more equal societies almost always do better*, Penguin, London.

WHO 2006, *Public health, innovation and intellectual property rights*, Report of the Commission on Intellectual Property Rights, Innovation and Public Health (CIPIH),

WHO 2008, *Closing the gap in a generation. Health equity through action on the social determinants of health*, http://www.who.int/social_determinants/thecommission/finalreport/en/

C5 | PUBLIC HEALTH IN THE EXTRACTIVE SECTOR IN EAST AND SOUTHERN AFRICA*

Equity and development in East and Southern Africa

Countries in East and Southern Africa (ESA) have significant biodiversity and considerable genetic, mineral and other natural resources. Resources available in this region are enough to satisfy the basic social determinants of health. However, the Human Development Index (HDI) improved in only five of the sixteen ESA countries between 1997 and 2005, despite growing economies in most of these countries (EQUINET, 2012). For example, the Democratic Republic of Congo (DRC), a global leader in strategic mineral reserves, hydroelectric power and other natural resources has one of the lowest official per capita GDPs in the region (EQUINET Steering Committee, 2007).

ESA countries with higher levels of aggregate wealth have also had higher levels of inequality in wealth, suggesting that growth paths are not addressing the inequality and may be intensifying it (EQUINET, 2012). In an analysis of trends in the 16 ESA countries, inequality, measured by the Gini coefficient, appeared to be a critical factor limiting household access to resources, a phenomenon that was observed to have been intensifying since 1995 (EQUINET Steering Committee, 2007). An analysis of 70 developing and transition economies in the 1990s similarly found rising relative inequality to be a barrier to poverty reduction (Ravallion, 2005). This makes equity a key issue for health and social development in ESA countries, raising a policy demand for more inclusive economic growth and a wider distribution of its benefits (AU Commission, 2015).

Such discourses on economic pathways are not unique to the ESA region. The significant structural asymmetries, social deficits and inequality in the global economy have led to debates over development in many parts of the world. They have sought to identify alternative relationships between society, economy and the environment to address universal rights and strengthen human capacities, build a more harmonious relationship with nature, balance the liberating qualities of work and leisure, reconstruct the public sector and build a representative, participatory democracy (Boron, 2015). The '*buen vivir*' paradigm in several Latin American countries, for example, critiques the equation of progress with economic growth, when this is at the cost of intense exploitation of nature and significant social inequality. It focuses on the well-being and quality of life of the individual and community, and integrates the social rights of current and future generations as a collective or common good and in a balance with nature (Gudynas, 2011). Health systems, and the choices, organization and implementation of public health services, play a role in achieving this common good.

Health in a region of increasing extractive activities[1]

Most ESA countries are richly endowed with mineral reserves, providing an important source of export earnings and investment (Yager et al., 2012). Africa accounts for 70 per cent of the world's cobalt production, 57 per cent of diamond production and 19 per cent of gold and uranium production (ibid.). African minerals have been sought after for centuries by high-income countries (HICs) and more recently by emerging economies (AU and United Nations Economic Commission for Africa, 2007; Besada and Martin, 2013). The ownership of mines, referred to as extractive industries (EIs), is highly concentrated. In South Africa, for example, five companies were reported to account for 85 per cent of the total mine ownership (Munnik, 2010).

Countries rich in mineral resources also experience high levels of inequality and poverty – a situation often referred to as 'the resource curse' (Global Witness, 2012). While the extraction and export of unprocessed raw materials may lead to rapid growth, it is often unsustainable and not accompanied by higher value-added processing activities in African countries (ibid.). Trade in unprocessed natural resources thus accounted for nearly 80 per cent of African exports in 2000, compared to 31 per cent for all developing countries (Commission for Africa, 2005). EI activities lead to periods of economic boom, but with equally fast declines when commodity prices fall (African Union, 2009). They are commonly 'enclave' activities, using imported equipment, and technical, financial and managerial services and with refinement and processing taking place outside ESA countries. They, thus, create limited linkages with the national economy and limited job opportunities outside the EIs themselves (Catholic Relief Services, 2011). While they contribute through taxes, they also get significant tax concessions, including exemptions on value-added tax on imports or export sales, waiver of customs duty on imports and exports, lower corporate income tax rates, lower withholding tax rates and reductions on taxes on profits and royalties (Lambrechts et al., 2009).

EIs present a number of benefits. The benefits largely come from the jobs, income security and other benefits for those directly employed, from the EI's tax contribution and from the social services some EIs provide to employees and their families. They may also contribute to local capacity-building and investment in infrastructure (Shelton and Kabemba, 2012).

They also bring health risks. Besides a high rate of accidents and risk to workers from hazardous working conditions, environmental and other ills affect the health of workers and of the wider community. Poor infrastructures and living conditions, degradation of ecosystems, air and water pollution and poor social conditions in communities living around mines raise the risk of

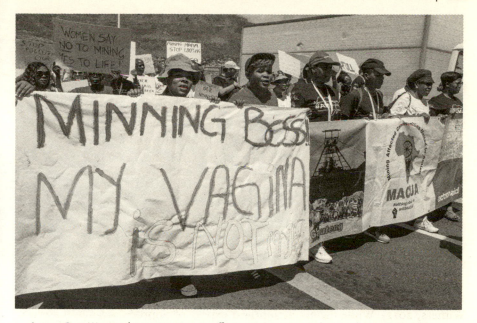

Image C5.1 Women demonstrate again effects on extractive industries (Louis Reynolds)

disease. Income differentials and insecure employment in some EI activities have been associated with increased alcohol consumption, commercial sex work and sexually transmitted infections (STIs).

The commencement of EI activity may displace local people, affecting their living and social conditions, their economic activities and health (Catholic Relief Services, 2011). Displacement has been reported, for example, of the San communities in Botswana to facilitate diamond mining; in Marange, Zimbabwe, to facilitate diamond-mining; in Tete province, Mozambique, of approximately 2,500 families, to facilitate coal mining (GEF, OSISA & UNDP, 2013; Human Rights Watch, 2013). Poorly planned involuntary resettlement of communities to enable EI activities has led to loss of livelihoods, loss of access to water, depletion of flora, arable land and pastures for livestock, and conflict between communities and the mining companies over unfulfilled commitments (Human Rights Watc,h 2013; Kabemba & Nhancale, 2012).

In addition, there are numerous health risks associated with specific EI processes (Table C5.1), quite apart from the risks of accident and injury at work and the ill-effects of noise pollution associated with mining.

Low-income communities living around the mines are particularly vulnerable to pollutants, given their poor living conditions. They are also least able to obtain reliable information on health risks or to register their concerns with decision-makers (Catholic Relief Services, 2011). A study of communities adjacent to 800 mines across 44 low- and middle-income countries, including countries in ESA, found that lead and heavy metals possibly present within a 5-kilometre radius of mines depressed blood haemoglobin in women, with a 3–10 per cent increase in the incidence of anaemia as compared to control groups in areas not close to the mines. It was found that the affected women recovered more slowly from blood loss during pregnancy and delivery, and their children had stunted growth due to in-utero exposure to lead and heavy metals (Von der Goltz and Barnwal, 2014).

TABLE C5.1: Risks to health in mining activities

Mining of	Potential risks
Coal	Inhalation of CO_2, nitrogen, sulphur oxides and hydrocarbons causes eye, nose and throat irritation. It can lead to black lung disease, silicosis and skin diseases and complicate TB. Radionuclides can lead to respiratory diseases, lung cancer and gastrointestinal problems. Communities living near mines are exposed to carbon, nitrogen gas, mercury, cadmium, copper, nickel, ammonia and fluoride, and to water, soil and air pollution from waste and fly ash spills. Abandoned mines can lead to sinkholes and heavy metal contamination.
Gold	Exposure to asbestos, silica dust and arsenic increases the risk of lung disease and lung, liver and oesophageal cancer. Mercury contamination of water, soil and food raises the risk of pulmonary, gastrointestinal, neurological and renal diseases, and reproductive risks in female workers. Health is also affected by mine contamination of water and stress to water tables. Unlined mine tailings and silicosis elevate the risk of TB.
Diamond	Illegal trading, money laundering, criminal activity and violence have been reported.
Uranium	Exposure to fine particles of uranium and to radon gas increases the risk of bronchial and lung cancer, leukaemia, stomach cancer, silicosis, chromosome mutations and birth defects. Radioactive and heavy metal contamination of groundwater, the use of waste rocks from mines to improve roads, and radioactive metal reuse by locals to make utensils and other goods raises the risk of birth defects, cancer and immune impairment. Water extraction can reduce the groundwater table, with risk of toxicity from pumping contaminated water back into rivers and lakes, and from arsenic in tailing ponds of abandoned mines.
Copper	Long-term exposure to copper dust causes respiratory irritation, headaches, dizziness, nausea and diarrhoea. Water with high levels of copper may cause nausea, vomiting, stomach cramps and diarrhoea.
Cobalt	There is risk of asthma, pneumonia, and metal lung disease due to chronic exposure to dust and fumes. Dermal exposure can result in contact dermatitis.
Oil and gas	Pollution and environmental destruction from oil spills, waste dumping and gas flares are damaging to soil fertility and agricultural productivity. Threats to food security may occur due to the shift away from agriculture.
Energy (hydro power)	There are health risks from asbestos dust, lubricants and insulation products, as well as electrical hazards and risks from equipment contaminated with polychlorinated biphenyls. Environmental changes increase risks of flooding, and reduction of water supply and of the fish population downstream.

Source: Adapted from Loewenson, R, Hinricher, J & Papamichail, A, 2016 pp 8–9

International norms to promote fair benefit from EI activities

For ESA countries, the contradiction between the EIs' potential economic contribution and the reality of poor returns for local communities and economies is driving demand to implement policy choices that link the finite stock of natural resources to wider well-being and a more sustainable development. The *African Mining Vision* (African Union 2009, p. 3), for example, seeks to make the mining sector contribute to growth and development in a way that is "sustainable and well-governed", that "effectively garners and deploys resource rents and that is safe, healthy, gender and ethnically inclusive, environmentally friendly, socially responsible and appreciated by surrounding communities" (ibid.). Various initiatives taken by Africa states have begun to strengthen and take forward this policy intention. The African Commission on Human and People's Rights has established a Working Group on Africa to examine and propose responses to the impact of the extractive industries on human rights and the environment (Manirakiza, 2012). The Economic Community of West African States (ECOWAS) has set a directive on the harmonization of guiding principles and policies in the mining sector, while the Southern African Development Community (SADC) with the UN Economic Commission for Africa (UNECA) is advancing the harmonization of mining policies, standards, legislative and regulatory framework in Southern Africa (African Union 2009; Murombo 2013, pp. 31–49; United Nations Economic Commission for Africa 2004)

"These policy initiatives are consistent with international standards, codes and guidance documents. Various United Nations (UN) instruments have elaborated upon the governance of EIs and natural resources, and the duties in relation to human rights principles set out in UN declarations, including the right to health in the International Covenant on Economic, Social and Cultural Rights (ICESCR). The Organization for Economic Co-operation and Development (OECD), covering the states in which many of the multinational enteprises (MNEs) operating in the sector are headquartered, has set the „Guidelines for MNEs and due diligence guidance for responsible supply chains of minerals from conflict-affected and high-risk areas". Financial institutions investing in EIs, such as the International Finance Corporation (IFC), have set performance standards for EI operations (Equator Principles, 2006; International Finance Commission, 2010). The International Council on Mining and Metals (ICMM), the organization of mining and metals companies, has established the 'ICMM 10 Principles' for sustainable development in the mining and metals industry (ICMM, 2017). Civil society, through the Natural Resource Charter „offers policy options and practical advice for governments, societies and the international community on how best to manage resource wealth" (Natural Resource Governance Institute, n.d.).

The health-related content of the standards is detailed in Loewenson, et al. (2016). Collectively, the standards provide for

- consultation, impact assessment and protection of health in the negotiation of prospecting rights, including rights to culture, identity, employment, education and fair benefit-sharing
- health and social protection in the resettlement/relocation of affected communities
- occupational health and safety (OHS) for employed workers and subcontractors
- health benefits for workers and their families
- environmental, health and social protection for surrounding communities, and access to remedy where harm has occurred
- EI fiscal contributions for health promotion and healthcare
- fair local benefit from EI activities, and
- transparent, democratic and accountable governance of these issues by government, civil society and affected communities and industry on an equal footing.

Efforts are under way to move some of these international norms into practice. For example, the Extractive Industries Transparency Initiative (EITI) has been actively promoted and used in many ESA countries, among others, Mozambique, the DRC, Zambia and Madagascar, to advance EI transparency and accountability, with public reporting of their activities (Moffatt and Haralampieva, 2014, pp. 4–13; Von der Goltz and Barnwal, 2014. In South Africa, the 2009 King Committee Report on Corporate Governance has sought to bring local companies in line with global best practices (GEF, OSISA and UNDP, 2013). Kenya has similarly sought to adopt the UN Guiding Principles on Business and Human Rights in its emerging oil and gas sectors by initiating 'The Nairobi Process: A Pact for Responsible Business' (Samuel, 2015).

Variable application of international standards

A comprehensive review of the national constitutions and their provisions for health and occupational health and of the environmental, labour, mining and company laws of the 16 ESA countries reveal that some elements of the international standards relating to health are found in different ESA countries, but no country covers them completely (Loewenson et al., 2016). The protection of health during negotiations on prospecting rights and EI agreements is largely pursued through environmental impact assessments (EIAs). Only a few countries, such as Kenya and Zambia, have explicitly included health or social impacts in EIAs, and none explicitly requires health sector approval of EIAs. There are weak *specific* provisions for health and social protection in relocating affected communities, with poor representation of directly affected communities in decision-making and grievance redressal. Occupational health and safety, and workers' compensation, is universally provided for in all ESA countries for employed workers and contractors in the mining sector. Fewer countries, however, include healthcare or medical surveillance for workers, their families and the larger community, as this is regarded as a matter for voluntary corporate social responsibility. Some countries, such as Angola, Kenya, Mozambique and the DRC, require that municipalities in mining areas benefit directly from a share of the taxes, and others such as South Africa and Zimbabwe have provisions for historically disadvantaged people to benefit from mining, potentially yielding resources for health services and infrastructures. Newer environment laws now cover healthy environments, including for the surrounding communities, but their 'polluter pays' remedy may leave public health harms unresolved. Further, while laws in most ESA countries include the obligation of ensuring environment and public safety after mine closure, none have provisions for the handing over of social service obligations post-closure with regard to occupational lung diseases and other chronic conditions (Loewenson et al., 2016).

Moreover, even where laws do exist, there may be gaps in their implementation. The World Health Organization has noted that health issues often trigger claims against EIs, but are not often the basis for corrective action, given difficulties in establishing the burden of proof in relation to health and environment and the lack of uniform interpretation of what health responsibilities imply, especially if there is no public sector implementation of health impact assessments (WHO, 2011). Shelton and Kabemba (2012, p. 197) note from studies in Angola, the DRC, Mozambique, South Africa, Zambia and Zimbabwe that "Legislative and policy shortcomings are...not the most important constraint...the most serious problem is the gap between what the law or policy says should happen and what does happen."

In many countries, and particularly in those with new mining operations, the state has appeared to be less well prepared to manage the social issues in the rapidly growing EI sector, and laws were often introduced after social reaction or pressure. In Mozambique, for example, the legal instrument to guide resettlement was introduced in 2012, following community unrest due to poor resettlement conditions. In Malawi, the churches and local non-governmental organizations (NGOs) took court action to block uranium mining until appropriate laws were in place (Catholic Relief Services, 2011).

Multinational EIs are often more highly resourced technically and financially than the states or communities they operate in, generating asymmetrical interactions, especially when actively supported by the governments of their source countries (African Union, 2009; Shelton and Kabemba, 2012). The volatility in the minerals market weakens the negotiating power of states to demand tax reforms and measures for social benefit, especially at times of falling commodity prices (Lambrechts et al., 2009; Lungu, 2008). The same executive who oversees the regulation of EIs also encourages their economic contribution, and a desire to set investor-friendly outcomes impacts on the willingness to enforce fair-benefit conditions (African Union, 2009; Murombo,

2013). This ambivalence has led civil society to express doubts as to whether the interests of citizens is ever prioritized over that of EIs and to demand the inclusion of community representatives in the oversight of agreements (Shelton and Kabemba, 2012; Ujamaa Centre and Institute for Law and Environmental Governance, 2010).

States face capacity deficits that weaken the regulation of EIs, including in relation to qualified staff, infrastructure, information, technology and financial resources (Human Rights Watch, 2013; Kabemba, 2014). Further, even when they do act, the fines imposed are reported in many cases to be too low to have a deterrent effect (Human Rights Watch, 2013).

Fiscal contributions for public sector interventions and voluntary corporate social responsibility thus often become the primary means, *de facto*, for addressing public health in EIs. With respect to fiscal contributions, a range of practices exist. Zambia, Zimbabwe and Tanzania have increased metal royalties to improve public revenues; Zambia has implemented a windfall tax on 'super-profits' from EIs; and South Africa has proposed a capital gains tax of 50 per cent on sales of prospecting rights (De Backer, 2012; Kabemba, 2014; Lambrechts et al., 2009). The DRC in 2014 introduced a micro-levy on EIs of US$ 0.10 on every barrel of oil sold by the state, with the funds to be used to fight chronic malnutrition (Innovative Finance Foundation, 2014). Some countries (South Africa and Zimbabwe) have set targets for a share of public revenues earned from operations of EIs for historically disadvantaged people, while others have obtained direct state ownership in EIs (such as Zimbabwe, the DRC, Zambia, Botswana, Namibia and Mozambique (Kabemba, 2014). Others, such as Botswana and Zimbabwe, have established a sovereign wealth fund, to build reserves from current resources for the well-being of future generations (Mutonhori, 2014).

As is the case for all fiscal contributions, these revenue flows may not go to health, especially given the poor performance in the ESA regions in meeting the Abuja commitment of 15 per cent of government spending on health (EQUINET Steering Committee, 2012). Financial contributions are more likely to have potential benefit for communities affected by mining if there are fiscal and investment rules that align with equity and avoid elite capture, are accompanied by clear responsibilities and ethical standards, and are subject to regular audits and public disclosure, and strong and independent oversight and enforcement of fund rules (De Backer, 2012; Mutonhori, 2014; Zimbabwe Environmental Law Association, 2011).

In practice, however, the significant tax incentives that many EIs get may reverse the public revenues gained from these initiatives, especially when there are 'no change' clauses in agreements with EIs that promise to not amend such incentives for substantial periods of time, regardless of law reforms (Lungu, 2008, pp. 403–15). In Zambia, for example, when the government introduced a windfall tax in response to protests over EI tax incentives, it remained bound

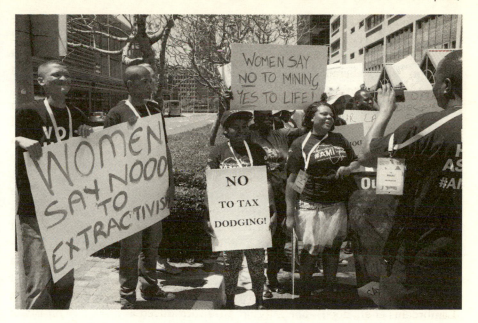

Image C5.2 Protest against mining and tax dodging in South Africa (Louis Reynolds)

to earlier incentives through such a 'stability period' in the existing agreements, restricting its policy space to act (ibid.). Poorly negotiated contracts, tax concessions and various creative accounting mechanisms by MNEs are estimated to have cost countries significant revenues, with annual estimates as follows: South Africa, US£ 359–499 million in 2006; Tanzania, US$ 29 million annually between 2002 and 2006; Malawi, US$ 16.8 million; and the DRC, US$ 0.36 million annually between 2001 and 2003 for a single-mine contract (African Union, 2009; Lambrechts et al., 2009).

As a second *de facto* approach, voluntary corporate social responsibility (CSR) takes various forms, such as through donating funds or technical resources to support health services and epidemic control; investing in non-mine social development programmes and providing grants for community health programmes, infrastructure and services (International Institute for Environment and Development, 2002; Lambrechts et al., 2009). The use of a share of profits for public good evidently has benefits. However such voluntary activity does not address the health determinants that arise from EI activities and may focus on visible and physical projects, reflecting corporate public relations concerns more than local community or national health system priorities (Lange and Kolstad, 2012). Left to decisions taken in corporate boardrooms, voluntary CSR has no commitment to involve affected communities or their representatives or state officials; nor does it set obligations that can be monitored, reviewed and publicly reported (Brereton, Owen and Kim, 2011).

The demand for more direct social voice and accountability

There is a recognition that those affected by EI activities have a right to participate in decisions that affect their health and livelihoods. Most ESA countries provide constitutional rights to information, association, assembly and participation and provide for tripartite consultation on occupational health. Newer laws include duties of public information and consultation, while some countries (the DRC, Mozambique, Kenya, Tanzania) provide for informed participation of the affected local communities in EI governance and resttlement plans, and prohibit public officers from acquiring mining interests to protect against conflicts of interest. Tanzania's Extractive Industries (Transparency and Accountability) Act has, for example, provisions for transparency, the inclusion of civil society in an independent oversight committee with disclosure obligations on EIs, and measures for public reporting and citizen awareness on agreements (Loewenson et al., 2016).

States and civil society institutions have cooperated in legal reviews and consultations in the EI sector (Massawe, 2010; Twesigye, 2010). Workers, unions and the government in Zambia have, for example, successfully exercised joint pressure for first aid kits and ambulances to be provided at mines (Human Rights Watch, 2013 Shelton and Kabemba, 2012). Environmental law reforms have led to representation from affected communities and civil society in the oversight of EI activities, with accompanying actions to build local community capacities to rightfully claim and use information and to participate in processes (Ujamaa Centre & Institute for Law and Environmental Governance, 2010).

In some countries, however, the state is formally assumed to represent the interests of the communities, weakening their direct formal voice (Murombo, 2013). This may involve only employed workers with a more direct and formal means of engagement with EIs, often around wage demands (De Backer, 2012). There is some debate as to who makes up the 'local community', and to what extent those identified as leaders or representatives can be trusted to put forth community views and claims. Further, civil society itself is noted to be weak in relation to the significant power of EIs (Kabemba, 2014; Murombo, 2010).

A gap between what *should* exist and what *does* exist in relation to the social and health impacts and obligations of EIs has led to social protest (Bambas-Nolen et al., 2013). For example in Mozambique in 2011, resettled communities in Tete province voiced their concerns about poor resettlement conditions in a letter to the company and local government. When they did not get a response a month later, they took part in a demonstration that blocked the railway transporting the coal, leading to police action and arrests (Human Rights Watch, 2013). Civil society has also protested against procedural issues. For example the Zimbabwe Environmental Law Association (ZELA) walked out of the Kimberley Process Intersessional Meeting in 2011 due to perceived executive disrespect towards civil society (Zimbabwe Environmental Law Association, 2011).

A demand for a meaningful voice in the face of perceived deficits in state protection has led to a range of civil society actions: for example, the People's Mining Indaba was organized as a counter-event to the Stakeholders' Mining Indaba (Bambas-Nolen et al., 2013). In Kenya, perceiving inadequate action by local state authorities, a coalition of a civil society organizations (CSOs) brought cases to the Kenya National Commission on human rights in the early 2000s. This legal action was taken on behalf of communities in Malindi district affected by forcible evictions, health and safety and worker's rights violations, environmental degradation, and harassment by companies undertaking salt mining in the area (Ujamaa Centre & Institute for Law and Environmental Governance, 2010). In Malawi, local CSOs took the government to court for constitutional and environmental law violations in the negotiations over a uranium mine in Kayalekere. The CSOs alleged that an environmental impact study had not been conducted, that the agreement had been kept a secret, and that the project should not have progressed in the absence of national laws to regulate uranium mining (Lambrechts et al., 2009).

While the demand for information and participation in decision-making by those affected is their right, it is also a matter of health equity. When local communities do not participate in decision-making or in acting on or preventing the impacts of mining, they "bear a disproportionate share of the costs of mineral development without adequate compensation, and receive an inappropriately small share of the economic and social benefits" (International Institute for Environment and Development, 2002, p. 208), particularly when there is poor response to their grievances (Human Rights Watch, 2013).

Steps to advance health equity in relation to extractive industries

The evident contradictions within the extractive sector in Africa has raised questions at all levels, from community to international, on what choices to make to generate wealth in a manner that does not sacrifice the health and well-being of future generations. The evidence of the health impacts of EI activities, of the gaps and variations in ESA country laws in relation to international standards, and the power assymetries between global corporate actors and the states and communities they interact with suggests that ESA countries may benefit from regional processes to strengthen their ability to protect health. The findings validate the policy intention to harmonize these standards at the regional level, to avoid a downward competitive push on standards and to support those countries with newly emerging or growing EI sectors. While no single ESA country addresses all the required standards of health and social welfare in EIs in their laws, in combination the laws across ESA countries can provide guidance (Loewenson et al., 2016).

At the same time, the evidence suggests the need to close the gap between law and practice, through raising public awareness of rights and duties in the sector, and building evidence and capacities for the implementation of these duties, such as through health impact assessments. Models of corporate social responsibility often promote public–private partnerships, partnering often weak local authorities with powerful EI companies. However, the evidence suggests a need for strengthened *public–public* partnerships, between affected communities, civil society and state institutions, and across different public sectors, to promote population health. The range of determinants of health in EIs point to the interconnections between the choices made on environment, employment, production, infrastructure, fiscal policy and trade, and their consequences for health.

What is the role then for health sectors in the ESA region? What expectation may communities have as they watch wagons carry their natural resources away, as they breathe air pollutants that leave them short of breath, watch huge infrastructures rise while they don't have access to safe water or sanitation, or are displaced from their cultural roots, homes and livelihoods?

Certainly, communities would expect the state to exercise the public health authority it has in law and to detect and prevent harm to health, no matter what institution is causing it. They would expect that their countries would collect the evidence and regulate commercial interests that are harmful to health, even if this means confronting their economic power. They would expect the public health sector to not only make commitments for what it will do, but also to move from the limited confines of disease programmes and medical care services to raise and advocate 'bottom lines' of what rights and obligations must be secured from others to protect public health. They would expect that in doing this, the health sector, as a people-driven sector, would build strong partnerships by involving the people.

* The evidence cited from literature on health in the extractive sector draws on Loewenson, Hinricher and Papamichail (2016). The chapter also draws on other evidence to offer analysis, discussion and conclusions that are the author's alone.

References

African Union 2009, *Africa mining vision*, AU, Addis Ababa.

AU Commission 2015, *Agenda 2063: the Africa we want*, AU, Addis Ababa.

AU & United Nations Economic Commission for Africa 2007, *Accelerating Africa's development through diversification*, Ethiopia.

Bambas-Nolen, L, Birn, A E, Cairncross, E 2013, *Case study on extractive industries*, prepared for *The Lancet* –University of

Oslo Commission on Global Governance for Health.

Besada, H & Martin, P 2013, *Mining codes in Africa: emergence of a 'fourth' generation?* The North–South Institute, Ottawa.

Brereton, D, Owen, J & Kim, J 2011, *Good practice note: community development agreements*, Centre for Social Responsibility in Mining, Brisbane.

Boron, A 2015, *Buen vivir (sumak kawsay) and the dilemmas of the left governments in Latin America*, http://climateandcapitalism.com/2015/08/31/buen-vivir-and-dilemmas-of-latin-american-left/

Catholic Relief Services 2011, *Extractives and equity: an introductory overview and case studies from Peru, Angola and Nigeria*, CRS, Baltimore, MD.

Commission for Africa 2005, *Our common Interest: Report of the Commission*

for Africa, London. http://www.
commissionforafrica.info/wp-content/
uploads/2005-report/11-03-05_cr_report.pdf

De Backer, S 2012, Mining investment and
financing in Africa: recent trends and key
challenges, Webber Wentzel, Johannesburg.

Equator Principles 2006, The equator
principles, viewed 1 May 2017 http://
equator-principles.com/resources/
equator_principles.pdf

EQUINET Steering Committee 2007,
Reclaiming the resources for health: a
regional analysis of equity in health in East
and Southern Africa, EQUINET, Weaver
Press, Zimbabwe; Fountain Publishers,
Uganda; Jacana, South Africa.

EQUINET 2012, Regional equity watch 2012,
EQUINET, Harare.

GEF (Global Environment Facility), OSISA
(Open Society Initiative for Southern
Africa) & UNDP (United Nations
Development Programme) 2013, Land,
biodiversity and extractive industries in
southern Africa: how effective are legal
and institutional frameworks in protecting
people and the environment? GEF,
Washington DC; OSISA, Johannesburg;
UNDP, New York.

Global Witness 2012, Extractive sector
transparency: why the EU needs a strong
set of rules, Global Witness, London.

Gudynas, E 2011, Transitions to post-
extractivism: directions, options, areas of
action, Uruguay. https://www.tni.org/files/
download/beyonddevelopment_transitions.
pdf

Human Rights Watch 2013, What is a house
without food? Mozambique's coal mining
boom and resettlements, HRW, New York.

ICMM 2017, ICMM 10 principles, https://
www.icmm.com/en-gb/about-us/member-
commitments/icmm-10-principles

Innovative Finance Foundation (IFF) (2014)
'Implementing an extractive industries
micro-levy to fight chronic malnutrition:
Executive summary', Innovative Finance
Foundation: Geneva.

International Finance Commission (IFC) 2010,
Performance standard 5 (rev. 1, 14 April
2010) – land acquisition and involuntary
resettlement, IFC, Washington DC.

International Institute for Environment
and Development 2002, Breaking new

ground: mining minerals, and sustainable
development, Earthscan Publications,
London and Sterling, VA.

Kabemba, C 2014, Myths and mining: the
reality of resource governance in Africa,
SARW and OSISA, Johannesburg.

Kabemba, C & Nhancale, C 2012, Coal versus
communities: exposing poor practices by
Vale and Rio Tinto in Mozambique, SARW,
Johannesburg.

Lambrechts, K, Darimani, A, Kabemba, C &
Olaleye, W 2009, Breaking the curse: how
transparent taxation and fair taxes can turn
Africa's mineral wealth into development,
SARW, TWN Africa, Tax Justice Network
for Africa, ActionAid and Christian Aid,
Johannesburg.

Lange, S & Kolstad, I 2012, 'Corporate
community involvement and local
institutions: two case studies from the
mining industry in Tanzania', Journal of
African Business, vol. 13, no. 2, pp. 134–44.

Loewenson, R, Hinricher, J & Papamichail, A
2016, Corporate responsibility for health in
the extractive sector in East and Southern
Africa, EQUINET discussion paper 108,
Training and Research Support Centre,
Harare, www.EQUINETafrica.org/sites/
default/files/uploads/documents/EQ%20
Diss108%20EIs%20and%20health2016.pdf

Lungu, J 2008, 'Copper mining agreements
in Zambia: renegotiation or law reform?'
Review of African Political Economy, vol. 35,
no. 117, pp. 403–15.

Manirakiza, P 2012, Report of the working
group on extractive industries, environment
and human rights violations in Africa,
African Commission on Human and
Peoples' Rights, Banjul.

Massawe, E S 2010, 'Securing rights of
communities against state and private
sector actions in the mining sector:
experiences from the Tanzania lake region
mining sites, in Mtisi, S (ed), Securing
environmental, economic, social and
cultural rights in the natural resources
sector, ZELA, Harare.

Moffatt, P & Haralampieva, V 2014, 'Through
the looking glass: the role of the Extractive
Industries Transparency Initiative (EITI) in
sustainable resource development', Law in
transition, Spring 2014, pp. 4–13.

Munnik, V 2010, The social and environmental

consequences of coal mining in South Africa, Environmental Monitoring Group, Cape Town; Both ENDs, Amsterdam.

Murombo T (2010) 'Conceptual framework for implementation and enforcement of environmental, economic, social and cultural rights in Southern Africa: Challenges and opportunities' in S Mtisi (ed) Securing environmental, economic, social and cultural rights in the natural resources sector. Zimbabwe Environmental Law Association (ZELA): Harare. 4-12.

Murombo, T 2013, 'Regulating mining in South Africa and Zimbabwe: communities, the environment and perpetual exploitation', *Law, Environment and Development Journal*, vol. 9, no. 1, pp. 31–49.

Mutonhori, N 2014, *A commentary on the Sovereign Wealth Fund Act of Zimbabwe*, ZELA, Harare.

Natural Resource Governance Institute n.d., *Natural resource charter*, https://resourcegovernance.org/sites/default/files/NRCJ1193_natural_resource_charter_19.6.14.pdf

Ravallion, M 2005, *A poverty–inequality trade off?* World Bank policy research paper 3579, World Bank, Washington.

Samuel, M 2015, *Mitigating the extractive industries resource curse in East Africa: adopting the UN Guiding Principles on Business and Human Rights*, AfricLaw, https://africlaw.com/2015/05/04/mitigating-the-extractive-industries-resource-curse-in-east-africa-adopting-the-un-guiding-principles-on-business-and-human-rights

Shelton, G and Kabemba, C (eds) 2012, *Win-win partnership? China, Southern Africa and the extractive industries*, SARW, Johannesburg.

Twesigye, B 2010, Oil, 'Environment and the people: key issues and considerations in the governance of oil resources in Uganda', in Mtisi, S (ed), *Securing environmental, economic, social and cultural rights in the natural resources sector*, ZELA, Harare.

Ujamaa Centre & Institute for Law and Environmental Governance (ILEG) 2010, 'Securing community assets in mining areas: case of salt mining in Kenya', in Mtisi, S (ed), *Securing environmental, economic, social and cultural rights in the natural resources sector*, ZELA, Harare.

United Nations Economic Commission for Africa 2004, *Harmonization of mining policies, standards, legislative and regulatory frameworks in Southern Africa*, UNECA, Addis Ababa; SADC, Gaborone.

Von der Goltz, J & Barnwal, P 2014, *Mines: the local wealth and health effects of mining in developing countries*, viewed 1 May 2017 http://cdep.sipa.columbia.edu/sites/default/files/cdep/von%20der%20Goltz%20and%20Barnwal%20Mines%202014%20with%20Appendices.pdf

WHO 2011, *Environmental law: an instrument to promote and protect health in extractive industries*, WHO, Geneva.

Yager, T R, Bermúdez-Lugo, O, Mobbs, P M, Newman, H R, Taib, M, Wallace, G J & and Wilburn, D R 2012, *2010 Minerals Yearbook – The Mineral Industries of Africa*, US Geological Survey, Reston, VA.

Zimbabwe Environmental Law Association 2011, *Update and analysis of extractive sector and mining issues in Zimbabwe*, ZELA, Harare.

C6 | THE WAR ON DRUGS: FROM LAW ENFORCEMENT TO PUBLIC HEALTH

"I believe that drugs have destroyed many lives, but wrong government policies have destroyed many more". Kofi Annan, speech to the World Health Assembly, 19 May 2015

Since the mid-twentieth century global drug policy has been dominated by strict prohibition, with the use of punitive law enforcement to try and reduce the illicit drug trade. This approach, which has come to be known as 'war on drugs', is not working. Not only has it failed to achieve its goals, it has also fuelled poverty, undermined health and failed some of the poorest and most marginalized communities worldwide.

Just like trade policy, tax avoidance and climate change, current global drug policies clearly undermine public health, yet campaigners on poverty and global justice, and to a lesser extent the health community, have remained largely silent on drug policy. Despite this, a growing recognition of the failure of the war on drugs and a move towards adopting a public health approach are gathering pace around the world.

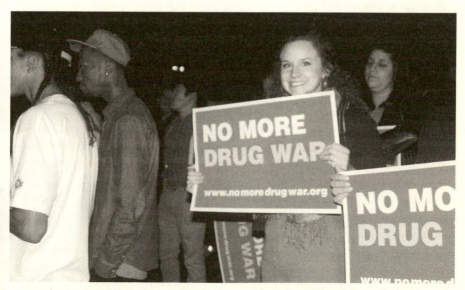

Image C6.1 A Rally & Concert to End the War on Drugs, MacArthur Park, Los Angeles, 3 November 2011 (Nikki David / Neon Tommy; License: CC BY-SA 2.0, https://creativecommons. org/licenses/by-sa/2.0/)

Drug policies – public health impacts

The war on drugs impacts health – in particular that of the poor and marginalized – in a number of ways. These include the following:

Direct health impacts By driving drug use underground and into criminal markets, strict prohibition means there are no controls on drug strength and purity, and criminal sanctions for the possession of drugs and drug paraphernalia mean that drug injection is frequently done with unsterile equipment in unsafe conditions. This increases the rates of overdose and infectious disease among people who use drugs (Keefer and Norman, 2010).

Enforcement activities such as aerial drug crop spraying, most prevalent with the chemical herbicide glyphosate (Guyton et al., 2015, pp. 490–91), which the WHO declared a likely carcinogen in 2015, have been identified as causing damage to eyes and skin, as well as miscarriages (Count the Costs, n.d.). Although Colombia suspended the dangerous practice of aerial spraying with glyphosate in 2015 (the last country in the Americas to do so), South Africa continues to spray harmful herbicides from the air on inaccessible areas of cannabis cultivation, endangering the health of some of the most marginalized communities in the country (De Greef, 2016).

Restricted access to medicines In a speech to the World Health Assembly on 19 May 2015, Kofi Annan said that "Under current drug control policies, African access to essential medication for pain management is highly restricted". Stringent implementation of the international drug control treaties restricts access to essential (mainly pain) medicines for the populations of entire countries. This is because unduly restrictive regulations aiming to combat the non-medical, illicit market have resulted in highly restricted access to controlled drugs for essential medical purposes.

Five and a half billion people, or 80 per cent of the world's population, living in countries largely in the Global South, have limited or no access to essential medicines such as morphine for pain relief (Hallam, 2014). Ninety per cent of the world's AIDS patients and 50 per cent of global cancer patients living in low- and middle-income countries, have access to only 6 per cent of the morphine used for pain management globally (West African Commission on Drugs, 2014).

A 2010 Human Rights Watch report found that hundreds of thousands of children in Kenya suffer from AIDS, cancer and other chronic or fatal illnesses that cause severe and debilitating pain, which could be easily alleviated by opioid medicines. Many of them were suffering in unnecessary pain due to the widespread unavailability of these medicines as a result of strict legal and regulatory barriers, despite the medicines being classified as essential by the WHO (Box C6.1) and the Kenyan government (Human Rights Watch, 2010).

Box C6.1: Inaccessibility of essential opioid medicines in India

Access to controlled essential medicines, such as morphine and other opioids for pain relief, became severely limited in India as a consequence of the 1985 Narcotic Drugs and Psychotropic Substances (NDPS) Act. The NDPS Act introduced highly cumbersome licensing procedures to obtain opioids and significant penal penalties for very minor infringements, leading to fear of penalization among pharmacists and medical professionals for even minor clerical errors. This has contributed to a widespread aversion to stocking or prescribing these drugs (Rajagopal, 2007, pp. 615–22).

Different norms exist across state-level legislations and policies on licensing, the maximum days' supply of opioids allowed in a single prescription (varying between six and thirty days), dispensing procedures for pharmacies and allowances for emergency prescriptions and corrections (Cleary et al., 2013). A 2014 amendment to the 1985 NDPS Act was intended to address the impact of these regulatory barriers and improve access to opioids for medical purposes. However, these legislative changes have not yet been properly implemented across the majority of Indian states, and many of the barriers to access, as well as the culture of fear stemming from the 1985 Act, still continue to limit access to controlled essential medicines across large regions of India. The availability of essential opioid analgesics in India is among the lowest in the world; according to data from the WHO and the International Narcotic Control Board (INCB), India was ranked 117 out of 144 for the availability of morphine in 2014 (Pain and Policy Studies Group, 2015).

The continuing disparity in the availability of essential opioid analgesics across the states and between urban and rural areas in India means that in many cases patients and their families must travel hundreds of kilometres to these medicines. Interviews conducted in New Delhi, Gujarat and Punjab in 2017 (Health Poverty Action, forthcoming) give first-hand accounts of advanced stage cancer patients and their family members being forced to travel very long distances every month, in some cases across multiple states, to access essential opioid pain relief medicines, with the travel alone costing 40–80 per cent of the family's monthly income and in several causing families to incur debts (this does not even account for the additional costs of purchasing the medicine itself). As one cancer patient interviewed in Ahmedabad, Gujarat, said:

"I have travelled 450 kilometres from my town called Bhilwara in the state of Rajasthan to come here because morphine is not [readily] available there...I have had pain before also, but I started to have pain so strong I could not bear it since March. It is very difficult for me to come here and also for my family to accompany me. It takes 10 hours to travel from my town to here and costs 800 rupees per person. As my family is accompanying, for four of us it costs 3,200 rupees per month to come by train. Our family's income in total however is only 5,000 rupees a month. We cannot pay for the travel costs from our income, so we have had to take loans with interest from other people in our town".

In a number of cases people have been forced to quit work to care for their family members, including to undertake these long journeys with them or on their behalf to collect medicines. Children are forced to give up school to take up wage labour to fill the gap in the family's income or pay off their debts. In some cases families making these journeys were also regularly forced to leave young children at home without anyone to take care of them. A 37-year-old female patient with stage 4 cancer, also interviewed in Gujarat, said:

"I travel to receive treatment for my disease and now also to ask for the prescription for morphine from a village that is 450 kilometres away from here...My husband is a labourer in construction works, but he quit his job to take care of me, so we had to take a loan. I have three children aged 16, 12 and 10, and the two oldest stopped going to school to go to work as labourers so that the family is able to pay back the loans".

Ketamine, an anaesthetic drug suitable for use in major surgeries performed in resource-poor settings without oxygen or electricity, is also in potential danger of being placed under the same restrictions internationally (International Committee of the Red Cross, 2015). Some anecdotal reports indicate that recent national restrictions in India are having an impact on its availability in health facilities in rural areas.

Restricted access to health services The criminalization of people who use drugs and the social stigma attached to drug use act as strong barriers to accessing medical care and other support services. Women who use drugs face particularly strong stigma, especially pregnant women who are often denied prenatal care and opioid substitution therapy, putting their life and that of their baby in jeopardy (Kensy, 2012; United Nations Office on Drugs and Crime, 2014). Social stigma also constrains state expenditure on narcotic substance abuse treatment services.

Some countries are also unwilling to fund or develop HIV/AIDS treatments for people who use drugs. Among people who inject drugs, less than 4 per cent of those living with HIV globally have access to antiretroviral treatment, which plays a key role in reducing HIV transmission (Harm Reduction International, 2012; Montaner et al., pp. 531–36). Harm reduction services, which provide access to sterile injecting equipment through needle and syringe programmes, are essential in reducing HIV transmission and prevalence (Global Commission on Drug Policy, 2012). Where harm reduction services have been established early on – such as in the UK, Switzerland and the Netherlands – this has curbed HIV epidemics among people who use drugs, whereas countries that continually refuse to implement these life-saving programmes – such as Russia – face elevated HIV prevalence among people who inject drugs (Global Commission on Drug Policy, 2011).

Diverting attention and resources from essential services Many governments are engaged in a constant civil war with drug cartels, a war they are ill-equipped to win. The costs of waging this war, both financial and in terms of dominating space on the political agenda, leave little room for state services and social improvements. Enforcing anti-drug policies costs at least US$ 100 billion a year globally, rivalling the US$ 130 billion worldwide aid budget (Count the Costs, 2012). Reforming drug policies could release substantial funds at both the national and international levels for basic services such as education and health. To take one example, the Overseas Development Institute (ODI) estimates that the additional financing needed to meet the Sustainable Development Goal of universal healthcare is US$ 37 billion a year.[1] Conversely, the annual estimated resource needed for harm reduction globally is just US$ 2.3 billion (Cook et al., 2014).

It is also important to remember that the US$ 100 billion spend on enforcement is only a part of the overall cost of the war on drugs. The extent of the damage inflicted by current drug policies on poor and vulnerable communities is impossible to calculate.

Escalating violence Between 2006 and 2009 at the height of the country's war on drugs, Mexico mobilized 45,000 military troops to combat drug trafficking gangs and increased its federal police force from 9,000 to 26,000 officers (Keefer and Norman, 2010). The Mexican government has estimated that from December 2006 to December 2010, the first four years following the launch of a major offensive against drug cartels, there were 34,612 violent deaths directly related to the war on drugs (Tuckman, 2011). Similarly, in February 2003 Thailand's war on drugs resulted in the extrajudicial killing of approximately 2,800 people, the arbitrary arrest of thousands and the use of extreme violence by the police (Human Rights Watch, 2004).

In recent years, the media in Ghana, Liberia and Sierra Leone has documented incidents of people using drugs being killed or injured by police officers during raids (International Drug Policy Consortium, 2017). More recently, we have seen the shocking extrajudicial killings of over 7,000 people in the Philippines as a result of the approach of President Duterte who ran on an anti-drugs platform (Human Rights Watch, 2017). In March 2016 prior to his election, Duterte had declared, "When I become president, I will order the police to find those people [dealing or using drugs] and kill them. The funeral parlours will be packed."

Undermining democratic governance and state services The power and influence of drug cartels severely weakens states. The corruption this fuels has a devastating impact on attempts to address poverty. It means that officials make decisions in the interests of those bribing them, and exclude ordinary citizens from having a say in holding their governments accountable. The culture of fear and corruption can make it almost impossible for citizens to exert democratic influence, access their rights or hold their officials to account for the quality and reach of essential services.

Increasing poverty and undermining local food production Prohibition has had a severe impact on small-scale farmers who grow drug-linked crops. In the opium growing areas of Southeast Asia and Afghanistan, and the coca growing areas of Latin America, forced drug crop eradication campaigns have led to the destruction of the only means of subsistence for these marginalized farmers and their families, further exacerbating their poverty and vulnerability. In many areas it has created a vicious cycle where illicit crop producers become increasingly dependent on cultivating drug-linked crops to counter the impoverishing effects of eradication (Transnational Institute, 2014).

This approach can also result in the contamination of water supplies and destruction of nearby food crops as a result of aerial spraying. A lack of sequencing in alternative development programmes, which places conditional crop eradication before the establishment of alternative livelihoods, also creates food insecurity and in some cases has led to humanitarian crises requiring emergency food aid (Jelsma and Kramer, 2008).

A turning tide

It is almost always the health of the poorest and most marginalized that bears the brunt of the war on drugs: whether small-scale farmers in Asia and Latin America whose sources of income are destroyed, non-violent drug offenders who make up a large share of people in the criminal justice system in Africa, or people – largely in the Global South – who have limited or no access to essential pain relief medicines (International Drug Policy Consortium, 2017).

Taking a public health approach to drug policy would mean that people who use drugs are no longer targeted for human rights abuses; they could access the health and support services they need. Thus a key barrier to accessing essential medicines currently faced by people across the world would be removed.

Further, if the money spent on enforcing failing drugs laws were to be freed up and spent on public services, it could enormously enhance the quality and reach of state services aimed at improving health.

The recognition of the failure of the war on drugs is growing. A number of countries in both the North and South are already pioneering alternative policies that emphasize harm reduction, public health and human rights. These range from de-penalization or decriminalization (reducing or eliminating penalties for low-level drug offences like possession and use, while trafficking remains illegal) as in the Netherlands and the creation of a market where some drugs are legal but strictly regulated, as with prescription medications, to health and education programmes to help reduce the potential harm drugs can do to people and communities.

An approach in which offences like drug possession or use are reduced from criminal to civil violations, is increasingly being pursued with regard to certain drugs, for example in Jamaica, Belize, Puerto Rico (Metaal and Ten Velde, 2014). In their report on drug decriminalization, Rosmarin and Eastwood (2013) note that around 25 countries have removed criminal penalties on personal possession of some or all drugs. Among others, Colombia, Chile, Mexico, Paraguay, Peru, Spain and Uruguay have decriminalized the possession of small amounts of certain drugs for personal use.

Portugal is perhaps the most cited example of decriminalization, having decriminalized the possession of all drugs in 2001. This was combined with an extensive public health programme aimed at people who use drugs. In spite of the initial fears, decriminalization did not lead to significant increases in drug use and the country has seen a decrease in HIV infections and drug-related deaths, although this has been attributed as much to the shift to a health-centred approach to drugs and its wider health and social policy changes as to its drug policy reforms (Transform, 2014).

The Organization of American States (2013) released a sweeping review of drug policies in the Americas, including a 'Scenarios Report', the first multilateral agency report to seriously consider drug policy reform and legal regulation. The governments of Mexico, Colombia and Guatemala openly called for a genuine discussion on reforming the United Nations' drug policies, which resulted in the 2016 UN General Assembly Special Session on Drugs. They have been joined by the World Health Organization and UNAIDS, both of which have called for the decriminalization of drug use (Bridge, 2014a, 2014b).

Perhaps the most widely discussed approach is the creation of a legal, regulated market for some drugs. Uruguay is now adopting this approach to cannabis, as are the US states of California, Colorado, Washington, Oregon, Alaska, Maine, Massachusetts, Nevada and the District of Colombia, which have all legalized cannabis for recreational use. A recent study from the Colorado Department of Revenue indicates that the presence of a legal market for cannabis has not led to a significant increase in the number of new users; most of the demand is coming from visitors to the state and from people who previously bought cannabis illegally (Light et al., n.d.). Canada will be next to take this approach; its new Cannabis Act plans to legalize and regulate cannabis and the act is anticipated to come into force by July 2018.

What next?

Paul Hunt (2008), special rapporteur on the Right to Health has observed, "I have no doubt that it is now time to develop a human rights based approach to drug policy." It is clear that the recognition that the current drug policy is causing immense suffering and is denying poor and marginalized people their right to health, is swiftly gathering pace.

The debate is often polarized between two extremes – prohibition on the one hand and free market legalisation on the other – and neither of these simplistic positions provides a viable solution to what is a complex public health problem. In reality, the choice is not limited to these two extremes. There is a third set of policy options, which is to use a combination of regulation and legal controls. This is the area that should now be explored.

Drug use should not be a criminal problem requiring law enforcement solutions. It is a public health problem requiring public health solutions. There is no one-size-fits-all approach to drug policy, as the failure of the war on drugs has demonstrated. Policies should be developed to fit the needs, and involve the active participation, of those who are most affected: impoverished drug crop cultivators, people who use drugs, and poor and marginalized communities who rely on non-violent involvement in the trade to meet their basic needs.

We urgently need research into new approaches and public health solutions, including an evidence-based assessment of all policy options. This must be approached innovatively and with a completely open mind, actively encouraging creative new approaches and trialling new policy options.

Note

This estimate covers childhood illnesses, immunization, maternal health, family planning, TB, malaria, HIV/AIDS and health system strengthening, but has some limitations (such as the omission of non-communicable diseases) that are discussed further in Greenhill and Ali (2013).

References

Bridge, J 2014a, *UNAIDS slams Russia and calls for decriminalisation of drug use*, International Drug Policy Consortium, 28 July, http://idpc.net/blog/2014/07/unaids-slams-russia-and-calls-for-decriminalisation-of-drug-use

Bridge, J 2014b, *World Health Organisation calls for the decriminalisation of drug use*, International Drug Policy Consortium, 16 July, http://idpc.net/blog/2014/07/world-health-organisation-calls-for-the-decriminalisation-of-drug-use?utm

Cleary, J, Simha, N, Panieri, A, Scholten N I, et al., 2013, 'Formulary availability and regulatory barriers to accessibility of opioids for cancer pain in India: a report from the Global Opioid Policy Initiative (GOPI)', *Annals of Oncology*, vol. 24, no. 11, https://doi.org/10.1093/annonc/mdt501

Cook, C, Bridge, J, McLean, S, Phelan, M & Barrett, D 2014, *The funding crisis in harm reduction*, International Harm Reduction Association, London.

Count the Costs n.d., *The war on drugs: undermining human rights*, Count the Costs

– 50 Years of the War on Drugs, http://www.countthecosts.org/sites/default/files/Human_rights_briefing.pdf

Count the Costs 2012, *The war on drugs: wasting billions and undermining economies*, Count the Costs – 50 Years of the War on Drugs, London, http://www.countthecosts.org/sites/default/files/Economics-briefing.pdf

De Greef, K 2016, *Cash crops poisoned in Pondoland*, http://www.groundup.org.za/article/cash-crops-poisoned-pondoland/

Global Commission on Drug Policy 2011, *War on drugs*, report of the Global Commission on Drug Policy, Rio de Janeiro.

Global Commission on Drug Policy 2012, *The war on drugs and HIV/AIDS – how the criminalization of drug use fuels the global pandemic*, report of the Global Commission on Drug Policy, Rio de Janeiro.

Greenhill, R & Ali, A 2013, *Paying for progress: how will emerging post-2015 goals be financed in the new aid landscape?* Overseas Development Institute, London.

Guyton, K Z, Dana L, Grosse, Y, E I Ghissassi, F, et al., 2015, 'Carcinogenicity of tetrachlorvinphos, parathion, malathion, diazinon, and glyphosate', *The Lancet Oncology* , vol. 16, no. 5, pp. 490 –91, http://www.thelancet.com/journals/lanonc/article/PIIS1470-2045%2815%2970134-8/abstract

Hallam, C 2014, *The international drug control regime and access to controlled medicines*, The International Drug Policy Consortium and the Transnational Institute, London.

Harm Reduction International 2012, *The global state of harm reduction: towards an integrated response*, Harm Reduction International, London.

Health Poverty Action, forthcoming

Human Rights Watch 2004, *Thailand – not enough graves: the war on drugs, HIV/AIDS and violations of human rights*, vol. 16, no. 8.

Human Rights Watch 2010, *Needless pain: government failure to provide palliative care for children in Kenya*, Human Rights Watch, New York.

Human Rights Watch 2017, *Licence to kill, Philippine police killings in Duterte's 'war on drugs'*, 1 March, https://www.hrw.org/report/2017/03/01/license-kill-philippine-police-killings-dutertes-war-drugs

Hunt, P 2008, *Human rights, health and harm reduction – states' amnesia and parallel universes*, International Harm Reduction Association, https://www.hri.global/files/2010/06/16/HumanRightsHealthAndHarmReduction.pdf

International Committee of the Red Cross 2015, *Joint position of the ICRC and International Federation on the placing of ketamine under international control*, ICRC, Geneva, https://www.icrc.org/en/document/joint-position-icrc-and-ifrc-placing-ketamine-under-international-control

International Drug Policy Consortium 2017, *Drug policy in Africa: towards a human rights-based approach*, 26 April, http://idpc.net/publications/2017/04/drug-policy-in-africa-towards-a-human-rights-based-approach

Jelsma, M & Kramer, T 2008, *Withdrawal symptoms, changes in the Southeast Asian drugs market*, Transnational Institute, Amsterdam.

Keefer, P & Norman L (eds) 2010, *Innocent bystanders: developing countries and the war on drugs*, The World Bank, Washington, DC.

Kensy, J 2012, *Drug policy and women: addressing the negative consequences of harmful drug control*, IDPC briefing paper, International Drug Policy Consortium, London.

Light, MK, Orens, A, Lewandowski, B & Pickton, T n.d., *Market size and demand for marijuana in Colorado*, prepared for the Colorado Department of Revenue, Marijuana Policy Group (MPG), Colorado.

Metaal, P & Ten Velde, L 2014, *Drugs and violence in the Northern Triangle: two sides of the same coin?* Transnational Institute, 8 July, viewed 21 August 2014, http://www.tni.org/article/drugs-and-violence-northern-triangle?context=595

Montaner, J S G, Hogg, R, Wood, E, Kerr, T, Tyndall, M, Levy, A R & Harrigan, P R 2006, 'The case for expanding access to highly active antiretroviral therapy to curb the growth of the HIV epidemic', *The Lancet*, vol. 368, pp. 531–36.

Organization of American States 2013, *Scenarios for the drug problem in the Americas, 2013 –2025*, Organization of American States, Washington, DC, www.oas.org/documents/eng/press/Scenarios_Report.PDF

Pain and Policy Studies Group 2015, *2015 global consumption of morphine (mg/capita)*, University of Wisconsin/WHO Collaborating Centre, http://www.painpolicy.wisc.edu/sites/www.painpolicy.wisc.edu/files/global_morphine.pdf

Rajagopal, M R 2007, 'India: opioid availability – an update', *Journal of Pain and Symptom Management*, vol. 33, pp. 615–22, http://www.painpolicy.wisc.edu/sites/www.painpolicy.wisc.edu/files/india07.pdf

Rosmarin, A & Eastwood, N 2013, *A quiet revolution: drug decriminalisation policies in practice across the globe*, Release, London.

Transform 2014, *Drug decriminalisation in Portugal: setting the record straight*, 11 June, http://www.tdpf.org.uk/blog/drug-decriminalisation-portugal-setting-record-straight

Transnational Institute 2014, *Bouncing back: relapse in the golden triangle*, Transnational Institute, Amsterdam.

Tuckman, J 2011,'Mexico drugs war murders data mapped', *The Guardian*, 14 January, http://www.theguardian.com/news/datablog/2011/jan/14/mexico-drug-war-murders-map#data

United Nations Office on Drugs and Crime 2014, *Women who inject drugs and HIV: addressing specific needs*, policy brief, UNODC, Vienna.

West African Commission on Drugs 2014, *Not just in transit: drugs, state, and society in West Africa*, West African Commission on Drugs, Dakar.

SECTION D

WATCHING

D1 | MONEY TALKS AT THE WORLD HEALTH ORGANIZATION

The World Health Organization (WHO) elected Tedros Adhanom Ghebreyesus as the new director-general at the World Health Assembly (WHA) in May 2017, marking the completion of two four-year terms of the current director-general, Margaret Chan.

The new director-general of the WHO inherits an organization beset with fundamental challenges that threaten the very foundations and founding principles of the organization. The WHO's capacity to intervene on issues related to international health and accomplish its basic norm-setting function has been seriously eroded over the years. The legitimacy of the WHO in affairs related to international health stands compromised. The organization's perceived failure to play a more decisive role in containing the Ebola epidemic in 2014 was met with widespread criticism (Kamradt-Scott, 2016, pp. 401–18). Underpinning the deficiencies in the WHO is its funding crisis, which does not allow the organization to carry out its normative activities. Previous editions of the *Global Health Watch* have referred to WHO's funding crisis. In this chapter, we analyse the roots and consequences of this crisis.

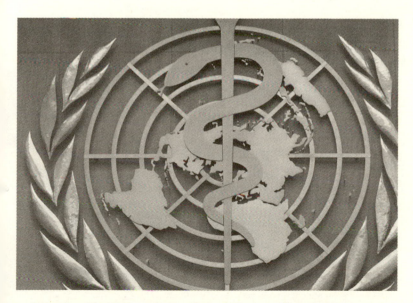

Image D1.1 The WHO Logo. WHO finds it difficult to effectively implement its norm setting activities (Thomas Schwarz)

Who finances WHO

For the last three decades at least, and increasingly, the WHO is burdened with a chronic funding crisis that has jeopardized its mandate and its ability to carry out all of its responsibilities with regard to global public health. The WHO's budget has always been fairly modest, increasing from approximately US$ 900 million in 1998 to about US$ 2,200 million in 2017 (Figure D1.1). The current annual budget of US$ 2,200 million is around 30 per cent of the annual budget of the US Centre for Disease Control (CDC); 4 per cent of Pfizer's turnover; 3 per cent of Unilever's turnover; and around 10 per cent of the annual advertising expenses of pharmaceutical corporations in the USA (WHA Today, 2017).

The WHO's budget is financed through a mix of assessed and voluntary contributions. As with other United Nations (UN) specialized agencies, assessed contributions are required 'membership' contributions to the budget of the WHO from member states, according to a formula based on the size of their economies and populations (Legge, 2011, p.23). Table D1.1 provides details regarding assessed contributions payable by the top 25 (in terms of their contribution) member states as assessed contributions to the WHO's general budget.

As Table D1.1 shows, the assessed contribution that countries are required to make in lieu of their membership in the WHO is extremely low. The gap is made up by voluntary contributions. Such contributions, in the form of either donations or grants, can come from public and private sources, or a blend thereof; they can vary substantially from year to year and lack the predictability needed for early warning disease preparedness and response, on-going standard-setting or capacity-building support.

In the early period after the WHO's formation, assessed contributions constituted the principal source of its budget. In 1971 of the US$ 100 million

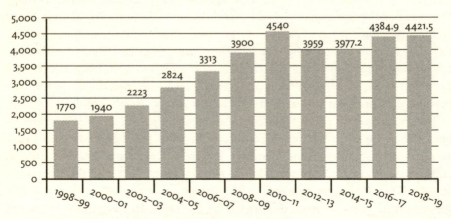

Figure D1.1: WHO biennial budget – 1998–2019 (in US$ million)

Source: Calculated from data for different years available at WHO's budget portal: http://open. who.int/

TABLE D1.1: Assessed contributions by top 25 member states

Country	Per cent of total assessed contributions	Amount of assessed contribution (in US$ million)
USA	22	115.4
Japan	9.7	50.8
China	7.9	41.5
Germany	6.4	33.5
France	4.9	25.5
UK	4.5	23.4
Brazil	3.8	20.1
Italy	3.7	19.7
Russian Federation	3.1	16.2
Canada	2.9	15.3
Spain	2.4	12.8
Australia	2.3	12.3
Republic of Korea	2	10.7
Netherlands	1.5	7.8
Mexico	1.4	7.5
Saudi Arabia	1.1	6.0
Switzerland	1.1	6.0
Turkey	1	5.3
Sweden	1	5.0
Argentine	0.9	4.7
Belgium	0.9	4.6
Norway	0.8	4.5
Poland	0.8	4.4
India	0.7	3.9
Austria	0.7	3.8

Source: Revised assessed contributions payable by member states and associate members 2017(n.d.)

budget, US$ 75 million came from assessed contribution; of the rest, three-quarters was provided by other UN agencies such as the United Nations Development Programme (UNDP) and United Nations Population Fund (UNFPA). By 1986–1987 (biennium), assessed contributions amounted to US4 543 million, matched by other contributions amounting to US$ 437 million. In 1988–1989, for the first time in the WHO's history, extra-budgetary resources exceeded assessed contributions and since then the former has progressively become the dominant source of the WHO's finances (Beigbeder et al., p. 165).

It is important to recall the chain of events that led to the WHO's increasing reliance on extra-budgetary resources. In 1980 the WHA voted to freeze assessed contributions from members in real dollar terms (subject only to currency fluctuations against the dollar) and this took effect with the 1982–1983 budget. This freeze on assessed contributions was applied across the UN system under pressure from donors led by the USA. In 1993 the WHA voted to further freeze assessed contributions by moving from zero real growth to zero nominal growth, removing the possibility of increasing the same based on currency fluctuations and inflation. In the early 2000s the UN General assembly voted to increase UN membership dues but the WHA continued to recommend a freeze on membership dues. Not only were assessed contributions frozen but through the 1980s and 1990s many members failed to pay the assessed membership dues. Thus, for example, in 1989 the WHO was able to collect just 70 per cent of assessed contributions from member states. The largest proportion of funds thus withheld was accounted for by the USA's refusal to pay its dues (Clinton and Sridhar 2017a, pp. 90–91). In 1985 the USA paid only 20 per cent of its assessed contribution to all UN agencies. This move by the USA was interpreted in many quarters as being related to its unhappiness regarding the formulation of the WHO's list of essential medicines, in sync with the opposition to the WHO's work on essential medicines by US pharmaceutical companies (Brown and Cueto, 2010, p. 22; Clinton and Sridhar, 2017b, p. 2). The then WHO director-general, Halfdan Mahler, called this practice 'financial hostage' (Clinton and Sridhar, 2017a, p. 91).

The original intent of the constitutions of specialized UN agencies (such as the WHO) was that approved budgets would be funded through assessed member contributions. Thus a 2007 report of the Joint Inspection Unit of the UN noted that "Notwithstanding the provision for some voluntary funding, the Inspectors believe that, for the most part, the intention in the constitutions was for approved budgets to be funded through assessed contributions of the

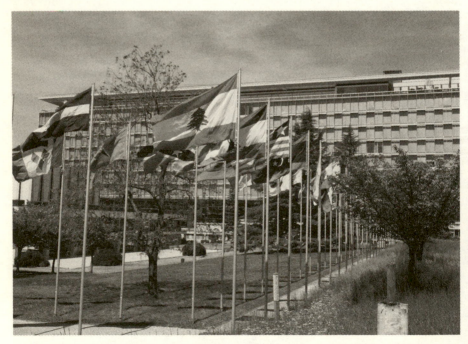

Image D1.2 National flags in front of the UN building in Geneva. WHO is increasingly captive to demands of donors (Thomas Schwarz)

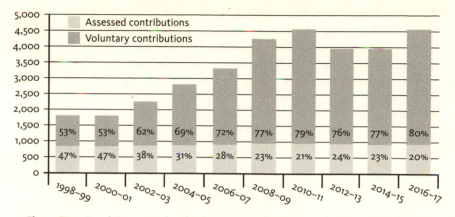

Figure D1.2: Trends in assessed and voluntary contributions, 1998–2017 (in US$ million)

Source: WHO's Financing Dialogue 2016 A proposal for increasing the assessed contribution, http://www.who.int/about/finances-accountability/funding/financing-dialogue/assessed-contribution.pdf?ua=1

Member States" (Yussuf, Larrabure and Terzi, 2007). However, the funding crisis that was precipitated in the 1980s forced UN agencies like the WHO to increasingly rely on voluntary funding from donors – countries, private foundations, other UN agencies and so on. While this succeeded in increasing overall revenue, it enormously increased the relative importance of voluntary contributions, which now make up about 80 per cent of the WHO's total budget (see Figure D1.2).

Voluntary contributions come from member states (in addition to their assessed contribution) or from other donors. These contributions can range from flexible to highly earmarked, that is, tied to a particular programme. Core voluntary contributions are funds provided to the WHO that are fully flexible at the level of the programme budget, or highly flexible at the category level, that is, only tied to a particular category of WHO's programme Core voluntary contributions allow flexibility and less well-funded activities benefit from a better flow of resources and ease implementation bottlenecks that arise when immediate financing is lacking. However, just 7 per cent of all voluntary contributions for the 2014–2015 biennium had been made to the Core Voluntary Contributions Account (WHO, 2016c). Of the total budget of approximately US$ 2.3billion in 2015, assessed contributions accounted for less than a quarter (US$ 463 million). Core voluntary contribution accounted for a meager US$ 116 million and was contributed to by just ten countries (the largest donors were the UK, Sweden and Australia). The remaining US$ 1.7 billion of the budget was contributed to by countries, other UN agencies, partnerships (like the Global Fund to Fight Aids, Tuberculosis and Malaria – the Global Fundor GFATM and Global Vaccines Alliance – GAVI) and foundations (mainly the Bill and Melinda Gates Foundation –the Gates Foundation or BMGF) in the

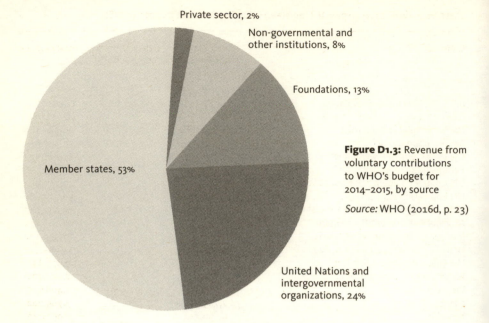

Private sector, 2%

Non-governmental and
other institutions, 8%

Foundations, 13%

Figure D1.3: Revenue from
voluntary contributions
to WHO's budget for
2014–2015, by source

Source: WHO (2016d, p. 23)

Member states, 53%

United Nations and
intergovernmental
organizations, 24%

form of specified (tied to a particular programme) voluntary contributions
(WHO, 2016d). About half of the voluntary tied funding was from countries
(with the USA and the UK accounting for the largest share – US\$ 305 million
and US\$ 157 million, respectively) and the rest from other donors, including
private foundations, intergovernmental organizations, partnerships and so on
(see Figure D1.3).

The imbalance of voluntary in relation to assessed contributions has resulted
in the WHO having less flexibility in its budget allocations, and thus in its ability
to respond to unexpected challenges and maintain its normative responsibilities.
This has been exacerbated as specified funds, those earmarked for particular
projects or programmes, increasingly dominate voluntary contributions.

Embracing philanthropic foundations and corporate engagement

Shortfalls in public funding (that is, from member states), both assessed and
voluntary, have obliged the WHO to turn to private sources, mainly private
and corporate philanthropic organizations. In addition, joint programming with
UN agencies, funds and programmes and contributions from pharmaceutical
companies are noticeable in the top 20 voluntary, non-state contributors (Table
D1.2). Notably none of the non-state contributors provide untied core funds.

As Figure D1.4 shows, the scale of this shift is evident in the fact that
after the US government, the Bill & Melinda Gates Foundation (or BMGF)
was the organization's largest voluntary contributor in 2015 (WHO, 2016c).

Since it began supporting WHO a decade ago, the BMGF has been contributing between US\$ 250 million and US\$ 300 million a year. In one year

TABLE D1.2: WHO's top 20 private (non-state) voluntary contributors 2015 (in US$)

Contributor	Voluntary, contributions specified	Other voluntary contributions[a]	Total revenue
Bill & Melinda Gates Foundation	181,820,644	3,451,881	185,272,525
GAVI Alliance	126,421,673		126,421,673
National Philanthropic Trust	86,252,168		86,252,168
Rotary International	56,302,924		56,302,924
UN Development Programme	46,746,622		47,221,524
European Commission	45,637,006		45,637,006
UN Central Emergency Response Fund	42,219,954		42,219,954
UN Population Fund	30,723,860		30,723,860
UN Fund for International Partnerships	19,276,440	705,687	19,982,127
African Development Bank Group	19,105,011		19,105,011
Joint UN Programme on HIV/AIDS	17,936,172		17,936,172
UNITAID – International Drug Purchase Facility	14,923,517		14,923,517
UN Office for Project Services	9,979,445		9,979,445
Bloomberg Family Foundation	8,424,000		8,424,000
Wellcome Trust	7,314,109	94,496	7,408,605
GlaxoSmithKline	7,769,202		7,769,202
Novartis	6,992,742		6,992,742
Carter Center	6,500,000		6,500,000
UN Children's Fund	6,337,126		6,337,126
Sanofi Pasteur	6,158,152		6,158,152

Source: WHO (2016d, p. 25)

Note: [a] Includes contributions to Contingency Fund for Emergencies; Special Programme of Research, Development and Research Training in Human Reproduction; Stop TB Partnership; and Special Programme for Research and Training in Tropical Diseases

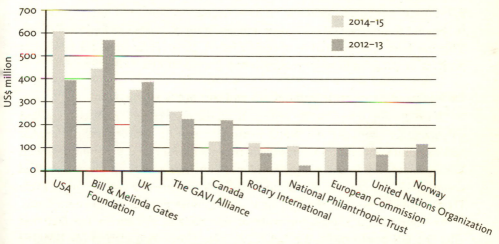

Figure D1.4: Top 10 voluntary contributors to the programme budget 2014–2015 and programme budget 2012–2013 (US$ million)

Source: WHO Programmatic and Financial Report for 2014–15, http://apps.who.int/gb/ebwha/pdf_files/WHA69/A69_45-en.pdf

– 2013 – it was the largest donor bar none, overtaking total contributions from the governments of both the USA and the UK.

The impact of funds from private donors is readily apparent in WHO's spending. One of the priorities of the BMGF is the eradication of polio. A breakdown of the WHO's finances reported in 2016 shows that its polio programme is by far the best-resourced, accounting for 23.5 per cent of the WHO's programme budget (Kelland, 2016).

The BMGF's interest in health is not limited to polio. As a founder and principal donor to GAVI, it has pumped money into massive vaccination programmes (see Chapter D4 on GAVI). It is also a substantial supporter of the health programmes of other UN entities by contributing to the UN Foundation, which in turn channels its resources through the United Nations Fund for International Partnerships (UNFIP). Moreover both GAVI and the UNFIP are listed among the top contributors to the WHO, thereby multiplying the channels of influence that the BMGF can leverage upon. The question remains: How does this relate to governance and accountability? Is there such a thing as governance double-dipping?

BMGF has also been criticized in the past for having a negative effect on research systems. In late 2007 in a highly critical memorandum, head of WHO's malaria programme, Dr Arata Kochi, complained to Dr Margaret Chan, the director general of the WHO, that the Bill and Melinda Gates foundation's money, while crucial, could have "far-reaching, largely unintended consequences." He warned that the growing dominance of malaria research by the foundation risks stifling a diversity of views among scientists and wiping out the world health agency's policy-making function. Many of the world's leading malaria scientists are now "locked up in a 'cartel' with their own research funding being linked to those of others within the group," Dr. Kochi wrote. Because "each has a vested interest to safeguard the work of the others," he wrote, getting independent reviews of research proposals "is becoming increasingly difficult." He added, the foundation "even takes its vested interest to seeing the data it helped generate taken to policy." Dr. Kochi, called the Gates Foundation's decision-making "a closed internal process, and as far as can be seen, accountable to none other than itself." He argued, the foundation's determination to have its favoured research used to guide the health organization's recommendations "could have implicitly dangerous consequences on the policy-making process in world health" (McNeil , 2008).

Partners or competitors for health?

The ever increasing role of private voluntary contributions has accelerated the so-called 'partnership model' (essentially involving partnerships between public entities and the private sector, including private foundations) in public health. The GFATM and GAVI are two examples of such mega partnerships and are discussed in other chapters in the volume (see Chapter D4). The partnership approach and its impact have been the subject of an increasing number of analyses.[1] Clinton and Sridhar (2017b, p.5) observe in this respect:

"The move towards the partnership model in global health and voluntary contributions...allows donors to finance and deliver assistance in ways that they can more closely control and monitor at every stage. [This shift] illustrates three major trends in global health governance more broadly: towards more discretionary funding and away from core or longer-term funding; towards multi-stakeholder governance and away from traditional government-centred representation and decision-making; and towards narrower mandates or problem-focused vertical initiatives and away from broader systemic goals sought through multilateral cooperation".

Targeted donor influence not only results in less flexibility, it also weakens support to leadership driven by independent health considerations and has had a marked effect on undermining the WHO's ability to sustain/maintain adequate expertise and staff capacity. This has been well documented in response to the Ebola crisis and is threatening to undermine the gains in HIV response. In September 2016, the WHO sounded the alarm that due to inadequate finances, the organization is likely to lose expertise and to struggle in providing countries the necessary technical guidance on a number of health issues, such as antimicrobial resistance and HIV/AIDS.

Further, it makes the WHO more vulnerable to influence by rich donor countries, many of them active in promoting the interests of powerful corporations within the health business, especially pharmaceutical companies (see Box D1.1). Margaret Chan (2013) spelled out the pressures faced from corporate influence and 'business interests of powerful economic operators' in the following manner:

"Research has documented these tactics well. They include front groups, lobbies, promises of self-regulation, lawsuits, and industry-funded research that confuses the evidence and keeps the public in doubt.

Tactics also include gifts, grants, and contributions to worthy causes that cast these industries as respectable corporate citizens in the eyes of politicians and the public. They include arguments that place the responsibility for harm to health on individuals, and portray government actions as interference in personal liberties and free choice.

This is formidable opposition. Market power readily translates into political power. Few governments prioritize health over big business...This is not a failure of individual will-power. This is a failure of political will to take on big business".

Impact of voluntary contributions on programme budget allocations

The WHO programme budget for 2016–2017 amounted to nearly US$ 4,400 million for the biennium. Table D1.3 provides details of how specified (earmarked) voluntary contributions are distributed over different programme

Box D1.1: Corporate influence on WHO policies and programmes: how does it work?

Shortly after the WHO had declared the swine flu outbreak (2009–2010) a pandemic, it was reported that some of the experts advising the emergency decision-making committee had ties to drug companies that were producing antivirals and influenza vaccines. The pandemic proved to be a trigger point for pharmaceutical companies to establish vaccine contracts with governments, many of which subsequently lay dormant due to overestimation of the severity of the virus by the emergency committee. This entailed significant costs for countries already facing tight health budgets, and raised serious concerns about potential conflicts of interest. It took the WHO more than one year after the declaration to reveal the names behind the decision-making processes of the committee, with the organization citing the need to protect the experts from external pressures. After a large number of reviews, the question remains: Was it the interests of pharmaceutical companies or concern for public health that was being prioritized? (Cohen and Carter, 2010)

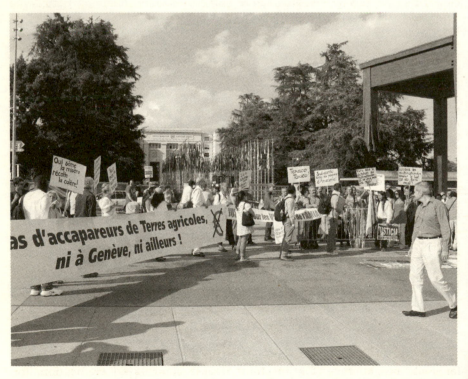

Image D1.3 Protest against land grabbing by TNCs at the UN in Geneva (Claudio Schuftan)

areas. Of the specified voluntary contributions, 84 per cent go to the top 10 technical programmes, while the bottom 10 areas receive just 1.4 per cent of the specified voluntary funds. Clearly donors are cherry-picking the areas they wish to fund. The WHO funnels funding from its core budget to fill the gaps in areas not funded by voluntary contributions, such as the areas of non-communicable diseases, social determinants of health, ageing and gender equity, and especially the new WHO Health Emergencies (WHE) Programme, requested and approved by member states at the WHA in May 2016.

TABLE D1.3: Percentage of specified voluntary contributions to WHO programme area, 3rd quarter, 2016–2017

Polio eradication	35.2
Outbreak and crisis response	15.8
Reproductive, maternal, newborn, child and adolescent health	7.7
Vaccine-preventable diseases	6.5
Access to medicines and other health technologies and strengthening regulatory capacity	4.2
Neglected tropical diseases	3.5
National health policies, strategies and plans	3.4
Malaria	2.8
HIV and hepatitis	2.7
Integrated people-centred health services	2.5
Tuberculosis	2.4
Country emergency preparedness and the International Health Regulations (IHR)	2.1
Health and the environment	1.8
Non-communicable diseases	1.8
Infectious hazard management	1.2
Health systems information and evidence	1.1
Emergency operations	1.0
Nutrition	0.8
Health emergency Information and risk assessment	0.6
Mental health and substance abuse	0.6
Antimicrobial resistance	0.3
Disabilities and rehabilitation	0.3
Food safety	0.3
Management and administration	0.3
Violence and injuries	0.3
Emergency core services	0.2
Leadership and governance	0.2
Social determinants of health	0.2
Ageing and health	0.1
Gender, equity and human rights mainstreaming	0.1
Strategic communications	0
Strategic planning, resource coordination and reporting	0
Transparency, accountability and risk management	0

Source: WHO (2016a)

It would be incorrect to infer from the data indicating better funding for some programmes (for infectious disease control and eradication, for example) that these are overfunded. Given the WHO's financial situation, all programmes are inadequately funded. What the data however suggests is that some programmes are grossly underfunded as a consequence of the donor chokehold on the WHO's finances. It is instructive to note that some programme areas, where the WHO has invested considerable effort and attention – such as social determinants of health and non-communicable diseases (NCDs) – receive very little donor support.

Overall, the programmes that donors choose to fund are those where tangible results are simpler to measure. Thus infectious disease programmes and infectious disease eradication receive a bulk of donor support. Donors are more inclined to support actions in areas where they are able to see that their money is 'well spent'. In contrast, areas in which it is difficult to measure outcomes in the short and medium term, irrespective of their importance to public health, receive no support from donors. It can be argued that attention to the social determinants of health or to better nutrition can, in many situations, contribute more to public health outcomes than interventions that focus on particular diseases.

Similarly areas of work that relate to strengthening of health systems are likely to have better long-term benefits than disease-focused programmes. However these are precisely the areas that are ignored by donors. The Burden of Disease (BoD) data is clear regarding the rising burden placed by NCDs, not just in high-income countries (HICs) but also in low- and middle-income

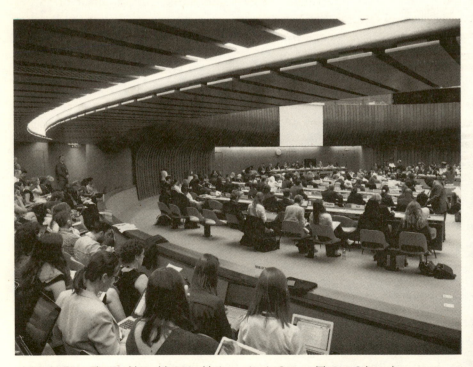

Image D1.4 The World Health Assembly in session in Geneva (Thomas Schwarz)

countries (LMICs). But work on NCDs involves systemic efforts related to health system strengthening and on a range of social determinants such as nutrition, exposure to environmental toxins and so on. Actions in these areas are less amenable to quickly measureable outcomes and hence largely ignored. Similarly the BoD data is unequivocal as regards the very large contribution of mental illnesses and injuries, yet they receive scant support from donors (WHO, 2004).

A telling example of how donor priorities override important decisions taken by member states at the WHO is that of the WHE Programme. It was set up in 2016 in recognition of the need for the WHO to better respond to health emergencies following its tardy response to the Ebola outbreak in 2014. It focuses on building capacity in the areas of early warning, risk assessment and emergency response in order to provide needed services to affected populations and at the same time tackle the root causes of their vulnerability. "Crucially these strategies must be integrated with health-systems strengthening. The health system as a whole provides the foundation on which to build the International Health Regulations (IHR) core capacities required to raise readiness and resilience across the board" (WHO, 2016b, p. 4).

Financing for the US\$ 485 million WHE Programme is drawn from core funds for baseline staff. The US\$ 100 million WHO Contingency Fund for Emergencies (CFE) has a funding gap of US\$ 68.5 million and the WHE is the most critically underfunded WHO programme, with a deficit of 56 per cent of requirement (WHO, 2016b, p. 13). At a special session in October 2016 to address the funding gap, Margaret Chan noted that "the organization has been asked to do more, specifically through WHE, while income from voluntary contributions has not increased and core voluntary contributions income has actually decreased".

The WHO has emphasized that the CFE has been critical in enabling the organization to quickly respond to emergencies, particularly in the early stages, rather than wait for humanitarian appeals. The problem with its design, based on front-loading funds and asking the WHO to fundraise to reimburse has not been successful, either because "appeals are not fully financed or donors do not agree to direct their funds to reimburse the CFE but only for additional activities" (WHO, 2016b, p. 14). Clearly, evidence from its limited tenure indicates that the new WHE Programme has suffered from many of the same flaws that it was designed to address, namely funding that is inadequate, highly specified and not sustainable.

Consequences beyond global public health

The WHO was set up as a global authority, so nations would "compromise their short-term differences in order to attain the long-run advantages of regularized collaboration on health matters" (Clinton and Sridhar, 2017b, p. 6). However, this approach is frequently challenged as member states have disagreed about the primary work of the organization. While some member states have prioritized the need for strong public health institutions and broad health coverage, others have argued for a more 'selective' approach, concentrating attention on eradicating specific diseases, through coordinated intervention by a number of sources, public and private.

In the resulting turmoil, the WHO has lost its political importance relative to new actors in the global health arena. From being the foremost – and virtually the only – authority on global health in the first decades of its existence, the WHO now stands amongst a growing number of public and private actors, initiatives and international partnerships in health, including the GFATM, GAVI, UNAIDS and especially BMGF. Some member states, led by the USA and other HICs, have been instrumental in driving health initiatives outside the WHO, such as to the problem-focused vertical funds (GAVI and the GFATM) and to some extent the World Bank, without consideration of the impact on the norm-setting role and importance of public and preventive health systems, which are intimately connected to human rights and to reducing inequalities (income and non-income). This phenomenon has affected many UN entities in the last 10 to 15 years. The resulting decline in effectiveness, most notably in the case of Ebola, has had a negative impact on the UN development system as a whole and has encouraged a myriad of special initiatives outside the UN. At the same time, other international organizations such as UNICEF and the World Bank have expanded their role in health and have at their disposal significant resources for programme implementation.

Shift in governance: member state-driven to multi-stakeholder

The shift in funding strategy – from assessed to voluntary to specified – has been instrumental in redirecting the work of the WHO. It also raises some important issues beyond public health: first and foremost those of policy coherence and democratic governance. Concern about this shift was echoed by Margaret Chan: "When private economic operators have more say over domestic affairs than the policies of a sovereign government, we need to be concerned" (WHO, 2014). The vicious circle evident in the WHO is also at play in many parts of the UN system. When unable to ignore the enormous gap between the demands placed on the UN system and the resources contributed, most governments (and non-state actors) have responded with earmarked funds or with partnership arrangements sometimes, thus diluting or ignoring the norms and standards that are the hallmark of the UN. Few governments follow the good practice evidenced by Sweden, which made a core voluntary contribution of US$ 25.88 million in 2016. This was over 30 per cent of the core voluntary contributions from all countries put together (WHO, 2017). Traditional donors seem to favour the partnerships approach and resource non-UN entities in areas that should be UN-led. This financing strategy further fragments programme design and delivery, undermines the normative authority of the UN, and not only encourages competition among UN entities, but sets up and nourishes programmes parallel to and competing with the UN programmes.

The growing dependence of the WHO on funding beyond core assessed contributions from member states and the increasing importance of contributions from non-state actors (foundations being the main source) has provided impetus to move towards a governance structure in the WHO that is able to accommodate entities other than member states. The modified strategy towards governance is evident in Margaret Chan's observation:

"If multisectoral collaboration and multi-stakeholder engagement are the reality for sustainable development in the post-2015 era, we need to debate what type of mechanisms are required to allow all stakeholders to make contributions and to protect against the influence of vested interest. We also need to consider the UN's role as an honest broker that promotes fair play" (WHO, 2014).

The WHO, thus, has clearly embarked on a path where, as in other UN agencies, a member state-driven governance system is being replaced by a 'multi-stakeholder governance' system.

The Framework for Engagement with Non-State Actors (FENSA), passed by the WHA in 2016 has been characterized as "opening the floodgates to corporate influence on global and national decision-making processes in public health matters" (Hawkes, 2011). A civil society statement raised the following concerns regarding how FENSA is poised to modify the governace of WHO (Civil Society Statement 2016):

"FENSA, in its overarching section puts private sector entities on an equal footing with other NSAs [non-state actors], failing to recognize their fundamentally different nature and roles. It uses the principle of 'inclusiveness' for all five 'types of interactions' (resources, participation, evidence, advocacy and technical collaboration) to all NSAs. When applied to major transnational corporations, their business associations and philanthropic foundations, this categorization of interactions, combined with an alleged right to inclusiveness, will once and for all, legitimize the framing of public health problems and solutions in favour of the interests and agendas of those actors.

FENSA, for example, proposes technical collaboration with the private sector, including capacity building, with no adequate safeguards. It seems that there is opposition from developed countries to a clause that would exclude private sector resources for activities such as norms and policies development and standard setting. FENSA removes the existing minimum restrictions on accepting financial resources from the private sector to fund salaries of WHO staff. If the WHO relies on funds from the private sector for any operational expenses, it risks showing favouritism towards those sectors in its standard-setting, expert advisory, and other public health functions."

Concluding observations

As has been outlined, the WHO has had a series of financing crises making it unable to fund its swelling mandate. Two shifts represent milestones in what has become a deep-seated undermining of the global health authority: the shift from assessed to voluntary contributions and the shift within voluntary to specified contributions.

While member states have agreed to a series of reform measures to address these shifts and to encourage increased funding, these measures have continued the pattern of fragmentation and resulted in pushing the WHO further from its core role as global health authority. Moreover, the shift in financing weight from assessed and flexible contributions to specified contributions, the overwhelming influence of a few donors, and the empowering of non-state 'partners' has undermined the importance and leadership of public health authorities.

As the health world is further fragmented, its institutions often competing rather than cooperating with each other, this has enhanced the influence of a few big donors, including powerful member states such as the USA and UK as well as private actors, notably the BMGF (Clinton and Sridhar, 2017b, p. 7).

There is an urgent need for a transition strategy to re-position the WHO as a primary and central health authority, and break donor control, public and private, of the health sector. The vital next steps are for member states and the WHO leadership to develop and implement a transition strategy to reconstitute assessed and core, supplemented by flexible financing.

Some elements of a transition strategy are as follows:

- Member states must reverse the trend towards voluntary specified contributions and reliance on private sector financing.
- Payment of assessed contributions must be in full and on time.
- The maximum of allowed voluntary specified contributions per donor must be established at 50 per cent (of the total contribution by the donor).
- There should be agreement on a multi-year strategy to move towards a 50/50 ratio for voluntary flexible and voluntary specified contributions.
- A threshold of assessed or voluntary flexible contributions must be set for eligibility to make voluntary specified contributions (VCS). For member states, no VCs should be allowed unless fully paid up on assessed contributions. For non-state partners, no VCs to be allowed unless an equal voluntary flexible contribution is made.
- Contributions from non-state 'partners' must be accompanied with signed agreements that guarantee commitment to UN standards, in particular to not engage in other programmes and funding that undermine the achievement of the WHO and UN mandates, including the achievement of the Sustainable Development Goals (SDGs). Violations would result in expulsion from partnerships and forfeiture of contributions, and non-eligibility for contractual and procurement options.

- FENSA must be refined to distinguish between non-state partners in general and dominant donors. The latter need to comply with a distinct agreement as befits their size and influence.

The WHO is not alone among UN agencies in needing to implement a strategy that 'contains' contributions from donors within the UN standards and ensures respect and support for norm-setting, multilaterally designed and accountable programmes, and democratic governance. With the shift to operational and implementation control by donors and their various stakeholder partners, rights-based approaches and the governing role of member states in the public interest are being undermined, often intentionally.

The size and power of some corporations and foundations and their national enablers drive the status quo from which they benefit, and make transformative changes in governance and financing more difficult. In addition to entity-specific strategies, member states and the UN leadership must be active promoters of the public interest and the replenishment of essential public resources.

The WHO, like other UN entities, has been a victim of the shift in funding patterns by member states. An organization struggling for finance is more likely to accept or cooperate with a variety of approaches that bring or promise resources. This further fragments programming, decision-making and capacity. The major challenge facing the UN development system is how to spark and sustain the political leadership needed to break the vicious circle whereby responses to the chronic financing situation are actually exacerbating it.

Note

1 See chapter on the Gates Foundation in this volume and the work of the Global Policy Forum at https://www.globalpolicy.org/

References

Beigbeder, Y, Nashat, N, Orsini, M & Tiercy, J F 1998, *The World Health Organization*, Martinus Nijhoff Publishers, Leiden, p. 165.

Brown, T M & Cueto, M 2010, 'The World Health Organization and the world of global health', in Parker, R & Sommer, M (eds), *Routledge handbook of global public health*, Routledge Handbooks Online, viewed 5 June 2017, https://www.routledgehandbooks.com/doi/10.4324/9780203832721.ch3

Chan, M 2013, *Opening address at the 8th Global Conference on Health Promotion*, Helsinki, 10 June, www.who.int/dg/speeches/2013/health_promotion_20130610/en/

Civil Society Statement 2016, *On the World Health Organization's proposed Framework of Engagement with Non-State Actors (FENSA) 69th World Health Assembly, May 2016*, http://www.ghwatch.org/sites/www.ghwatch.org/files/Civil%20Society%20Statement%2060.pdf

Clinton, C & Sridhar, D 2017a, *Governing global health: who runs the world and why?* Oxford University Press, New York, pp. 90–91.

Clinton, C & Sridhar, D 2017b, 'Who pays for cooperation in global health? A comparative analysis of WHO, the World Bank, the Global Fund to Fight HIV/AIDS, Tuberculosis and Malaria, and Gavi, the Vaccine Alliance', *The Lancet*, January 27, p. 2, http://www.

thelancet.com/journals/lancet/article/
PIIS0140-6736(16)32402-3/fulltext

Cohen, D & Carter, P 2010, 'WHO and the
pandemic flu 'conspiracies', *British Medical
Journal*, vol. 340, http://www.bmj.com/
content/340/bmj.c2912

Hawkes, N 2011, 'Irrelevant' WHO outpaced by
younger rivals', *British Medical Journal*, vol.
343, http://www.bmj.com/content/343/bmj.
d5012/rr/697686

Kamradt-Scott, A 2016, 'WHO's to blame? The
World Health Organization and the 2014
Ebola outbreak in West Africa', *Third World
Quarterly*, vol. 37, no. 3, pp. 401–18, DOI:10.1
080/01436597.2015.1112232.

Kelland, K 2016, *The World Health
Organization's critical challenge: healing
itself*, Reuters Investigates, 8 February,
http://www.reuters.com/investigates/
special-report/health-who-future/

Legge, D 2011, 'Future of WHO hangs in the
balance', *British Medical Journal*, vol.
345, http://www.bmj.com/bmj/section-
pdf/187674?path=/bmj/345/7881/Analysis.
full.pdf

Mcneil, 2008, 'Gates Foundation's Influence
Criticized', *The New York Times*, Feb. 16,
2008 http://www.nytimes.com/2008/02/16/
science/16malaria.html

Revised assessed contributions payable by
member states and associate members
2017 n.d., http://www.who.int/about/
financesaccountability/funding/2017_AC_
summary.pdf?ua=1

WHA Today 2017, *A civil society perspective
on the 70th World Health Assembly*,
no. 3, http://g2h2.org/wp-content/
uploads/2017/05/WHA-TODAY-No.3-24-
May-2017.pdf

WHO 2004, *Part 4 – burden of diseases:
DALYs*, http://www.who.int/healthinfo/
global_burden_disease/GBD_
report_2004update_part4.pdf?ua=1

WHO 2014, *WHO director-general addresses
the UN Economic and Social Council*,
http://www.who.int/dg/speeches/2014/
economic-social-council/en/

WHO 2016a, *Taking steps towards a fully-
funded programme budget 2016–2017*,
http://www.who.int/about/finances-
accountability/funding/financing-dialogue/
Presentation-Financial-Situation.pdf

WHO 2016b, *Update – WHO Health
Emergencies Programme: progress and
priorities*, http://www.who.int/about/
finances-accountability/funding/financing-
dialogue/whe-update.pdf

WHO 2016c, *Voluntary contributions by fund
and by contributor, 2015*, http://www.who.
int/about/finances-accountability/reports/
A69_INF3-en.pdf?ua=1

WHO 2016d, *WHO programmatic and financial
report for 2014–2015 including audited
financial statements for 2015*, http://apps.
who.int/gb/ebwha/pdf_files/WHA69/
A69_45-en.pdf

WHO 2017, *WHO mid-term programmatic and
financial report for 2016–2017 including
audited financial statements for 2016*,
http://apps.who.int/gb/ebwha/pdf_files/
WHA70/A70_40-en.pdf?ua=1

Yussuf, M, Larrabure, J L & Terzi, V 2007,
*Voluntary contributions in United
Nations system organizations: impact
on programme delivery and resource
mobilization strategies*, Joint Inspection
Unit, United Nations, Geneva, https://
www.unjiu.org/en/reports-notes/archive/
jiu_rep_2007_1_english.pdf

D2 | PRIVATE PHILANTHROPIC FOUNDATIONS: WHAT DO THEY MEAN FOR GLOBAL HEALTH?

Over the last two decades, the philanthropic sector has grown in terms of the number of foundations, the size of their annual giving and the scope of their activities. While detailed information about their total annual spending on international development (including health) is not available, estimates range from US$ 7 billion to more than US$ 10 billion per year. Spending is concentrated in certain selected areas, especially the health sector (Edwards, 2011; Martens and Seitz, 2015).[1]

Today, there are more than 200,000 foundations in the world. Over 86,000 foundations are registered in the USA; another estimated 85,000 foundations are based in Western Europe and 35,000 in Eastern Europe (Foundation Center, 2014). The philanthropic sector is also growing in the Global South, with, for example, approximately 10,000 foundations in Mexico, nearly 2,000 in China and at least 1,000 in Brazil, largely due to the rapidly increasing number of wealthy individuals in countries in the Global South (UNDP, 2012). Philanthropies located in the South are largely engaged in supporting activities at the national level.

The number of foundations and the amount of philanthropic spending will, in all probability, increase in the coming years. As a consequence of the global campaign 'The Giving Pledge' (2017), initiated by Bill Gates and Warren Buffett in 2010, more than 158 billionaires have committed to spend large parts of their wealth to philanthropic purposes, among them Michael Bloomberg, Mark Zuckerberg and Saudi Arabia's Prince Alwaleed Bin Talal Bin Abdulaziz Alsaud. A large part of this is likely to flow as development assistance for health, though the precise route of spending is left to individual donors.

By far the largest foundation is the Bill & Melinda Gates Foundation (Gates Foundation or BMGF), established in the year 2000 by Microsoft co-founder Bill Gates, with an endowment of US$ 39.9 billion (augmented in 2006 by a US$ 30.7 billion pledge of company stocks from Bill Gates' billionaire friend of long standing, Warren Buffet) and an annual grant-making of US$ 4.2 billion as at December 2015, of which an estimated US$ 2.9 billion was allocated for health (Bill and Melinda Gates Foundation, n.d. b; Dieleman et al., 2016; USA Today, 2006). The Gates Foundation provides more aid to global health than any country donor and is the fifth largest donor to agriculture in developing countries. In 2013, only 11 countries spent more on aid than the Gates Foundation, making it the world's 12th largest donor (Curtis, 2016).

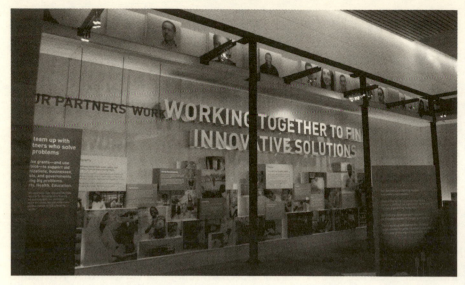

Image D2.1 Bill & Melinda Gates Foundation Visitor Center in Seattle, Washington, USA (By Jacklee - Own work; License: CC BY-SA 4.0, https://commons.wikimedia.org/w/index.php?curid=42308013)

An alternative notion of welfare

In recent years, civil society organizations, scientists and the media have focused attention on the growing influence of philanthropic foundations in global development and the risks and side-effects of this trend.[2] Critics have argued that philanthropy is aimed at preserving rather than redistributing wealth and a way for elites to pursue and legitimate their actions (McGoey, 2015).

In *Global Health Watch 3* we had unpacked the term 'philanthrocapitalism' as 'harnessing the power of the market to achieve social outcomes', to denote the operations of private foundations (People's Health Movement, Medact and TWN, 2011). It is important to underline that the philanthrocapitalist model is proposed as an alternative to the notion that public goods such as health are most efficiently provided by the state and funded through public money, that is money generated through taxation measures. It is an alternate notion of welfare embedded within the structures of capitalism. This is not a recent notion, though the rapid ascent of private foundations and the power that mega foundations such as the Gates Foundation wield is more recent. Over a century back, US steel tycoon Andrew Carnegie, often identified as the richest man ever, suggested that: "[Philanthropy would enable the] problem of rich and poor to be solved. The laws of accumulation will be left free, the laws of distribution free. Individualism will continue, but the millionaire will be but a trustee of the poor, entrusted for a season with a great part of the increased wealth of the community, but administering it for the community far better than it could or would have done for itself". (McGoey, 2016)

Carnegie essentially argued that laws (including laws regarding labour rights and taxation) should not hinder the ability of a few individuals to accumulate huge sums of money. Such individuals, whom he called 'trustees of the poor' (and not governments) were best placed to attend to the needs of the poor. In 'The Gospel of Wealth' (1889) he argued that the wealthy could undermine social protest by donating to worthy causes and rejected demands to raise wages and living standards because that would cut into profits. Instead of giving money to governments, Carnegie advised the rich to establish charitable foundations so they could shape society (Rosenthal, 2015).

Modern day philanthropic foundations such as the Gates Foundation work on the very principles that Carnegie enunciated. Well-endowed foundations exist because they receive endowments from super profits accumulated by a variety of means. One of them is by not paying taxes commensurate with profits earned. Bill Gates, for example, made all his money as the founder of Microsoft (and he continues till date on its board and is the company's largest individual shareholder). A 2012 US Senate report calculated that Microsoft was able to shift offshore nearly US$ 21 billion (in a three-year period), or almost half of its US retail sales net revenue, saving up to US$ 4.5 billion in taxes on goods sold in the USA. The US$ 4.5 billion in taxes lost to the US Treasury each year is greater than the Gates Foundation's annual global spending. Important to note is the fact that contrary to the widely held belief that Bill Gates is donating all his money to charity, his personal wealth has actually risen from US$ 56 billion in 2011 to US$ 78.9 billion in 2015 – an increase of US$ 23 billion in four years, roughly the same amount of money that the BMGF has disbursed since its inception (Curtis, 2016, p. 8).

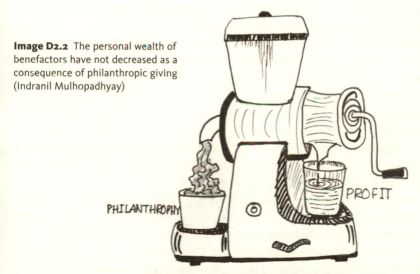

Image D2.2 The personal wealth of benefactors have not decreased as a consequence of philanthropic giving (Indranil Mulhopadhyay)

PHILANTHROPHY

PROFIT

PHILANTHRO CAPITALISM

Further, with the setting up of the Gates Foundation, more taxes are foregone by the state, as in the USA (also in several other countries) philanthropic foundations are exempt from paying most taxes, and contributions to philanthropies benefit from tax deductions. Up to a third or more, depending on the tax rate, of the endowment monies of private philanthropies are thus subsidized by public money (Birn, 2014). It would thus not be incorrect to conclude that foundations, such as Gates Foundation, channelize public money to support their 'philanthropic' activities. Logically the public in such a situation should be party to decisions regarding how this money is spent. In practice, however, in the case of the Gates Foundation, important grant-making decisions are the purview of three people (the trustees of the foundation): Bill Gates himself, his wife Melinda Gates and his friend Warren Buffet! To this august list one can add Bill Gates' father, William H Gates, who is the co-chair of the BMGF (Bill & Melinda Gates Foundation, n.d. a).

Risks and side-effects

Several criticisms of the model of philanthropy promoted by the Gates Foundation have been articulated. A major concern is that such a model exacerbates growing inequality rather than mitigate it, by depriving treasuries of tax revenues that could be spent on redistributive welfare policies. A related concern is that philanthropy is used to thwart demands for higher taxation, protecting and expanding assets rather than redistributing wealth. It has been noted that philanthropy often opens up markets for US- or Europe-based multinationals that partner with organizations such as the Gates Foundation in order to reach new consumers (McGoey, 2016). The Gates Foundation's lack of accountability and real-time transparency (over what are, after all, taxpayer-subsidized dollars) as well as the fact that it encourages the partnership model over the public good model are other points of criticism (Birn, 2014, pp.10, 17). The fact that it both invests in and champions corporate actors that have had a detrimental impact on health outcomes has also been criticized. This concern parallels an underlying criticism of the Gates Foundation, which is that its main funding source, revenues accrued from Microsoft, was amassed through labour practices and monopolistic intellectual property strategies that are contrary to its stated health aims (People's Health Movement, Medact and TWN, 2011).

However, despite this, a rosy picture of philanthropic engagement is still predominant and possible risks and side-effects are still ignored by most governments, the media and many civil society organizations.

With the adoption of the United Nations' (UN) 2030 Agenda and its Sustainable Development Goals (SDGs), governments have attributed an ever more prominent role to partnerships with corporations, philanthropic foundations and international organizations in order to achieve the new goals and to close the identified funding gap (UN, 2015). Thus, for example, SDG 17.16 seeks to: "Enhance the global partnership for sustainable development, complemented by multi-stakeholder partnerships that mobilize and share knowledge, expertise, technology and financial resources, to support the achievement of the sustainable development goals in all countries, in particular developing countries." SDG 17.17 strives to: "Encourage and promote effective public, public-private and civil society partnerships, building on the experience and resourcing strategies of partnerships."

Facing stagnating public spending for global development purposes, politicians are putting their hopes in philanthropy. In the Addis Ababa Action Agenda of July 2015, governments declared: "We welcome the rapid growth of philanthropic giving and the significant financial and non-financial contribution philanthropists have made towards achieving our common goals. We recognize philanthropic donors' flexibility and capacity for innovation and taking risks, and their ability to leverage additional funds through multi-stakeholder partnerships. We encourage others to join those who already contribute". (UN General Assembly 2015, para. 42)

It is Important to note that at the 2015 Financing for Development Conference in Addis Ababa, many developing countries called for targeting illicit financial flows and ensuring efficient and fair taxation of transnational corporations (TNCs) and domestic elites, which would have enabled far more public spending on development, but large donor countries blocked any formal mechanisms (Birn, Pillay and Holtz, 2017, p. 557).

The trend of partnering with corporations and philanthropic foundations is based on the assumption that the UN and its member states would not be able to solve today's global problems alone. Partnerships with the private sector are seen as pragmatic, solution-oriented, flexible, efficient and un-bureaucratic – attributes that the proponents of partnerships allege are lacking in intergovernmental projects and processes.

However, as we have argued earlier, there is a "direct correlation between increased wealth accumulation, regressive tax measures, and funding towards philanthropic activities. Philanthropy may be growing, but only in the context of rampant inequality" (Hinnovic.org, 2013).

Beyond the more fundamental problems with regard to the rise of philanthropic foundations, which are related to ineffective or misdirected economic and fiscal policy and the attempt to deflect criticism away from the growing and rampant inequity engendered by capitalism, there are several areas of concern that are related to their functioning and activities. The concerns cannot be generalized as foundations differ in type, purpose, the way they are funded, their thematic focus and geographic scope, and their priorities, approaches and political orientation. However, there are main points of criticism that can be summarized under the following five headings:

1. Applying a business model to the measurement of results One prominent feature of many private foundations is their practice of applying business and often market-based approaches to development. This includes a strong emphasis on results and impact that donors want to see. While this approach is beneficial to donors as they are able to report these to their boards, it obligates grantees to demonstrate donor-defined results, privileging

---

Box D2.1: How BMGF 'manages' public opinion

The BMGF runs an aggressive self-promotion campaign (Birn, 2014). The public doesn't see much coverage of the media's collaboration with the Gates Foundation; yet it is substantial and influential (Paulson, 2013) The foundation has spent more than one billion dollars on what it calls 'advocacy and policy' – essentially an attempt to influence decision-makers and sway public opinion. The foundation has provided direct funding for global health and development coverage to British newspaper *The Guardian*, Spain's El País, the African Media Initiative, and in the USA to the Public Broadcasting Service, National Public Radio, and other broadcasting outlets, and through the Kaiser Family Foundation, which runs a leading global health portal that has been accused of soft-pedaling its postings on the Gates Foundation.

The foundation has invested millions in training programs for journalists. Gates-backed think tanks turn out media fact sheets and newspaper opinion pieces. Magazines and scientific journals get BMGF money to publish research and article (Doughton and Helm, 2011). All of this coverage directly or indirectly generates positive publicity for the BMGF's approach to global health and development (Birn, 2014). The foundation's grants to media raise obvious conflict-of-interest questions. Critics fear foundation funding of media will muffle debate on the foundation's approaches that are controversial, such as its embrace of genetically modified crops and emphasis on technological fixes for health problems. This is evident in the fact that few of the news organizations that get Gates money have produced any critical coverage of foundation programmes (Doughton and Helm, 2011).

Personal relationships also play a part. Bill and Melinda Gates deal directly with the leading scientific, business and political elites, establishing important ties, and often privileged access. In November 2014, for instance, when Bill Gates visited Berlin to campaign for the GAVI Alliance, he met the German Chancellor Angela Merkel, various ministers and parliamentarians, in an effort to prepare for the January 2015 Berlin meeting to replenish the GAVI Alliance resources. At this event, the German Chancellor announced a massive increase in Germany's contribution to the Alliance and pledged EUR 600 million for GAVI over the period 2016–2020.

interventions that produce short-term and narrow gains at the expense of investing in initiatives where benefits may be visible only in the longer term. Consequently, foundations tend to neglect investments in areas where impact becomes evident only over time.

Given the power that foundations with deep pockets wield, augmented by active political lobbying (see Box D2.1), public resources tend to be shifted to quick-win approaches, such as developing vaccines or disseminating insecticide-treated bed nets, while structural and political obstacles to development (for example, weak public health systems) remain neglected.

Grant-making on the basis of cost-benefit analyses and social return on investment analyses risks not supporting those in real need, but rather those who are able to deliver apparently successful and cheap interventions. Foundations following merely business logic, have been criticized for 'managing' the poor rather than empowering them (People's Health Movement, Medact and Global Equity Gauge Alliance, 2008, p. 245).

2. Reliance on technical solutions The Gates Foundation actively promotes the notion that better technologies can offer lasting solutions to combat diseases and global hunger (Bill & Melinda Gates Foundation, 2010). Through its strategic mix of grant-making, funding of specific research and scientific publications, personal networking and advocacy, it has successfully positioned itself in the centre of an epistemic community that is promoting market-based techno-fix solutions to the complex global problems of hunger and malnutrition. Such an approach veers away from addressing important and fundamental underlying structural impediments, most notably the trade and financial agreements that restrict their support to local agricultural firms and smallholder farmers (Martens and Seitz, 2015, p. 58).

Similarly, in the health sector, a major emphasis of the Gates Foundation has been on promotion of vaccines. In May 2011, in his address to the World Health Assembly Bill Gates said: "As we think about how to deploy our resources most effectively, one intervention stands out: vaccines. Today, I would like to talk about how you can provide the leadership to make this the Decade of Vaccines" (Bill and Melinda Gates Foundation, 2011). Gates argued that "Vaccines are an extremely elegant technology. They are inexpensive, they are easy to deliver, and they are proven to protect children from disease. At Microsoft, we dreamed about technologies that were so powerful and yet so simple." Clearly the Gates Foundation applies the same logic to global health policy as it did to building a computer empire. Yet a public health evaluation of the emphasis on technological fixes, especially on vaccines, would show that such an approach ignores a range of issues, such as the necessity to build functional health systems and the need to attend to a range of social determinants. Thus, for example, in many situations a vaccine against rotavirus to prevent diarrhoea may appear 'elegant' but cannot replace required action

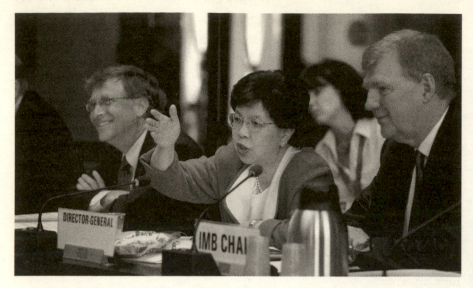

Image D2.3 WHO Director General Chan and Bill Gates lead discussion on polio at WHA (By United States Mission Geneva - Flickr; License: CC BY 2.0, https://commons.wikimedia.org/w/index.php?curid=15328920)

on the fundamental causes of diarrhoea – sanitation, safe drinking water and better nutrition.

3. Influence on policymaking and agenda-setting In 2013, in an op-ed in *The New York Times*, Peter Buffet, Warren Buffet's son, commented on his experience of working in the charity sector: "Because of who my father is, I've been able to occupy some seats I never expected to sit in. Inside any important philanthropy meeting, you witness heads of state meeting with investment managers and corporate leaders. All are searching for answers with their right hand to problems that others in the room have created with their left" (Curtis, 2016).

Philanthropic foundations have enormous influence on political decision-making and agenda setting. This is most obvious in the case of the Gates Foundation and its role in global health policy, especially given the sheer size of its grant-making (Birn, 2014, p. 9). Though its practice of providing matching funds and active advocacy, it influences priority setting in the World Health Organization (WHO) and promotes an emphasis on vertical, diseases-specific programmes.

Between 2014 and 2017, the Gates Foundation has granted more than US$ 1 billion to the WHO (2016b). The BMGF is the second largest funder of the WHO for the biennium 2016–2017,after the USA (WHO, n.d.). Most of the Gates Foundation's grants to the WHO have been dedicated to polio eradication, global policy and advocacy, and maternal, newborn and child health. (See Chapter D1 for a discussion on the influence of the Gates Foundation on the WHO.)

In addition, the Gates Foundation contributes to global public private partnerships that sit outside the UN framework, such as the Global Fund to Fight AIDS, Tuberculosis and Malaria (GFATM) and the vaccine and immunization alliance GAVI. The Gates Foundation sits on the boards of both GAVI and the GFATM (it is one of only four permanent members on GAVI's board along with the WHO, UNICEF and the World Bank). With an allocation of more than US$ 478 million in 2015,the GFATM has become the largest funder of UNDP (2016). GAVI contributed US$ 179.67 million to the WHO in the biennium 2014–2015 (WHO, 2016b). The GFATM and GAVI have also given significant contributions to the United Nations Children's Fund (UNICEF).

The Gates Foundation's increased influence on the priorities and operations of the WHO have increased in a situation where Northern countries led by the USA have imposed a 'zero-growth doctrine' on mandated assessed contributions by countries. (See Chapter D1 for a discussion on the WHO's funding crisis.)

4. Fostering privatization, fragmentation and weakening of global governance The Gates Foundation makes the involvement of the private sector and the support of public–private partnerships a prerequisite for their cooperation with individual governments, for example, the German government (Martens and Seitz, 2017). BMGF funded projects often lead intentionally or *de facto* to privatization of basic services in the health and education sectors. This is the case not only in countries of the global South but also in the USA. The Gates Foundation has been a major funder in the campaign to promote 'Charter' schools, that is, schools that are taxpayer-funded but privately run and exempt from many of the regulations governing public schools. Charter school proponents raised US$ 3.9 million after 2004 for a campaign on the issue in Washington state, and most of it came from three 'philanthropists' who donated about US$ 1 million each: Bill Gates, who had recently made education reform the main focus of his domestic philanthropy; Walmart heir John T. Walton and Donald Fisher (Barkan, 2016). The International Finance Corporation (IFC) – the World Bank's arm that promotes private sector development – is a major recipient of BMGF funds. It has awarded 11 grants to the IFC worth over US$ 40 million (Curtis 2016, p. 36).

Philanthropic foundations, particularly the Gates Foundation, the Rockefeller Foundation and the UN Foundation are not only major funders but also the driving forces behind global multi-stakeholder partnerships (partnerships that involve countries sharing decision-making powers with private enterprises and private foundations). Many of these partnerships, like the Children's Vaccine Initiative, GFATM, GAVI, and Scaling up Nutrition (SUN), have been initiated by these foundations. The Gates Foundation has also been active in silencing critiques of such partnerships. A Gates-funded evaluation report of the Scaling Up Nutrition multi-stakeholder initiative portrayed those who raised conflict-of-interest concerns as harbouring "phobias" and "hostile feelings" towards industry, which could "potentially sabotage the prospects of multi-stakeholder efforts to scale up nutrition" (Birn & Richter, forthcoming).

The mushrooming of global partnerships and vertical funds, particularly in the health sector, has led to isolated and often poorly coordinated solutions. These initiatives have not only contributed to the institutional weakening of the UN and its specialized agencies such as the WHO, but have also undermined the implementation of integrated development strategies at the national level. Supporters of see the variety of global initiatives as a strength and as a possibility to maintain political flexibility and mobilize a broad range of different actors. However, this in fact results either in duplication and thematic overlap or in high transaction and coordination costs at international and national levels.

As the private sector and private foundations acquire almost as much power (through partnerships) as sovereign nation states, they erode and dilute the political and legal position hitherto legitimately occupied by public bodies. Multi-stakeholder partnerships implicitly devalue the role of governments, parliaments and intergovernmental decision-making bodies, and overvalue the political status of private actors, including transnational corporations, philanthropic foundations, and sometimes even wealthy individuals like Bill Gates and Ted Turner.

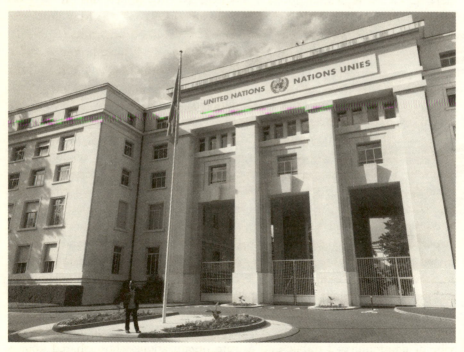

Image D2.4 The UN Building in Geneva. Philanthropic foundations are replacing UN institutions in global governance (People's Health Movement)

5. Lack of transparency and accountability mechanisms While foundations like the Gates Foundation and the Rockefeller Foundation have significant influence on development policies, they are not accountable to the 'beneficiaries' of their activities, be it governments, international organizations or local communities. Generally, they are only accountable to their own boards or trustees. This can be a quite limited number of people, as in the case of BMGF, where three family members and Warren Buffett act as trustees and co-chairs.

Lack of political will to limit influence of philanthropic foundations

Governments are realizing the risks related to the growing influence of corporate philanthropy only gradually. In the Addis Ababa Action Agenda they stated: "We call for increased transparency and accountability in philanthropy. We encourage philanthropic donors to give due consideration to local circumstances and align with national policies and priorities" (UN General Assembly 2015, para. 42).

This call reflects their concerns about the lack of transparency and accountability and the often uncoordinated and unaligned project activities of philanthropic donors. Though, it should be noted, the call also 'encourages' philanthropies to continue donating.

Following the pressure of civil society organizations, international organizations and a few individual governments have initiated discussions on the risks of engagement with private actors and possible safeguards. In May 2016, the WHO adopted its Framework of Engagement with Non-State Actors (FENSA), including a specific section on the engagement with philanthropic foundations (WHO, 2016a). In summer 2016, the German Ministry for Economic Cooperation and Development began to develop a strategy for engagement with philanthropists and private foundations.

However, the political will to effectively limit the influence of corporate philanthropy is still lacking. FENSA has several deficiencies, including as regards its basic design and its approach to the prevention of conflict of interests. It thus remains far from being an effective fence against private sector influence (Seitz, 2016). Critics of FENSA argue that the framework has been crafted to accommodate private foundations and for-profit entities in WHO's decision-making processes rather than to effectively manage conflict of interest issues when WHO engages with for-profit non-state actors. Instead of being a step towards member countries reclaiming leadership over decision-making in the WHO, FENSA could well become the instrument for legitimizing the interference of private entities in the governance of the WHO. It is thus not surprising that the International Federation of Pharmaceutical Manufacturers and Associations welcomed the framework as giving "an equitable voice to a vibrant community of public and private organizations whose shared goal is to make this world healthier" (Buse and Hawkes, 2016).

The frailties embedded in FENSA were in evidence in January 2017, when the WHO's executive board granted official relation status to the Gates Foundation amidst serious concerns related to conflict of interests in financing and staffing of the foundation. Civil society organizations protested against the decision as the Gates Foundation invests its endowment in polluting and unhealthy food and beverage industries and in corporations that benefit from its support of particular global health and agriculture initiatives.[3] Although the Gates Foundation sold many of its pharmaceutical holdings in 2009 (Hodgson, 2009), its financial interest in Big Pharma, as well as in food and beverage companies remain, particularly through its Berkshire Hathaway holdings.

Need for clear rules and criteria for cooperation with private foundations

Rules, standards and red lines for cooperation with private foundations are mostly lacking at national and international levels. They are urgently needed. Existing principles and rules can be used as a starting point, such as the principles of the Paris Declaration on aid effectiveness and the Accra Agenda for action (2005/2008) and the revised guidelines on a principle-based approach to the cooperation between the United Nations and the business sector (UN Secretary-General, 2015).

The required rules should define the normative base for the interaction between the government or the international organization and philanthropic foundations; they should spell out the different types of cooperation; and they should include minimum requirements for the cooperation, conflict of interest policies, provisions for due diligence assessments, and rules for transparency, accountability, independent evaluation, monitoring and review.

The development of such rules would be a prerequisite for any cooperation between international organizations or individual governments and philanthropic foundations. But this does not mean automatically, that international organizations and governments should actively pursue such cooperation. There are a number of questions to be answered first: Does any such cooperation absorb scarce public resources for development? Can these public resources be used in other projects in a more sustainable and effective way? Does the cooperation contribute to strengthening civil society organizations and take into account sufficiently the interests of civil society and affected communities? Does the cooperation foster the development of democratic public structures and institutions, for example, in the education and health sectors, or does it rather undermine the provision of public goods? Does it support multilateral organizations such as the WHO in fulfilling their mandate or does it instead weaken them by establishing parallel structures?

As long as these questions cannot be clearly answered with a 'yes', international organizations, individual governments and also civil society organizations should reconsider their cooperation with philanthropic foundations. In April 1938, President Franklin Roosevelt warned the US Congress: "The liberty of a democracy is not safe if the people tolerate the growth of private power to a point where it becomes stronger than their democratic state itself. That, in its essence, is fascism" (Monbiot, 2017). Given the power and influence of private foundations, it is a warning that resonates today regarding real concerns about the chokehold of private interests and influence on public affairs.

Notes

The OECD estimates philanthropic giving for development purposes of US$ 6.5 billion per year on average, according to a survey covering more than 70 private philanthropic foundations (OECD, 2017).

See, for example, Baby Milk Action (n.d.).

See the open letter to the executive board of the World Health Organization regarding 'Conflict of interest safeguards far too weak to protect WHO from influence of regulated industries (the case of the Bill and Melinda Gates Foundation)' (Centre for Health, Science and Law 2017).

References

Baby Milk Action n.d., Viewed 12 April 2017, www.babymilkaction.org/archives/3361

Barkan, J 2016, 'How Bill Gates and his billionaire pals used their enormous wealth to start privatizing schools in Washington State', *Nonprofit Quarterly*, vol. 23, no. 1, http://www.alternet. org/education/how-bill-gates-and-his-billionaire-pals-used-their-enormous-wealth-start-privatizing

Bill & Melinda Gates Foundation n.d. a, *Who we are – executive leadership team*, http:// www.gatesfoundation.org/Who-We-Are/ General-Information/Leadership/Executive-Leadership-Team

Bill & Melinda Gates Foundation n.d. b, *Who we are – foundation fact sheet*, www. gatesfoundation.org/Who-We-Are/General-Information/Foundation-Factsheet

Bill & Melinda Gates Foundation 2010, *Global health strategy overview*, https://docs. gatesfoundation.org/documents/global-health-strategy-overview.pdf

Bill & Melinda Gates Foundation 2011, *World Health Assembly: keynote address*, http:// www.gatesfoundation.org/media-center/ speeches/2011/05/world-health-assembly

Birn, A 2014, 'Philanthrocapitalism, past and present: the Rockefeller Foundation, the Gates Foundation, and the setting(s) of the international/global health agenda',*Hypothesis*,vol. 12, no. 1, http:// www.hypothesisjournal.com/wp-content/ uploads/2014/11/HJ229%E2%80%94FIN_Nov1_2014.pdf

Birn, A, Pillay, Y & Holtz, TH 2017, *Textbook of global health*, 4th edn, Oxford University Press, Oxford.

Birn, A & Richter, J forthcoming, 'U.S. philanthrocapitalism and the global health agenda: the Rockefeller and Gates Foundations, past and present', in Howard Waitzkin and the Working Group for Health Beyond Capitalism (eds), *Health care under the knife: moving beyond capitalism for our health*, Monthly Review Press, http://www. peah.it/2017/05/4019/

Buse, K & Hawkes, S 2016,'Sitting on the FENSA: WHO engagement with industry', *The Lancet*, vol. 388, http://www.thelancet. com/pdfs/journals/lancet/PIIS0140-6736(16)31141-2.pdf

Centre for Health, Science and Law 2017,*Open letter to the executive board of the World Health Organization January 2017*, http:// healthscienceandlaw.ca/wp-content/ uploads/2017/01/Public-Interest-Position. WHO.FENSAGates.Jan2017.pdf

Curtis, M 2016, *Gated development. Is the Gates Foundation always a force for good?* 2nd edn, Global Justice Now, London, www. globaljustice.org.uk/sites/default/files/files/ resources/gjn_gates_report_june_2016_web_final_version_2.pdf

Dieleman, J L, Schneider, M T, Haakenstad, A, Singh, L, et al., 2013, 'Development assistance for health: past trends, associations, and the future of international financial flows for health', *The Lancet* 2016, vol. 387, no. 10037, http://dx.doi.org/10.1016/ S0140-6736(16)30168-4

Doughton S, Helm K. 2011 Does Gates funding of media taint objectivity? The Seattle Times [Internet]. 2011 Feb 19. http://seattletimes.nwsource.com/html/localnews/2014280379_gatesmedia.html

Edwards, M 2011, *The role and limitations of philanthropy*, Commissioned by the Bellagio Initiative, http://opendocs.ids.ac.uk/opendocs/bitstream/handle/123456789/3717/Bellagio-Edwards.pdf?sequence=1

Foundation Center 2014, *Key facts on US foundations*, New York, http://foundationcenter.org/gainknowledge/research/keyfacts2014/

Hinnovic.org 2013, *Philanthrocapitalism, the Gates Foundation and global health – an interview with Linsey McGoey*, www.hinnovic.org/philanthrocapitalism-gates-foundation-globalhealth-with-linsey-mcgoey/

Hodgson, J 2009, 'Gates Foundation sells off most health-care, pharmaceutical holdings', *The Wall Street Journal*, 14 August, https://www.wsj.com/articles/SB125029373754433433

Martens, J & Seitz, K 2015, *Philanthropic power and development: who shapes the agenda?* https://www.globalpolicy.org/images/pdfs/GPFEurope/Philanthropic_Power_online.pdf

Martens, J & Seitz, K 2017, *Gestiftete Entwicklung? Die Kooperation zwischen der deutschen Entwicklungspolitik und privaten Stiftungen*, https://www.globalpolicy.org/images/pdfs/Gestiftete_Entwicklung_final.pdf

McGoey, L 2015, *No such thing as a free gift: the Gates Foundation and the price of philanthropy*, Verso, London.

McGoey, L 2016, 'Does philanthrocapitalism make the rich richer and the poor poorer?' *Evonomics*, 23 February, http://evonomics.com/does-philanthropy-actually-make-the-rich-richer-and-the-poor/

Monbiot, G 2017, 'How corporate dark money is taking power on both sides of the Atlantic', The Guardian, 2 February, 2017 https://www.theguardian.com/commentisfree/2017/feb/02/corporate-dark-money-power-atlantic-lobbyists-brexit?CMP=share_btn_fb.

OECD 2017, *Global private philanthropy for development: preliminary results of the OECD Data Survey*, viewed 12 April, Paris, www.oecd.org/dac/financing-sustainable-development/development-finance-data/Preliminary-results-philanthropy-survey.pdf

Paulson T. 2013 'Behind the scenes with the Gates Foundation's strategic media partners'. 2013 Feb 13. http://www.humanosphere.org/2013/02/a-personal-view-behind-the-scenes-withthe-gates-foundations-media-partners/

People's Health Movement, Medact & Global Equity Gauge Alliance 2008, *Global Health Watch 2: an alternative world health report*, Zed Books, London, www.ghwatch.org/sites/www.ghwatch.org/files/ghw2.pdf

People's Health Movement, Medact & TWN 2011, 'Conflicts of interest within philanthrocapitalism', in *Global health Watch 3*, Zed Books, London, http://www.ghwatch.org/sites/www.ghwatch.org/files/D3_0.pdf

Rosenthal, S 2015, 'Philanthropy: the capitalist art of deception', *Socialist Review*, http://socialistreview.org.uk/402/philanthropy-capitalist-art-deception

Seitz, K2016, '*FENSA – a fence against undue corporate influence? The new framework of engagement with non-state actors at the World Health Organization*, viewww.globalpolicy.org/images/pdfs/Briefing_0916_FENSA.pdf

The giving pledge 2017, https://givingpledge.org/

The Paris Declaration on Aid Effectiveness and the Accra Agenda for Action 2005/2008, http://www.oecd.org/dac/effectiveness/34428351.pdf

UN 2015, *Transforming our world: the 2030 Agenda for Sustainable Development*, UN Doc. A/RES/70/1, New York, www.un.org/ga/search/view_doc.asp?symbol=A/RES/70/1&Lang=E, accessed 12 April 2017.

UNDP 2012, *Evaluation of UNDP partnership with global funds and philanthropic foundations*, New York, http://erc.undp.org/evaluationadmin/downloaddocument.html?docid=5943

UNDP 2016,*Funding compendium 2015*, New York, www.undp.org/content/dam/undp/library/corporate/Partnerships/Funding%20Compendium%202015.pdf

UN General Assembly 2015, *Outcome document of the Third International Conference on Financing for Development:*

Addis Ababa Action Agenda, UN Doc. A/RES/69/313, Annex, New York, www.un.org/ga/search/view_doc.asp?symbol=A/CONF.227/L.1

UN Secretary-General 2015, *Guidelines on a principle-based approach to the cooperation between the United Nations and the business sector*, New York, https://business.un.org/en/documents/guidelines

USA Today 2006, *Warren Buffett signsover $30.7B to Billand Melinda Gates Foundation*, http://usatoday30.usatoday.com/news/nation/2006-06-25-buffett-charity_x.htm

WHO n.d., *The WHO programme budget portal*, viewed 12 April 2017, http://extranet.who.int/programmebudget/Biennium2016/Contributor

WHO 2016a, *Framework of engagement with non-state actors*, WHO, Doc. WHA 69.10,Geneva, http://apps.who.int/gb/ebwha/pdf_files/WHA69/A69_R10-en.pdf?ua=1

WHO 2016b, *Source and distribution of funds 2014–2015*, viewed 12 April 2017, http://extranet.who.int/programmebudget/Biennium2014/Contributor

D3 | MANAGEMENT CONSULTING FIRMS IN GLOBAL HEALTH

When Anthony Banbury was appointed at the helm of the newly established UN Mission for Ebola Emergency Response (UNMEER) in September 2014, he made a series of expected decisions and one surprising move: he called the Boston Consulting Group (BCG) (The Boston Consulting Group, 2015a). "The risks to the world were significant. We needed to move fast. This challenge was so complex that I knew I needed to call BCG," Banbury recalls. BCG consultants took part in planning meetings in New York, and flew to Accra with him to assist with the set-up, strategy and deployment of the mission. They would accompany his every move for the following period.[1] How BCG was chosen, what the basis of its legitimacy was, the details of what the consultants recommended or who they were accountable to in this process – none of this information is available in public domain.

The involvement of management consulting firms in the Ebola response is the tip of the iceberg. While many global health actors have been carefully examined, the role of management consulting firms, which can be linked to all significant global health institutions over the past decade and to critical junctures in countries in crises, has remained by and large hidden from public eye. Drawing from desk research and interviews with global health practitioners, former and current consultants, and health advocates,[2] this chapter describes the growing role of management consulting firms in global health and the impact of their involvement. It also explores the questions of governance, accountability and transparency that arise.

How management consulting firms became ubiquitous in global health

The entry of consultants into the field of global health and their engagement in crises predates the West African Ebola crisis. HIV/AIDS advocate and activist Gregg Gonsalves remembers when the penny dropped for him in the early 2000s. A young Harvard graduate who had been working for McKinsey & Company for no more than a couple of years showed up at a Global Fund (Global Fund to Fight Aids, Tuberculosis and Malaria – GFATM) meeting on anti-retroviral drugs, and "gave a presentation on what needed to happen for scale up. No one knew who he was, but everyone was transfixed"[3] The timing is corroborated by other observers, who note that management consultants began to enter the health arena over a decade and a half ago, at a time when the market for management consulting showed signs of saturation in the USA and in the rest of the Global North. With the scope for further domestic growth becoming limited, consulting firms needed to look elsewhere. As Duff McDonald (2013) recounts, "[B]y the early 2000s, McKinsey had not seen meaningful growth in the US and [was seeing] dramatically slower growth in Europe, and started turning to Africa, India [and] then China." This was the time when AIDS brought to global health the attention that it had lacked; a time when, to use the phrase coined by Allan Brandt (2013, pp. 2149–52), "AIDS invented Global Health."

In the wake of the HIV/AIDS crisis came the Millennium Development Goals (MDGs), the upsurge in development funding for health and the rise of global philanthropists led by the Bill & Melinda Gates Foundation (BMGF). There were suddenly significantly more resources and opportunities than ever before in global health.[4] "Huge amounts of money flew into the field – a field where there was not enough capacity," says Gonsalves.[5] There were demands to rethink the traditional models and public institutions (seen by many to self-serving and inefficient), to bring in new actors and to transcend traditional public–private divides. Public–private partnerships (PPPs), which would come to characterize the health field in the subsequent decade, were born with the blessing of the then Director General of the World Health Organization (WHO), Gro Brundtland, who famously stated in 1998: "When public and private sectors combine intellectual and other resources, more can be achieved." Global health institutions began proliferating outside of the UN system and traditional international organizations. The shift was not only in terms of the number of actors in the health field but in qualitative terms as well, with a redistribution of roles. Setting priorities and formulating policies on particular health matters ceased to be the sole prerogative of institutions such as the WHO that had until then held the mandate (McCoy et al., 2009, pp. 1645–53).

The evolving landscape also meant global health became a wedge to enter new markets. In a 2011 video, BCG's senior partner and managing director, Wendy Woods, reflected on the dramatic growth in the amount of funding going into global health and the tremendous "opportunities for improving the situation that the individuals in the developing world are facing regarding their health" (The Boston Consulting Group, 2011). The phenomenon did not escape McKinsey either, who saw in the creation of "high-aspiration founda-tions and new global entities...large, complex entities that are servable by the Firm".[6] Providing advice to "governments around the world the same way [as to] corporate clients" was an idea whose time had come (McDonald, 2013).

Entry by invitation Consultants were often brought to the discussion table by like-minded individuals, at times former consultants themselves, frustrated by perceived public-sector sluggishness, lack of impact and corrupt practices. They shared the belief that what the public sector needed was an injection of private-sector efficiency, cost effectiveness, project management skills and monitoring frameworks. With the exponential growth of new institutions, there was a capacity gap that the consultants filled. "Here were the management consultants saying this is what we do; we can show you how to run programmes, spend money," observes long-term health policy advocate Rohit Malpani.[7]

Consulting firms often participated in the creation of new public–private partnerships (PPPs), as was the case with BCG, whose initial foray into global health included building new organizations and developing their strategies (The Boston Consulting Group, 2011). Many of the senior leaders in the early days of public–private partnerships were themselves from consulting circles, as the example of the Global Fund illustrates. Rajat Gupta, McKinsey's managing director between 1994 and 2003, was a founding board member and subsequently became the chairman of the Board of the Global Fund. In February 2002, one month after the Global Fund Board met officially for the first time in Geneva, the services of McKinsey were "solicited to bolster the staff of the Secretariat, with management consultants working alongside the Secretariat staff for much of the year" (GFATM, 2003). The way in which the firm was selected raised eyebrows, as memorialized in the minutes of the third board meeting: "[Q]uestions regarding the use of competitive bidding processes to contract McKinsey and the currently confirmed LFAs [local fund agents] were raised by some delegations. It was emphasized that transparent procedures should be used in future which [would] result in cost-effective selection of LFAs and other contractors." (GFATM, 2002)

When UNITAID was set up in 2006, the BMGF funded McKinsey's engagement from the onset, and McKinsey developed key policy documents on "added value, procurement policy, market dynamics, monitoring & evaluation system, corporate key performance indicators and expertise requirements" (UNITAID, 2006).

Filling a capacity gap, reassuring boards Management consulting firms rapidly made themselves indispensable. Tactically offering their services (pro bono, at a reduced rate or paid for by a donor) at the onset of relationships, they were welcomed by new institutions in need of capacity but struggling to hire staff. The example of UNITAID is telling: the organization wrestled with the complex and lengthy procedures of its host, the WHO, to hire much-needed personnel. The executive board discussed the issue repeatedly in its meetings, acknowledging that "WHO rules made it very difficult for the Secretariat to recruit" and encouraged its team to hire consultants as a stopgap measure (UNITAID, 2007).

Management consulting firms also played an important function in building the confidence of board members and donors that contributions would be well spent, and operations efficiently conceived and overseen. According to a Geneva-based interviewee, a point was reached when you could only put

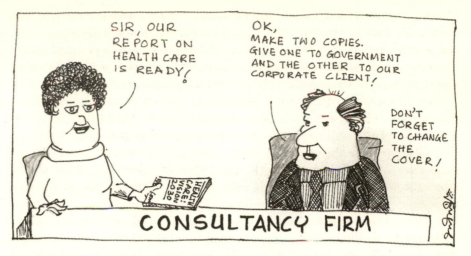

Image D3.1 There are huge conflicts of interest inherent in the way management consultancy firms operate (Indranil Mukhopadhyay)

in bids to persuade donors and boards if, at some stage, you had brought in management consultants to show that you had "understood the math, sums and costs".[8] The initial pro bono or secondment arrangements at the beginning of a relationship also meant that the engaging of consultants had no effect on headcounts or operating ratios, keeping board satisfaction high with what appeared to be lean structures.

Consultants not only established themselves as key features of these new institutions, but also gradually moved from providing organizational advice to offering strategic guidance. By the ninth session of the UNITAID Executive Board in November 2008, McKinsey was the one presenting the UNITAID strategy to its board (UNITAID, 2008). Once in a relationship, consultants would meet people, go to board meetings, get to know all stakeholders and their agendas, and gather privileged insights. The next time around, when a tender went out, they would have far more experience from within and be better positioned than anyone else might be. What was remarked with respect to the corporate sector generally seemed to be true in the global health field too: "Once they get the wedge end of a relationship into a company in the form of one engagement, they usually manage to hammer in the rest" (McDonald, 2013).

Becoming ubiquitous Today, management consulting firms have become ubiquitous in global health institutions and in countries in crises, with McKinsey and BCG being most prominent. They are known to operate on a mixed revenue model, which includes *pro bono*, secondments, discounted rates (traditionally 50 per cent of the rate charged to private clients) and full rates, with full fees for a senior consultant in a prestigious firm reaching US$ 10,000 a day.[9] Discounted or *pro bono* support often turns into further lucrative engagements, either with the institution initially supported or within the field. The Ebola crisis offers an interesting illustration of how firms capitalize on initial investments: BCG, which estimates that it invested a total of US$ 2.2 million in *pro bono* professional fees and expenses to support UN Mission to support Ebola Emergency Response (UNMEER), went on to produce background reports for the World Economic Forum (WEF) on 'Managing the risk and impact of future epidemics: options for public–private cooperation' and to shape debates on epidemic responses at high-profile convenings of world leaders and policymakers. They also undertook research on behalf of the Swiss-based Foundation for Innovative New Diagnostics (FIND), to better understand the gaps and opportunities in diagnostics in the wake of Ebola (including the role of diagnostics in the outbreak; diagnosis preparedness for unknown pathogens during outbreak situations; and semi-open platforms for product development and delivery).[10] In May 2015, McKinsey, whose staff initially supported the WHO Ebola response, went on to win a 9-month contract from the Department for International Development (DfID), worth GBP 2.9 million, to support Sierra Leone in its post-Ebola early recovery efforts (Gov.UK 2015), followed by an additional 15-month contract for GBP 8.8 million in May 2016 for Phase II (Gov.UK, 2016). McKinsey positioned itself as a key adviser within the President's office in Sierra Leone in this time of reconstruction. McKinsey was also contracted in mid-205 by the Foundation for the National Institutes for Health (FNIH), with the support of the BMGF, to assist in a review of the response to the Ebola crisis, with the view to improving future preparedness (Wellcome Trust, 2015).

Revenues of consulting firms come from both public and private sources, including bilateral donors, public–private partnerships and philanthropic institutions. In the past decade, both BCG and McKinsey have benefited from lucrative contracts from the BMGF, underlining the alignment in vision and approaches between management consulting firms and philantro-capitalist ventures. Firms retained by the BMGF support both its own programmes and that of its grant recipients (Holtzman, 2009). BMGF spends millions of dollars on BCG and McKinsey contracts (Table D3.1).

It appears from the (scarce) publicly available information, that both McKinsey and BCG have worked with the GFATM and WHO over the years, in addition to each having worked closely with multiple other significant global health institutions. BCG has, for instance, been associated with Roll Back Malaria (Winsten and Woods, 2011); World Food Programme (The Boston Consulting Group, 2015c; UNICEF, 2015); and GAVI, the global vaccine alliance (The Boston Consulting Group, 2013). The fingerprints of McKinsey can be found on UNITAID (UNITAID, 2006); the World Bank's International

TABLE D3.1: Bill & Melinda Gates Foundation contracts with McKinsey & Co. and BCG (in US$)

	McKinsey	BCG
2014	23,357,590	24,937,541
2013	22,936,500	13,850,816
2012	30,571,834	12,901,927
2011	19,472,506	18,051,829
2010	19,672,631	12,063,397
2009	14,357,648	8,109,531
2008	17,064,659	15,345,909
2007	6,696,149	7,352,820
2006	7,300,236	N/A
	161,429,753	112,613,770

Source: BMGF Internal Revenue Services I-90 forms

Finance Corporation (The World Bank, 2008); and the Stop TB partnership (McKinsey & Company, 2008), to name only a few. This is by no means an exhaustive list, but gives a sense of the depth and breadth of engagement of management consulting firms – from Ukraine to West Africa, and Haiti to Nigeria – making good on Winston Churchill's astute words: "Never let a good crisis go to waste." It should come as little surprise that by 2010, the public-sector practice of McKinsey was one of the fastest growing in the firm, with work spanning the USA, Europe, Asia and Africa (McDonald, 2013).

Applying a management consulting frame to the health field

Faced with the omnipresence of management consulting firms in global heath it is necessary to reflect on the impact of applying a management consulting frame to health. Many interviewees note that consulting firms have helped to professionalize the field. Their contribution to figuring out meaningful organizational processes, as well as their ability to translate ideas into marketable business terms for boards and for donors sensitive to such discourses, have been repeatedly highlighted as powerful assets. These positive observations notwithstanding, the questionable implications of using management consultants warrant examination.

Tendency to undermine systemic, root-cause interventions Management consultants tend to be generalists, who pride themselves in being able to solve problems in any area, regardless of the complexity of the issue at hand. A 2006 McKinsey report stated: "[I]n many ways, McKinsey seems ideally suited for tackling certain cross cutting issues. We solve problems for a living."[11] They analyze problems through an organizational management lens, and use this as the basis upon which their proposed response to a problem is built. This prompted David Oliver (2014), a British hospital consultant, to observe: "They are going to resort to what they know, which is consultancy approaches based on an industrial model."

This has far-reaching consequences. When an international organization or a bilateral donor chooses or presses its partners to choose for-profit management consultants over not-for-profit groups or academic institutions to advise a country or carry out work on its behalf, the choice that is made is not neutral. By choosing to frame issues primarily as things to be solved through problem-fixing and 'efficiency' gains, combined with a focus on immediate results, management consulting firms and those they advise, tend to collapse health and human development into a technical exercise.

Consequently, choosing a consulting firm to inform organizations and shape strategies often means weeding out upstream, alternative pathways and solutions, which may be more fundamental or long term, and not focusing on the systemic dimension of a problem or its root causes. It also often means, observes Malpani, that "[F]rom the start, you assume that there is a market-based solution".[12] Thus for example, the challenge of medicine pricing is addressed through PPPs or advanced market commitments, rather than by addressing issues related to the patent system, monopoly pricing or other issues. Lack of access to care is to be solved through assessment of infrastructure and logistical barriers, leaving aside questions of discrimination, rights and power, which might stand in the way of care.

The pathway to solving some of the most intractable health challenges is never merely technical, but requires engaging the power dynamics underpinning exclusion and marginalization. Health policymaking also requires that political choices and trade-offs be made, based on societal values, which in turn demands democratic participation. Such considerations are absent from consultants' playbooks. "I never heard a discussion of inequality or diversity, ever, led by consultants and yet clearly those are the challenges we face today," notes Roxana Bonnell, and once interventions aimed at the root causes are crowded out, it often means "entrenching the status quo when it comes to systems and power, rather than challenging power".[13]

Impact of leading with 'value for money' metrics Building on their for-profit private-sector expertise, management consultants bring with them tools, vocabulary and metrics emblematic of their ways of operating. Thus we see the widespread use in the global health arena of such terms as 'value for money', 'results-based financing' or 'high-impact interventions'. Having introduced these ideas, they move to implement them, working with not-for-profit entities or public–private partnerships to help them streamline their operations, get more out of their scarce resources or hone in on interventions whose impact would be more immediate and measurable. Such approaches have often been lauded by donors.

They have, however, received less than universal praise from health advocates, particularly when 'value for money' or impact analysis have caused the demise of efforts considered by many as essential, but whose metrics do not fit the framework and criteria set out by consulting firms. 'Value for money' approaches are often presented as intrinsically positive or as propositions no one can argue against. But as experiences in the humanitarian field have taught us over the years, it will almost always be more expensive to reach out and respond to those with the greatest needs: 'value for money' pushes in the direction of the easier wins and biggest bang for the bucks – not the greatest needs. The recent transition at the GFATM offers an interesting illustration of this phenomenon (Box D3.1).

Box D3.1: The transition at the Global Fund

Following the departure of Michel Kazatchkine from the GFATM (Rivers, 2012), Gabriel Jaramillo, a former chairman and chief executive officer of Sovereign Bank, was named as general manager by a board concerned with the alleged fund mismanagement and unmet fundraising goals. Jaramillo made no secret of the fact that he wanted to bring his "private-sector experience to addressing the problems of global health" and wholeheartedly embarked on "preparing a plan to save a crucial financial institution in trouble" by "re-engineering its internal systems, bringing greater efficiency to its operations, refocusing its management and creating a new investment strategy" (The Global Fund to Fight AIDS, Tuberculosis and Malaria, 2013).

With the support of Levitt Partners, BCG, McKinsey and Results for Development (R4D), Jaramillo initiated a set of ambitious reforms, in the areas of, tracking and investing of the funds of the GFATM, managing its grants, interacting with recipients and partners, and providing assurance on its investments. To address what were seen as issues with the funding model that the Global Fund had been using, the GFATM Board gave the green light to "explore new options that might lead to more strategic investment of resources, focusing on highest-impact countries and allowing for greater predictability". BCG and R4D were engaged in this process, completing various phases of work, including benchmarking, building models and simulating results for different options, and splitting the resources envelope among the three diseases. Some staff seconded by BCG to the GFATM worked on how 'qualitative' criteria, such as past performance, impact, risk, absorptive capacity and co-financing amounts would impact a country's funding allocation, and subsequently helped as 'change managers' to assist with the transition to the new model. Some went on to be hired by the Global Fund as staff.[14]

Julia Greenberg, who conducted the evaluation of the GFATM's partnership forum in 2011, remembers the central role of BCG in the development of the new funding model: "BCG is responsible for the new funding model—Round 10 has been cancelled. BCG was seen as a legitimate back-up to a dwindling leadership. It was believed that they would be able to produce more documentation and increase the accountability to the donors, who were questioning the way the Fund was being run".[15]

The final model, approved by the board in November 2012 and rolled out in 2014, assigned totals to countries, no longer calling on them to estimate their own needs, and used country disease burden and gross national income (GNI) per capita in eligibility formula, *de facto* kick-starting a shift of resources to interventions in low- or lower middle-income countries.

Though this certainly satisfied the donors eager to get "the most bang for their buck" (*Devex*, 6 September 2012), it also meant a focus on low-hanging fruits and in practice reducing support for key prevention activities, cutting support for high-risk groups such as injection drug users in upper middle-income countries, or reducing funds available for organizing civil society – all activities whose usefulness in controlling the HIV/AIDS epidemic have been documented over the years, but which failed to fit the new business-inspired approach. In several upper middle-income countries such as Romania, the gap in funding led to a drastic increase in HIV cases, specifically in key populations. The proportion of new cases of HIV related to injection drug use in Romania soared from 3 per cent in 2010 to 29 per cent in 2013. Much of this increase is linked to the lack of funds to provide basic prevention such as condoms and syringes (Health GAP, n.d.).

Undermining civil society and communities The impact of consulting language is also being felt in spaces where civil society is meant to engage. The very language used in documents, meetings and deliberations has evolved. Everyone is expected to master advanced market commitment or fiscal space discourses, and be able to engage on those technical issues, as opposed to contributing their rights-based or practical viewpoints. "By forcing them to engage in that frame, they become so driven by wanting to understand the details that they fail to see the bigger picture", observes Greenberg who adds: "It creates a language paradigm that you have to engage in. Why? Because there is a sense that that is where the power is, and you need to talk in the language of power. That language is given top credibility, and you have to challenge it on their terms".[16]

With the introduction of obscure jargon, management consultants have turned discussions on health into elitist debates, diminishing the space for people with different, practical experiences, and downgrading consideration for how change actually happens. As Gonsalves observes, "[T]his changes the nature of activism and advocacy. They are now filtered through the efficiency model."[17] Often vocal civil society groups from the South and representatives of partner governments tend to be pushed to the margins.

This also plays out upstream, in the groundwork consultants are often mandated to carry out, such as scoping and drawing up lists of people to interview. "Civil society is last. They will come up with a few names, such as MSF [Médecins Sans Frontières]. Very few organizations that work primarily at the country level or have limited resources will ever be included," remarks Malpani.[18] If an NGO is chosen for an interview, it tends to be a well-established group in the North. Very rarely would a local Ministry of Health (MoH) staff be included. As they define who the key stakeholders are, management consulting firms further the imbalance of representation, with represented voices tending to speak from a similar viewpoint.

Governance issues that ought to be explored

The evidence base While a systematic exploration of management consulting recommendations in the health field is made difficult by the lack of comprehensive, publicly accessible information, it is quite clear that consulting firms consistently champion the public–private model of cooperation as the quasi-universal solution to health challenges: from the response to epidemics (The Boston Consulting Group, 2015b) to the construction and operation of secondary and tertiary hospitals (Sharma, 2012) or access to medicines. While such recommendations may be straightforward and meaningful in business and financial terms, they are not necessarily backed by evidence when it comes to public health outcomes.

Consider the specific example of PPP model for hospitals. The evidence remains, at best, mixed. Research conducted by Martin McKee et al., (2006) on models in which a public authority contracts with a private company to design, build and operate an entire hospital seems to indicate that such new facilities, though more likely to be built within agreed-upon timeframes "have, in general, been more expensive than they would have been if procured using traditional methods". The experience on health PPPs indicates that "[E]scalating costs are a common feature of the model itself—some inherent and some due to serious oversights in the contracts underpinning them" (Marriott, 2015). PPP models for hospitals are nonetheless being promoted in places ranging from Sub-Saharan Africa to India. In 2012, McKinsey & Company recommended the public–private partnership route for improving healthcare delivery in India by 2022 (Sharma, 2012). In its 2008 report 'The business of health in Africa: partnering with the private sector to improve people's lives', produced for the World Bank with BMGF funding, McKinsey also laid the ground for PPPs to become a central strategy of the bank's International

Finance Corporation (IFC) (The World Bank, 2008). The 425-bed Queen Mamohato Memorial hospital, which replaced Lesotho's national referral hospital, was set up. Today, 51 per cent of the national health budget is being spent on payments to South Africa-based Netcare (one of the biggest private healthcare providers in the UK), which has built the hospital and runs it. The MoH is locked in an 18-year contract signed in 2009; this is siphoning off large amounts of the national health budget, while Netcare receives a 25 per cent return rate on its investment (Oxfam, 2014).

Consultants' briefs and presentations, when they are publicly accessible, rarely reference peer-reviewed articles or build on research on public health. While there may be evidence of the failure of public health systems to deliver, systematic research is lacking to support the opposing claim that the private sector can do better. Proprietary data, financial and otherwise, is rarely made available for public/academic scrutiny, rendering such claims difficult to sustain.

Confidentiality trumps transparency Management consulting firms are not bound to disclose the names of their clients or the products they generate for them. This practice is set to continue; in June 2016 McKinsey successfully weathered a court case that would have forced the firm to reveal the names of scores of its clients (Kary and Schoenberg, 2016). In fact, the firm prides itself on guarding the confidentiality of its clients and not publicizing their work (McKinsey & Company, n.d.), and "build[s] into its contract language that prevents clients from mentioning that the firm [has] been hired"(McDonald, 2013). Thus even when funding is public, the identity of their clients, the nature of the deals they enter into or the advice they provide remain largely hidden from public scrutiny. The issue becomes further murky when private foundations, which benefit from tax exemptions if they advance charitable purposes, second consultants to public or public–private institutions; or when consultants work *pro bono* for international organizations that seem to escape public scrutiny. There is currently no easy access to information on contracts awarded and amounts received by consulting firms for health-related work with PPPs or public health institutions, or details about the nature of the work. Those are neither made public by consulting firms themselves nor by institutions relying on their services. Consider the following:

- The *value of individual contracts*, such as the one granted to McKinsey & Company by the WHO-hosted Special Programme for Research and Training in Tropical Diseases for work on pooled funding for voluntary contributions towards research and development (R&D), is not made public. (In this case, informants privately revealed that the bill amounted to CHF 2 million and was borne by the Swiss Development Cooperation.)
- The absence of transparency extends to the *nature of the advice given* and the influence firms may have as a result. James Love, founder and direc-

tor of Knowledge Ecology International (KEI) recalls how, at some point, consultants began offering advice that he felt were policy recommendations. In the context of WHO's vaccine work, they recommended "shutting down government production of vaccines in favour of private production. If there is an emergency, the country that manufactures will get it first. How is this not a policy recommendation".[19] As Knowledge Ecology Initiative (KEI) noted in 2015 in a statement delivered at the session of 'WHO framework of engagement with non-state actors': "We believe the WHO has been discouraged from advancing very important reforms...sometimes this happens through the in-kind services the Gates Foundation provides to the WHO, such as through the consulting services of firms [like] the Boston Consulting Group (BCG) or McKinsey & Co., two firms hired by Gates that have recommended staff changes at the WHO." (Cassedy, 2015)

• Products generated by management consulting firms are generally kept private as well, unless it is otherwise negotiated in advance. Many interviewees described how, because of contractual agreements, detailed consultants' reports that they contributed to as informants, at times extensively, were never made available to them. "You often hand over very sensitive information, and yet you do not get access to the results. Nobody ever sees the data. You are only ever, at best, given the final overall picture," remarks Malpani.[20] The very stringent terms they impose often mean that not only is the textured analysis they produce not shared, but often the consultants are entrusted to filter the raw data and information and shape recommendations on the basis of assumptions they cannot disclose.

This opaque way of operating both limits the contribution consultants can make to public knowledge and debates, and enhances the consultants' own position in the field through the amassing of intelligence and proprietary information. Predictably, this often leads to consultants being hired time and time again on issues they have already worked on. This allows them to capitalize on the unique information and networks they have been paid to tap into, while their engagement in the public sphere and connections with decision-makers contribute to their enhanced reputation as informed and efficient counterparts in new fields. As they say in the business world: "Want to know what the competition is up to? Hire McKinsey" (McDonald, 2013).

Effectiveness and accountability The lack of robust transparency in the working of global health institutions, combined with the typical practice of management consulting firms to neither take blame nor credit for how their advice is used, creates major stumbling blocks for accountability. As the WHO's own 2015 procurement strategy document highlights, the current approach raises questions of business ownership, accountability and reporting, with particular risks identified in the areas of monitoring and governance, transparency,

Box D3.2: UNITAIDS funding scheme: 'massive' failure

Following its creation in 2006, UNITAID was universally acclaimed for establishing a new sustainable funding stream (through a small tax on airlines tickets in some countries), generating close to US$ 300 million in revenues in its very first year of operations. By 2007, though, bringing new countries with significant airline markets on board was proving much harder than anticipated. UNITAID's chairman, Philippe Douste-Blazy, and some of his close allies in the tourism business came up with an alternative idea: why not work with the industry directly and offer travellers the possibility to make voluntary micro-contributions every time they purchased travel services?

In December 2007, he presented the concept to the UNITAID Board, urging it to "make voluntary contributions the focus of the year 2008". Board members registered interest, and suggested that a feasibility study be conducted to validate the approach and add credibility to the endeavour. McKinsey & Company estimated that it could undertake the three-month study for US$ 1 million. The price tag made some supporters gasp, but Douste-Blazy was himself convinced that "it would be easier to get the UK, the BMGF and the WHO to sign off if such a document existed."

The BMGF had been contributing to UNITAID from its inception through the funding of McKinsey's involvement (UNITAID, 2006), and agreed to financially support the modelling of the initiative and the development of its business plan. The McKinsey study on the voluntary solidarity contribution was presented to the UNITAID Board in April 2008 and suggested that the new mechanism could raise between US$ 500 million and US$ 1 billion annually from private sources within five years, almost doubling UNITAID's budget from the airline-ticket tax and other contributions. The Board endorsed the plan and allocated a provisional budget of US$ 9 million for the first year, and US$ 12 million for the second year.

A director was appointed to set up the Millennium Foundation, which would host the project, and the team rapidly grew to be over 20-people strong. By July 2010, as the *Financial Times* reported, the foundation had fallen drastically behind schedule by year 1, "raising about [US$] 14,000 directly from the public while spending [US$] 11 [million] given to it by governments on salaries, advertising and legal expenses" (Jack, 2010). Several members of the board expressed "concerns that UNITAID has invested such a large amount of funds with very little return so far" (UNITAID, 2010), and it was decided that the initiative, plagued by recurring problems and failing to get on track, should be independently assessed. To do so, UNITAID went on to hire another firm, Dalberg.

Its study, whose costs were not made public, was damning and pointed at flaws in the assumptions and initial revenue modelling produced by McKinsey. In December 2012, UNITAID's chair reported that the Millenium Foundation had failed to reach its objectives and that, consequently, its board had passed a resolution to approve its dissolution (UNITAID, 2012). And so it – and millions of US dollars – was gone.

It is striking that McKinsey and its consultants were never held to account for the loss of public resources, in which their work played a large role. This naturally points to one of McKinsey's methods, whereby it takes neither responsibility nor credit for how an institution uses its advice. The UNITAID Board itself remained mostly silent about the incident, mindful of its own failure to appropriately scrutinize the proposal and oversee the efforts. While it might have had an opportunity to demand accounts, it chose not to, unwilling to create further backlash against funding for health and expose UNITAID to the types of criticism for wastefulness once levelled against traditional health institutions from which they were supposed to differ.

quality assurance and cost-effectiveness (WHO, 2015). The impact of the recommendations made by management consultants is rarely, if ever, evaluated. This lack of systematic research or evaluation is particularly ironic given how often consulting firms are invited into the health sphere based on claims of increased impact or value for money. And paradoxically, governments and bilateral donors, otherwise committed to transparency and accountability, de facto overlook these considerations when they employ consultants. At the country level, the situation is rarely much better as the "nomads of McKinsey or BCG have no formal commitments to the countries they work in, no connection with communities. It drains their engagement of any political accountability."[21]

The story of Massive Good, which was launched by UNITAID in 2009 and faded from the public eye by 2012, offers a telling example of the gap between the rhetoric of efficiency gained through management consulting advice and the reality, and the lack of accountability surrounding consulting firms' engagement (Box D3.2).

Revolving doors and conflicts of interest

Another set of questions regarding consulting firms pertain to networks, revolving doors and conflicts of interest. It is no secret that one of McKinsey's assets is its far-reaching alumni network. The firm's website proudly states that McKinsey counts over 30,000 alumni, who work in "virtually every business sector in 120 countries. Through formal events and informal networking, former McKinsey consultants make and sustain professional relationships." Alumni can open doors, provide a source of insider information, and act as future contracts; they also "tend to hire from old stomping grounds" (McDonald, 2013).

This phenomenon has been extensively documented in the UK, with evidence presented to the UK Public Administration Committee, prompting voices such as David Oliver's to state that "[T]here is far too much traffic between government bodies and consultancies and private health providers and lobbying companies which does verge on a form of institutional corruption" (Oliver, 2014). This phenomenon also comes into play with global health institutions, when former consultants take on positions with the institutions they have been advising, as was witnessed when Global Fund consultants who worked on the new funding model subsequently joined the fund as staff. This is also seen when staffers from global health institutions go on to work with consulting groups, at times staffing portfolios of clients that include their former employers.[22]

Conflict of interest considerations need scrutiny when consultants advise global institutions in areas where they also have, or are believed to have, private clients. Although 'Chinese walls' are allegedly put in place in a firm as soon as a perception of conflict might arise, the absence of publicly available information feeds doubts about potentially unstated conflicts. In February 2011, at the consultation with civil society during the "WHO open-ended working group of member states on pandemic influenza preparedness: sharing of influenza viruses and access to vaccines and other benefits" KEI asked a number of questions pertaining to the role of McKinsey in the preliminary findings for the technical studies conducted under the World Assembly Resolution WHA63.1 on pandemic influenza preparedness (Knowledge Ecology International, 2011a). The study itself notes, in its 'process' section, that "Given the significant breadth of the areas under study, and the limited human and financial resources of the Organization to carry out the full studies, the Secretariat sought external support. The Bill & Melinda Gates Foundation agreed to provide support through a contract with McKinsey & Company, which was selected on the basis of its broad expertise in public health, financing, health economics, and influenza vaccines; its ability to start working on the project quickly; and its global team". (WHO, 2010)

KEI formally enquired as to what the process of selection for McKinsey had been, and whether the WHO had used a competitive bidding process. It also asked whether the WHO had required the firm to disclose any conflicts of interest. WHO, in its response to KEI, (Knowledge Ecology International, 2011b) explained that member states had been informed at the onset about the BMGF offer of in-kind assistance to the WHO in the form of the services of McKinsey, and that since the practice of the WHO was to treat consulting firms as companies, no formal declaration of interest had been required.

How much McKinsey received for its work was not disclosed, nor was the arrangement between McKinsey and the BMGF.

KEI was motivated by its interest in having disclosure of possible conflicts, in particular where McKinsey might have had clients in the vaccine business. This would seem a legitimate concern in a context where publicly available information indicates that McKinsey has done work for at least three of the five top vaccines manufacturers in the world: Novartis, Merck and Sanofi (Bouchard, 2001; *Consultor.fr*, 24 April 2012; Cristofari, 2011); it has also been involved in the development of the business plan of GAVI (GAVI Alliance, n.d.); and it has had other vaccine-related engagements, including the preparation of a report for the Organization of Pharmaceutical Producers of India titled 'Transforming India's vaccine market' (McKinsey & Company, 2012).

Whether consulting firms' inroads into public institutions or PPPs get translated into enhanced engagements with private-sector clients remains in the realm of speculation. But the fact that consulting firms make recommendations that create a climate favourable to businesses, while bringing to the field of health a set of private sector–inspired methods and tools, and connecting with the entire health spectrum (from pharmaceutical companies to the WHO; from the largest private hospitals chains in India to the Global Fund, the BMGF, the NHS and the Food and Drug Administration) contributes to feeding the worry that the issue could range from simple connivance to outright conflict of interest.

Conclusion

The mix of private and public, state and non-state, for profit and not-for-profit actors has become a definitional trait of today's global health field. The legitimacy and efficiency of public institutions to tackle crises continue to be tested, including at the height of crises such as Ebola. Progress in entire swathes of the health field is now spearheaded by private-sector actors, who have become *de facto* prescribers of public health policy priorities.

In the past decade and a half, management consulting firms have also risen to prominence. Yet although they contribute to shaping the functioning and direction of public institutions, international organizations and PPPs, their influence has remained largely unexamined.

They bring to the health field the same principles that govern how they work in the business realm: a premium on confidentiality and the policy of not taking blame or credit for the advice they provide. This might be perfectly fine in case of wholly private endeavours, where corporations choose to employ management consultants to improve their bottom lines, with their shareholders' support and scrutiny. But when the work of consultants is subsidized, at least in part, by public funds, or when it influences the direction of public institutions, the public ought to have a greater sense of what is being proposed and the possible impact.

Management consulting firms seem by and large exempt from publicly articulating the basis upon which they ground their legitimacy in the health field or from providing evidence in terms of health outcomes that underpins their views. In the absence of both publicly available information and solid research, management consultants' forays into global health may be understood as well-choreographed profit-seeking endeavours. Through the engagements may often appear free of cost initially to the recipients, consultants gradually attach themselves to key stakeholders and gain access to information and funding streams. More often than not, the engagements get translated into lucrative dependencies. These engagements bring the additional benefit of burnishing a firm's reputation with conventional clients, as well as with leaders and policymakers. Health is, for consultants, a low-risk enterprise: an opportunity to learn and become familiar with a large field, using someone else's money, with no accountability and very few strings attached. Not unlike the pharmaceutical companies they serve, consultants appear to have mastered the art of socializing risks and privatizing benefits.

There is no evidence that the ascent of consulting firms in the health sector has led to approaches and solutions to radically improve health outcomes for the poor and most marginalized. The framing of health as a technical exercise and the related focus on value for money, efficiency gains and rapid results has led to the exclusion of those most in need; the sidelining of systemic long-term solutions and the downgrading of community voices. We must urgently ask whether we have examined closely enough the impact of choosing management consulting firms to support and guide institutions in their search to improve health outcomes. Public interest is seldom served by secrecy; and in the absence of robust participatory processes, transparency and accountability mechanisms, we risk letting go of functions essential to preserve health as a public good – without even realizing we are doing so.

Notes

1 WHO response team and UNMEER coordination member (2015), interview, September.

2 Interviews were conducted between August and December 2015. While interviewees were eager to provide first-hand accounts of their experience with management consulting firms, most were reluctant to be quoted by name, either due to confidentiality agreements or because of concerns about their professional development.

3 Gregg Gonsalves (2015), interview, September.

4 It was estimated that in the USA alone, individuals had donated US$ 5.5 to 7.4 trillion to charitable causes between 1998 and 2017. See Schervish (2005), pp. 15–37.

5 Gonsalves (2015), interview.

6 McKinsey & Company's reflection paper about the firm's possible increased engagement in global health.

7 Rohit Malpani (2015), interview, October.

8 Health access advocate (2015), interview, September.

9 Former consultant (2015), interview, December.

10 A number of leaders in the field received emails asking for their participation in this study.

11 McKinsey & Company's reflection paper

about the firm's possible increased engagement in global health.

12 Malpani (2015), interview.

13 Roxana Bonnell (2015), interview, October.

14 Global Fund employee (2015), interview, September.

15 Julia Greenberg (2015), interview, September.

16 Ibid.

17 Gonsalves (2015), interview.

18 Malpani (2015), interview.

19 James Love (2015), interview, September.

20 Malpani (2015), interview.

21 Gonsalves (2015), interview.

22 Malpani (2015), interview.

References

Basu, S, Andrews, J, Kishore, S, Panjabi, R & Stuckler, D 2012,'Comparative performance of private and public healthcare systems in low-and middle-income countries: a systematic review', *PLoSMedicine*, 19 June, https://doi.org/10.1371/journal. pmed.1001244

Boston University 2013, *Evaluation of the Queen Mamohato Memorial Hospital public private partnership (PPP) in Lesotho*, Center for Global Health &Development, Boston University, viewed 7 February 2017, https://www.bu.edu/cghd/our-work/ projects/evaluation-of-the-queen-mamohato-memorial-hospital-public-private-partnership-ppp-in-lesotho/

Bouchard, F 2001,'Novartis: le marketing prend le pas sur les scientifiques, c'est la victoire de Sandoz', *LesEchos.fr*, 1 January, viewed 7 February 2017, http://archives.lesechos.fr/ archives/2001/Enjeux/00165-049-ENJ.htm

Brandt, A M 2013,'How AIDS invented global health', *New England Journal of Medicine*, vol. 368, no. 23, pp. 2149–52.

Cassedy, C 2015, *Engagement with non-state actors*, 8 May, viewed 7 February 2017, http://keionline.org/sites/ default/files/DHHSListeningSession-Engagementwithnon-stateactors_0.pdf

Cristofari, J J 2011,'Sanofi se détached'Aventis', *Pharmanalyses*, 13 May, viewed 7 February 2017, http://pharmanalyses.fr/sanofi-se-detache-daventis/

GAVI Alliance n.d., *Part I overview – GAVI Alliance strategy and business plan*

2011–2015, viewed 7 February 2017, http:// www.gavi.org/library/gavi-documents/ strategy/gavi-alliance-strategy-and-business-plan-2011-2015/

Gilligan, A 2012. '"Poverty barons" who make a fortune from taxpayer-funded aid budget', *The Telegraph*, 15 September, viewed 7 February 2017, http://www.telegraph.co.uk/ news/politics/9545584/Poverty-barons-who-make-a-fortune-from-taxpayer-funded-aid-budget.html

Gov.UK 2015, *DFID 7168 support to the presidential delivery team – Sierra Leone, contract*, viewed7 February 2017, https://www.contractsfinder.service.gov. uk/Notice/89cc9f3d-a63b-4665-aa2e-5f9c7482cb62

Gov.UK 2016, *DFID 7424 support to Sierra Leone president's delivery team – phase II, contract*, viewed 7 February 2017, https://www.contractsfinder.service.gov. uk/Notice/92e8db9b-1d81-4c21-abc3-94ec2662b66b

Health GAP n.d., *Myths & facts: donor funding for the global AIDS response*, viewed 7 February 2017, https://d3n8a8pro7vhmx. cloudfront.net/healthgap/pages/1092/ attachments/original/1472838612/Myths___ Facts_Donor_Funding_for_Global_AIDS. pdf?1472838612

Holtzman, C 2009,'Gates Foundation spends big on consulting', *Puget Sound Business Journal*, 11 June, viewed 7 February 2017, http://www.bizjournals.com/seattle/ stories/2009/06/15/story7.html

Jack, A 2010, 'Health charity spent millions to raise thousands', *Financial Times*, 6 July, viewed 7 February 2017, https://www. ft.com/content/8e85f9fa-8914-11df-8ecd-00144feab49a?mhq5j=e2

Kary, T & Schoenberg, T 2016, *In battle to name McKinsey clients, discretion carries day*, 29 June, viewed 7 February 2017, https://www. bloomberg.com/news/articles/2016-06-29/ in-battle-to-reveal-mckinsey-clients-discretion-carries-the-day

Knowledge Ecology International 2011a, *KEI letter to WHO regarding McKinsey, vaccine policy and competing interests*, 15 February, viewed 7 February 2017, http://keionline. org/node/1078

Knowledge Ecology International 2011b, *Response of WHO to KEI letter regarding*

McKinsey, vaccine policy and competing interests, 2 March, viewed7 February 2017, http://keionline.org/node/1084

Knowledge Ecology International 2016, *TDR releases report on a health product research & development fund: a proposal for financing and operation*, 17 March, viewed 7 February 2017, http://keionline.org/node/2447

Marriott, A 2015, *Why is the World Bank group dragging its feet over its disastrous PPP policy on funding healthcare?* 20 November, viewed 7 February 2017, https://oxfamblogs.org/fp2p/why-is-the-world-bank-group-dragging-its-feet-over-its-disastrous-policy-on-funding-healthcare/

McCoy, D, Kembhavi, G, Patel, J &Luintel, A 2009,'The Bill & Melinda Gates Foundation's grant-making programme for global health', *The Lancet*, vol. 373, no. 9675, pp. 1645–53.

McDonald, D 2013, *The firm: the story of McKinsey and its secret influence on American business*, Simon and Schuster, New York

McKee M, Edwards N, Atunc R 2006, Public–private partnerships for hospitals, Bulletin of the World Health Organization, November 2006, 84 (11), WHO, Geneva https://www.researchgate.net/publication/6656463_Public_Private_Partnerships_for_Hospitals

McKinsey & Company 2008, *Independent evaluation of the Stop TB partnership*, 21 April, viewed 7 February 2017, http://www.stoptb.org/assets/documents/resources/publications/achieve_eval/Stop%20TB%20Evaluation%20Final%20Report_Exhibits_Annexes.pdf

McKinsey & Company2012, *Transforming India's vaccine market: saving lives, creating value*, viewed 7 February 2017, http://www.mckinsey.com/global-themes/india/transforming-indias-vaccine-market

McKinsey & Company n.d.,*What we do*, viewed 7 February 2017, http://www.mckinsey.com/about-us/what-we-do

'McKinsey misen concurrence', *Consultor.fr*, 24 April 2012, viewed 7 February 2017, https://www.consultor.fr/devenir-consultant/breves/470-mckinsey-mis-en-concurrence.html

Oliver, D 2014.'Stop wasting taxpayers' money on management consultancy for the NHS', *British Medical Journal*, vol. 349.

Oxfam 2014, *A dangerous diversion – will the IFC's flagship health PPP bankrupt Lesotho's Ministry of Health?* 7 April, viewed 7 February 2017, https://www.oxfam.org/sites/www.oxfam.org/files/bn-dangerous-diversion-lesotho-health-ppp-070414-en.pdf

Rivers, B 2012, 'Global Fund executive director Michel Kazatchkine to resign', *Aidspan*, 24 January, viewed 7 February 2017, http://www.aidspan.org/gfo_article/global-fund-executive-director-michel-kazatchkine-resign

Schervish, P G 2005,'Today's wealth holder and tomorrow's giving: the new dynamics of wealth and philanthropy', *Journal of Gift Planning*, vol. 9, no. 3, pp. 15–37.

Sharma, R 2012, 'PPP is the way forward to improve healthcare in India: McKinsey', *Down To Earth*, 29 December, viewed 7 February 2017, http://www.downtoearth.org.in/news/ppp-is-the-way-forward-to-improve-healthcare-in-india-mckinsey-39883

The Boston Consulting Group 2008, 'Making a difference 2008: BCG's partnerships and projects for social impact', 5 December, viewed 7 February 2017, https://www.bcgperspectives.com/content/articles/public_sector_making_a_difference_2008/

The Boston Consulting Group 2011, *Global health: BCG's Wendy Woods on the current situation, dynamics, and trends*, online video, viewed 3 February 2017, https://www.youtube.com/watch?v=JYZbAWDCY3E

The Boston Consulting Group 2013, *Report to the GAVI Alliance board – benchmarking of GAVI's vaccine procurement arrangements*, 21–22 November

The Boston Consulting Group 2014,*BCG's approach to achieving social impact*, 14 October, viewed 7 February 2017, https://www.bcgperspectives.com/content/articles/investing_for_impact_health_bcgs_approach_achieving_social_impact/?chapter=4

The Boston Consulting Group 2015a, *BCG wins award for pro bono work with the United Nations*, http://www.bcg.com/d/press/11september2015-bcg-wins-social-investment-award-16509.

The Boston Consulting Group 2015b, *Managing the risk and impact of future epidemics*, 4 June, viewed 7 February 2017, https://www.

bcgperspectives.com/content/articles/
health-public-sector-managing-risk-impact-
of-future-epidemics/

The Boston Consulting Group 2015c,*UNICEF/
WFP return on investment for emergency
preparedness study*, viewed 7 February
2017, https://www.unicef.org/publications/
files/UNICEF_WFP_Return_on_Investment_
for_Emergency_Preparedness_Study.pdf

'The Global Fund and value for money', *Devex*,
6 September 2012, viewed 7 February 2017,
https://www.devex.com/news/the-global-
fund-and-value-for-money-79075

The Global Fund to Fight AIDS, Tuberculosis
and Malaria2002, *Report of the third
Board meeting*, viewed 7 February 2017,
http://www.theglobalfund.org/documents/
board/03/BM03_BoardMeeting_Report_en/

The Global Fund to Fight AIDS, Tuberculosis
and Malaria2003, *Annual Report
2002/2003*, viewed 3 February 2017, http://
www.theglobalfund.org/en/archive/
annualreports/

The Global Fund to Fight AIDS, Tuberculosis
and Malaria2013, *Report and
recommendations by the outgoing general
manager*, 18–19 June, viewed February 2017,
http://www.theglobalfund.org/documents/
board/29/BM29_05-GeneralManager_
Report_en/

The World Bank 2008, *The business of health in
Africa: partnering with the private sector to
improve people's lives*, 1 January, viewed 7
February 2017, http://documents.worldbank.
org/curated/en/878891468002994639/
The-business-of-health-in-Africa-partnering-
with-the-private-sector-to-improve-
peoples-lives

UNICEF 2015, *UNICEF's strategy for health
(2016–2030)*,viewed 7 February 2017,
https://www.unicef.org/health/files/
UNICEF_Health_Strategy_Final.pdf

UNITAID 2006, *2nd UNITAID Board meeting,
Geneva, 29–30 November 2006 ,minutes*,

viewed 7 February 2017, http://www.
unitaid.eu/images/governance/eb2en/
minutes_eb2_en.pdf

UNITAID 2007, *Chair's summary, UNITAID
Executive Board meeting 9–10 July 2007*,
viewed 7 February 2017, http://www.
unitaid.eu/images/governance/eb5en/
utd_eb5_chairs-summary_en.pdf

UNITAID 2008, *UNITAID Executive Board, 9th
session 24–25 November 2008, Geneva,
chair summary*, viewed 7 February 2017,
http://www.unitaid.eu/images/governance/
EB9/eb9_chairsummary_en.pdf

UNITAID 2010, *12th meeting of the UNITAID
Executive Board, 8–9 June*, viewed 7
February 2017, http://www.unitaid.eu/
images/EB12/EB12_Approved-Minutes.pdf

UNITAID 2012,*Minutes of UNITAID's 17th
Executive Board session 3–5 December*,
viewed 7 February 2017, http://www.unitaid.
eu/images/Resolutions/EB17/Minutes_EB17.
pdf

Wellcome Trust 2015, *Generating evidence
for infectious diseases with epidemic
potential – meeting report*, 20 October,
viewed 7 February 2017, http://www.who.
int/medicines/ebola-treatment/meetings/
MeetingReport_GEIDEP.pdf

WHO 2010, '*Preliminary findings for the
technical studies under resolution WHA63.1*,
10 December, viewed 7 February 2017,
http://apps.who.int/gb/pip/pdf_files/
OEWG2/PIP_OEWG_Preliminary-findings-
en.pdf

WHO 2015,*WHO procurement strategy*, 27
April, viewed 7 February 2017, http://
www.who.int/about/resources_planning/
WHO_Procurement_Strategy_April2015.pdf

Winsten, J & Woods, W 2011,'Guest column:
resetting the Roll Back Malaria campaign
has had powerful lessons and results,'
Financial Times. 21 April, viewed 7 February
2017, https://www.ft.com/content/ca2ab162-
6753-11e0-9bb8-00144feab49a

D4 | GAVI AND GLOBAL FUND: PRIVATE GOVERNANCE STRUCTURES TRUMP PUBLIC OVERSIGHT IN PUBLIC PRIVATE PARTNERSHIPS

Global Public Private Partnerships (PPPs) have emerged as the new medium of global governance, replacing over time the nation state driven governance system which was embodied in the UN system. In other chapters (D1 and D2) we have commented on the process and motivation underlying this shift in global governance for health. In this chapter we examine, arguably, the two largest PPPs in the health sector, the Global Alliance for Vaccines and Immunization (GAVI) and the Global Fund to Fight AIDS, Tuberculosis and Malaria (GFATM). Both these organizations were deliberately positioned outside the UN system and provide a space for private entities in their governance structures. It is interesting to note that the Bill and Melinda Gates Foundation (BMGF) is closely linked with both these partnerships. Specifically the chapter looks at distortions in global governance that arise as a result of such partnerships. The chapter also focuses on how private actors appear to have hijacked both these partnerships and utilize them to expand the space for a range of private entities to intervene in areas of activities which are essentially public in nature. This is particularly problematic given that both these partnerships are largely funded from public sources – mainly through contributions from countries.

GAVI: Publicly funded with a private vision

Formation, objectives and governance The Global Alliance for Vaccines and Immunization (GAVI) was launched in 2000 with an initial grant of US$ 750 million over five years from the Bill and Melinda Gates Foundation. Countries are eligible to apply for support from GAVI when their Gross National Income (GNI) per capita is below a certain level (currently US$ 1,580) on average over the past three years (according to World Bank data published every year on 1 July)[1].

GAVI owes its existence to a meeting hosted by the World Bank President James Wolfensohn in March 1998 that brought the prospective GAVI board members together. GAVI's objectives, outlined in the first board meeting were: affordable prices for governments; adequate investment in capacity to supply global needs; and private investment in research and development of high priority vaccines for developing countries[2].

GAVI has a hybrid governance structure that involves non-state actors, such as pharmaceutical corporations, in its decision-making processes. The

Bill & Melinda Gates Foundation (BMGF), as a founding member, has played a key role in shaping GAVI's policies. The BMGF holds one of the four permanent seats on GAVI's Board (the others are UNICEF, WHO, and the World Bank). Beside thirteen members from governments and international organizations, two representatives from the vaccine industry (currently Sanofi Pasteur and Serum Institute of India, Ltd.) sit on GAVI's board[3]. In addition, several representatives from auditing companies, banks, investment companies, and foundations are among the nine 'independent board members' who have no connection with GAVI's technical work[4]. 79% of GAVI's funding comes from governments and the rest from foundations, corporations and individuals[5].

GAVI places emphasis on technological solutions to achieve quantifiable, quick, short-term results (see Chapter D2 about how this is the hallmark of BMGF supported initiatives) (Wirgau et al., 2010). Through its way of working which we discuss later, GAVI's strategies are geared towards promoting the interests of private vaccine manufactures. This is reflected in GAVI's adoption of Advanced Market Commitments and Tiered Pricing as the organization's fundamental approach towards promoting access to vaccines. GAVI does not promote local production and technology transfer.

GAVI follows the key strategies of market shaping and co-financing[6]. 'Market shaping' is understood as a strategy where both the demand and the supply of a vaccine are intentionally altered (Castro et al 2017) GAVI promotes this strategy on the ground that it will lead to lower prices: while countries gain bargaining power by pooling and guaranteeing demand, vaccine manufacturers realize economies of scale. However, GAVI's 'market shaping' strategy is entirely non-transparent. Through this strategy GAVI has been able to create a captive market for new vaccines for a small set of vaccine manufacturers by pushing these on national immunization schedules of the countries it supports. GAVI's Co-financing strategy involves cost sharing of vaccines by participating countries.

Contrary to what GAVI would like to project, there are serious doubts regarding GAVI's real impact on the promotion of public health goals. The Strategic Advisory Group of Experts on Immunization (SAGE), in the Midterm Review of the Global Vaccine Action Plan (2012–2020), observed that while the global rate of new vaccine introduction has remained strong, the progress towards the goals to eradicate polio, eliminate measles, rubella, maternal and neonatal tetanus, and increase equitable access to lifesaving vaccines remained slow. Since 2010, global average immunization coverage has increased by only 1 per cent. However, new or under-utilized vaccine introductions have overshot their target. Between 2010 and 2015, 99 low- or middle-income countries (LMIC) introduced one or more new or under-utilized vaccines. GAVI had provided support to 64 of these countries (SAGE, 2016).

Advanced Market Commitments An 'Advance Purchase Commitment', rebranded by GAVI as 'Advanced Market Commitment' (AMC) is GAVI's key strategy. Essentially AMC involves purchasers (in this case countries) committing to buy a certain quantity of a product (in this case vaccines) in advance, that is well before the product is supplied. It is a concept developed by Michael Kremer, the Bill and Melinda Gates Professor of Developing Societies and Economics at Harvard University (Light, 2009). From conception to execution the motivation to promote AMC has changed to accommodate pharmaceutical industry needs. Initially, the purpose of an AMC was to motivate private vaccine industry to conduct research and development for 'neglected diseases' that primarily afflict low-income countries. The logic being that vaccine manufacturers would be incentivized to develop new vaccines if they were guaranteed a market for their product. However, in GAVI's first major foray, an AMC was used to guarantee the purchase of new 'blockbuster' vaccines for pneumococcal diseases. It was clearly designed to benefit four multinational giants in vaccine development and manufacturing. It has been argued that AMCs promoted by GAVI "deliberately favour large pharmaceutical firms over small and new biotechs and not-for-profit, university-based, and developing-country-based research. Yet, they present no empirical evidence that such firms are the most efficient at vaccine research" (Farlow, 2004). The goal of developing regional vaccine production capacity through technology sharing was on GAVI's early agenda, but was quietly dropped. Instead, the economics, structure, legal terms, and handling of GAVI's AMCs favour a few multinational corporations. This is in spite of the widely accepted fact that more than four-fifths of all money for basic research to discover new vaccines or medicines comes from public sources (Light, 2006).

In AMCs the price and volume of purchase are pre-set by a committee, and companies promise to make their product available at a low initial price, while keeping their intellectual property (IP) rights intact (Light, 2009). AMCs include no arrangement for acquiring IP rights, technology transfer or promoting local production – all key components of improving and sustaining access to medical products (Sell, 1998). The legal advisers for drafting the legal terms of the purchase commitment were Covington & Burling, one of the most powerful international firms offering IP related services to the pharmaceutical industry[7]. Kremer's design of AMCs draws on industry-supported studies that exaggerate R&D costs for developing a new drug – industry driven estimates of product R&D are many times higher than what independent evidence suggests. This results in donors paying much more for development costs than the actual cost of research (Light, 2007).

An AMC was first applied by GAVI for the procurement of the pneumococcal conjugate vaccine (PCV). Contrary to the stated principle that AMCs would incentivize new vaccine development, the AMC had nothing to do with R&D as pneumococcal vaccines had already been developed, and were looking for lucrative markets (which the AMC provided) (Johns Hopkins, 2006). Prevnar by Pfizer-Wyeth was already in the market and two other versions of the vaccines by Pfizer-Wyeth and Merck, were close to gaining market approval (Balasubramaniam et al., 2014).

The entire market of pneumococcal conjugate vaccine, worth US$ 30 billion until 2016, is served by just two companies: Pfizer and GlaxoSmithKline (Cooper, 2016). An independent economic analysis of the 2006 PCV AMC pricing, commissioned by Médecins Sans Frontières (MSF), concluded that US$ 600 million would go as extra profits above the "regular" profits built into the pricing structure (Schoen-Angerer, 2008). Tore Godal, the former executive director of GAVI, conceded that the AMC price of US$ 5 a dose was too high (Gjerde, 2008). Despite this the price was raised to US$ 7 under pressure from private vaccine manufacturers (GAVI, 2008). By March 2015 Pfizer and Glaxo Smith Kline (GSK) had received US$ 1.095 billion from the AMC funds. Despite the discount it has negotiated, GAVI also recognizes that pneumococcal vaccine costs more than GAVI-eligible countries can afford (Johns Hopkins, 2006).

While the number of diseases against which a child is immunized has doubled between 2001 and 2014, the cost of the vaccines to fully immunize a child (after introduction of the new vaccines) has disproportionately multiplied 68-fold. This estimate represents a theoretical, best-case scenario, based on the lowest available prices for the UNICEF Supply Division and restricted to a select group of developing countries, usually only GAVI-eligible countries. The cost will be higher for countries not eligible for GAVI support (MSF, 2015).

If AMCs had really been designed to incentivize R&D by the private sector for requirements of low- and middle-income countries (LMICs), then R&D activities would have focused on real needs in these countries. Vaccine delivery can be extremely difficult and expensive, especially in countries where health systems are poorly developed. Most vaccines have stringent cold chain requirements, posing a challenge in places without uninterrupted power supply. Investments are required on R&D designed to develop products that are free of strict cold-chain requirements (ibid.).

GAVI and tiered pricing In the first board meeting in 1999, GAVI's Board endorsed use of differential or 'tiered pricing' as a pricing strategy. Tiered pricing[8] is a business strategy of charging different prices for the same product in different markets or consumer groups. It could be applied in different geographical segments: high and low income countries; and within a country across different consumer groups: private and public sector. This strategy allows pharmaceutical companies to maintain market monopoly by blocking generic competition, preventing use of TRIPS flexibilities and maximizing profits by selling at different prices to different market segments. It also helps skirt criticism of overpricing in low income country markets (Modi Pandav, 2014). Tiered pricing is a strategy that allows pharmaceutical MNCs to continue to charge monopoly prices, tailored to what different markets can absorb. The prices set are based on what markets can absorb and not on the actual cost of manufacture (even after factoring in research costs). Companies retain their monopoly Patent rights and continue to bar generic manufacturers from manufacturing and selling the products. While companies reduce prices in low income settings when they apply tiered pricing, the price set is still much higher than what would have obtained if competition from generic manufacturers was allowed.

Tiered-pricing policies of GAVI are voluntary, arbitrary, ad hoc and conditional (GAVI and non-GAVI countries) and pricing decisions lack transparency. Companies may offer discounts on some drugs but not others, to some high-burden countries but not others, for a limited time or subject to conditions attached (ibid). For example, in case of the 10-valent pneumococcal conjugate vaccine, GAVI negotiated an initial price of US$ 7/dose with GSK. The Pan American Health Organization (PAHO) could not obtain the same price and initially opted not to purchase the vaccine. Brazil independently negotiated an initial price of US$ 16/dose. PAHO subsequently settled for a price of US$ 14.85/dose (ibid.). In 2010, India's Serum Institute was offering the pentavalent vaccine at US$ 1.75 per dose as compared to US$ 3.2 paid with GAVI funds for a single dose vaccine from Crucell and US$ 2.95 for a two dose vaccine from GSK. GAVI justified this on grounds it could only rely on Western companies to provide uninterrupted supplies on a large scale. Till 2011 only GSK and Pfizer had qualified for GAVI's support with their pneumococcal vaccines (Arie, 2011).

Often the prices offered by GAVI, even after application of tiered pricing, are not affordable in LMICs. When Gardasil, the first vaccine against the Human Papilloma Virus (HPV) that is implicated in cancer of the cervix, was launched in 2006, it cost between US$ 100 and US$ 233 per dose in developed countries and between US$ 30 and US$ 100 per dose in developing countries. In 2011 PAHO negotiated a price of US$ 14 per dose for its member countries. Despite this decrease in price, it is still too expensive for many LMICs (Castro, 2017).

Robust generic competition, and not tiered pricing, offers a sustainable solution to the problem of higher prices of new medicines and vaccines. Tiered pricing only offers a short-term option to increase access to a product only when market volumes are very small or highly uncertain and/or multisource production capacity is lacking. Experience demonstrates that entry of additional manufacturers with WHO-prequalified vaccines, in particular developing-country manufacturers, stimulates competition and drives down prices (MSF, 2015). Policies which encourage technology transfer and promote competition should be adopted, which are not yet part of GAVI's strategy.

As has been argued (Balasubramaniam, 2001): "[T]he problem of lack of access to the two billion people who have no access to essential drugs cannot be solved by negotiating discounts country by country, company by company and drug by drug. Negotiations take place in total darkness since the real costs of production of drugs are not known to the negotiators. All pricing information is kept in confidence by the manufacturers. These are not therefore fair negotiations".

GAVI's bargaining power helps vaccine manufacturers A rationale for the setting up of GAVI was that it would, as a large pooled purchaser of vaccines, curb the monopoly power of large vaccine manufacturers to set high monopoly prices for new vaccines. However, evidence suggests that the reverse seems to have happened and vaccine manufacturers utilize the leverage they have in GAVI's governance to milk the system and accumulate super profits (see Box D4.1).

It is estimated that by 2025, 29 of the original 73 eligible countries will have lost Gavi support entirely. These countries will then face the dual challenge of meeting the higher cost of new vaccines and fully self-financing their national immunization programmes. They may have to pay up to six times more for pneumococcal conjugate vaccine, for example (GAVI Alliance, 2015). It is estimated that currently 'graduating' Honduras (meaning that it would no longer receive support from GAVI) will need to cover US$ 5 million paid annually by GAVI for new vaccines, a 38 per cent increase in the government's present expenditures for immunization (Government of Honduras, 2013). Other estimates of increase in immunization budgets to cover cost of new vaccines are: 197 per cent for Sri Lanka between 2012 and 2018, 801 per cent for Congo, 1,523 per cent for Angola and 1,547 per cent for Indonesia (Ryckman et al., 2014). The ultimate beneficiaries are vaccine manufacturers, largely situated in the North, who secure access to a large market through GAVI's AMCs and tiered pricing mechanisms.

Five companies control 80 per cent of the vaccine market – GSK, Merck, Sanofi-Pasteur, Pfizer and Novartis (Balasubramaniam, 2014). The business of vaccines is slated to become a major source of profits for the world's largest pharmaceutical corporations and the profits from vaccines are projected to reach US$ 61 billion by 2020 (Guzman, 2016).

GAVI's role in attempting to undermine the principles of the Pan American Health Organization's (PAHO) revolving fund for vaccines is particularly illuminating as regards the role GAVI plays vis-à-vis vaccine manufacturers. The PAHO Revolving Fund for Vaccine Procurement is a mechanism introduced in 1977 that facilitates timely access to high-quality vaccines at the lowest prices for national immunization programs of Member States. It offers vaccines to all participating Member States at the same single price. "Furthermore, the Fund establishes contractual terms and conditions in its international tenders in order to guarantee that the prices of the procured products are the lowest globally"[9].

Box D4.1: MSF Rejects vaccine donation from Pfizer

In October 2016 MSF refused a donation of one million PCV13 vaccine doses from Pfizer. MSF called this a principled stand against the extremely high cost of many vaccines. MSF while refusing the donation pointed out that while they value donations, this was not straightforward philanthropy. Donations from pharmaceutical companies are ineffective against a problem of massive dimensions. MSF said that while the donation would benefit people receiving care from MSF, accepting it could mean problems for others, and longer-term problems. "By giving the pneumonia vaccine away for free, pharmaceutical corporations can use this as justification for why prices remain high for others, including other humanitarian organizations and developing countries that also can't afford the vaccine" (Hamblin, 2016).

PCV13, sold under the name Prevnar 13 is among the best-selling vaccines on the market. In 2015 alone, Pfizer's revenue from its sale was US$ 6.245 billion. Its technology is protected by multiple product and process patents preventing generic competition. A South Korean company SK Chemicals came close to producing an analogue, but Pfizer sued the company and won (ibid.).

Even after five years of negotiations MSF has failed to secure lower prices from GSK and Pfizer for pneumococcal vaccines. MSF notes that "The GAVI price is still expensive when you compare it to other traditional vaccines where there is actual competition in the market (Cooper, 2016)." What these companies charge governments is shrouded in secrecy and the only price known is the price negotiated by GAVI – US$ 10 per child. MSF has been calling on both companies to reduce the price to US$ 5 per child for all developing countries, regardless of GAVI status, and to all humanitarian organizations. While Pfizer and GSK are happy to talk about the discounts they provide to GAVI, neither company was willing to give a breakdown of their international sales, disaggregated by 'GAVI-price' and 'non-GAVI price (ibid.).

Since 2007, the fund had come under pressure from GAVI and BMGF to pay higher prices, while they themselves procured the new vaccines at lower prices. The Fund conceded three exceptions (to the principle that the revolving fund would negotiate the lowest price obtainable globally) for the prices of pneumococcal, rotavirus and HPV vaccines in expectation of obtaining reduced prices for its Member States. Despite negotiations the price reduction offered to the revolving fund was minimal compared to the prices obtained by GAVI. GAVI, BMGF and some vaccine manufacturers continued to exert pressure

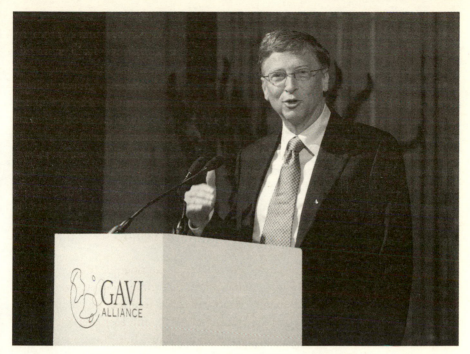

Image D4.1 Bill Gates addresses meeting of the GAVI alliance (Ben Fisher/GAVI Alliance; License: CC BY 2.0, https://creativecommons.org/licenses/by/2.0/)

for additional exceptions for other vaccines like the inactivated polio vaccine (IPV) (PAHO, 2013).

In 2013, PAHO adopted a resolution to ensure that the PAHO Revolving Fund is administered without exceptions. Member States also requested review of the previously conceded exceptions[10]. PAHO Member States were concerned about the continued erosion of the Revolving Fund's principles and the significantly higher prices it paid[11]. They overwhelmingly voted in favour of a Resolution that ratified the principles of the Revolving Fund and requested the PAHO Secretariat to ensure that the Revolving Fund is administered, without exception (PAHO, 2013).

GAVI's close association with BMGF raises further concerns regarding conflict of interest. Since 2008, the BMGF has been supporting establishment of National Vaccine Advisory Committees in Africa and Asia. In 2008, the French agency, Agence de Médecine Préventive (AMP), received a grant of 10 million dollars from the Gates Foundation to support the development of National Vaccine Advisory Committees in Africa and Asia. These committees help the national health authorities of GAVI-eligible countries to implement vaccination policy and programmes.

Conflict of interest is obvious. The Gates Foundation plays a key role in GAVI and simultaneously finance the National Vaccine Advisory Committees that guide Governments on immunization policies. The National immunization technical advisory groups are expert groups who provide guidance to national governments and policy-makers to develop and implement evidence-based, locally relevant immunization policies and strategies that reflect national priorities. These should be independent and should be funded by national governments to maintain autonomy.

GAVI and Health System Strengthening Despite the undisputed increase in the number of immunized children, GAVI has been criticized for following a "Gates-approach", focusing on disease-specific vertical health interventions (through vaccines) over a holistic approach of health system strengthening (Martens et al., 2015). Responding to the criticism, in 2005, GAVI included a health system strengthening (HSS) component in its programme portfolio[12]. However, only 10.6 per cent (US$ 862.5 million) of GAVI's total commitments between 2000 and 2013 have been dedicated to health system strengthening, whereas more than 78.6 per cent (US$ 6,405.4 million) have been used for vaccine support (Storeng, 2014).

The WHO defines Health System Strengthening (HSS) as "improving these six health system building blocks (Service Deliver; Health Workforce; Information; Medical Products, vaccines and Technologies; Financing; and Leadership/Governance) and managing their interactions in ways that achieve more equitable and sustained improvements across health services and health outcomes" (WHO, 2007). In practice, however, GAVI's interpretation of HSS is very different. GAVI's main emphasis as regards HSS is on resources such as cars, boats, bikes, kits for community health workers and cold chain equipment. The interconnectedness between the 'building blocks' is not part of GAVI's approach to HSS.

For example, GAVI funds a HSS programme in Kenya, with the aim to convince the population to vaccinate children. However, given weaknesses in the local health system, the demand for vaccination is not adequately met. Thus while GAVI creates a demand, in practice it remains challenging to vaccinate all children, thus eroding public trust in the health system. Further, even when immunization services are available, the absence of other care services in primary care settings erodes public trust in the system. This in turn decreases uptake of public immunization programmes. However GAVI appears satisfied with its HSS work as progress is measured (and reported) by vaccination follow up rates and other 'measurable' indicators directly related to vaccination[13]. (See Chapter D7 on the politics of measurement.)

GAVI's claimed focus on health systems has, however, *enhanced* GAVI's political appeal, to its more 'systems-oriented' donors. This has provided donors further justification for diverting ever-greater proportions of their development budgets to GAVI at the cost of crowding out other, and more flexible, funding for health systems (Storeng, 2014).

The Strategic Advisory Group of Experts on Immunization (SAGE), in the Midterm Review of the Global Vaccine Action Plan (2012–2020), pointed to the persistent disconnect between immunization and the broader health system agenda (SAGE, 2016). The weakness of a vertical disease based approach is highlighted by the measles outbreaks that have occurred in numerous countries – a result of sub-optimal immunization coverage through both routine services and campaigns, along with increased susceptibility in older age groups. Surveillance for measles remains weak in many countries. Rubella control lags even further behind.

Global Fund's demand for Immunities and Privileges

Global Fund: governance structure The Global Fund to Fight AIDS, Tuberculosis and Malaria (GFATM), a global public–private partnership, was launched in 2002 with a US$ 100 million grant from the Bill and Melinda Gates Foundation (BMGF) (Birn, 2014). It is an international public–private development finance organization that relies on voluntary financial contributions from all sectors: governments, private sector, foundations and individuals. In September 2016, the Global Fund Fifth Replenishment Conference secured pledges of financing for the 2017–2019 period[14]. Of the total US$ 12.9 billion raised at the conference, US$ 12 billion was pledged by donor governments. Thus, 93 per cent of all Global Fund support comes from donor governments[15]. These are held in a trust account at the International Bank for Reconstruction and Development (ILO, 2008).

It incorporates non-state actors as equal players in its core governance structures (Aziz, 2009; Schoofs and Philips, 2002; Yamey, 2002; The Economist, 2001). The private sector influence on the Global Fund is disproportionately large compared to its 7 per cent contribution. The Global Fund Board consists of eight "constituencies" comprising of 20 voting and eight non-voting members. All voting constituencies participate equally[16]. Private sector is one of the voting constituencies[17]. While, WHO and UNAIDS have no vote on the board of the Global Fund, the private sector does, represented by pharmaceutical Merck/MSD, and private foundations such as the BMGF (Birn, 2014).

The Global Fund's definition of private sector is broad. It includes interested corporations including pharmaceuticals, oil and gas, banking, management consulting, food and beverage, etc[18]. Many of these industries, such as pharmaceuticals, food and beverage, have interests that often conflict with public health policies. The remit of private sector influence also extends through funding to other Global Fund constituencies: Foundations and Civil Society. The Global Fund lacks an independent and accountable decision-making process as decision making is entrusted to a small group of representatives. Global Fund's policy is that public sector monies are not 'earmarked' for specific countries or programs, and that the allocation of funding is the responsibility of the Board of the Global[19]. Therefore, private sector with only 7 per cent contribution plays an equally important role in deciding the allocation of funding.

Immunities and privileges sought by Global Fund Since 2009 the Global Fund has been asking for blanket immunities and privileges from the grant recipient countries. Until 31 December 2008, under an Administrative Services Agreement with the World Health Organization (WHO), all those working in the Global Fund's Secretariat were WHO officials. This meant that Global Fund staff was employed on WHO contracts with all the immunities and privileges of United Nations employees. On 1 January 2009, the Global Fund became an administratively autonomous international financing institution, employing staff directly under its own policies, regulations, and procedures (ILO, 2008). The Global Fund justified this move as a means of attaining greater flexibility as an institution and at the same time retaining status as an international institution with privileges and immunities similar to UN organizations in Switzerland and the United States[20]. Staff obtained new contracts governed by Global Fund rules and regulations, and their UN privileges and immunities were terminated[21].

In 2009 itself, the Global Fund started asking States to consider granting it blanket privileges and immunities either by: a) Applying legislation to confer upon the Global Fund the privileges and immunities ordinarily provided to international organizations; or by b) Signing an Agreement on Privileges and Immunities (the "P&I Agreement")[22]. It argued that the blanket privileges and immunities would assist it in fulfilling its mandate and in securing its investments in countries supported by it.

Under the P&I Agreement, described by the Global Fund as an *international instrument*, blanket privileges and immunities extend to the Global Fund, its assets, archives and officials acting in their official capacity. All goods, supplies, materials, equipment, services or funds introduced into, acquired, or used in a country as part of, or in conjunction with, funding provided under a Global Fund grant are exempt from taxation[23]. This raises a fundamental question: how can an agreement involving a public private partnership (PPP) be an international instrument, when the PPP itself was not established by an international treaty?

Switzerland and the USA had already granted privileges and immunities to the Global Fund, but under different legal arrangements. The Global Fund signed a Headquarters Agreement with the Swiss Federal Council on 13 December 2004 under the terms of which it enjoys privileges and immunities in Switzerland. In addition, the Government of the United States has conferred privileges and immunities on the Global Fund by Executive Order of the President of the United States[24]. These privileges and immunities have been extensively used as examples by the Global Fund to secure privileges from other countries without clarifying the differences.

Gülen Atay Newton, Head Legal and Compliance Department, in a 2014 press release on accelerating efforts to secure privileges and immunities writes, that "...The Global Fund's dual legal status has been recognized as representing an innovation in public international law. This unique legal status reflects the nature of the organization as a public-private partnership, distinct from traditional international organizations. Through establishment as a foundation under Swiss law, the Global Fund was able to ensure the equal standing of public and private sectors in the organization's governance, and avoid the transaction costs and delays associated with treaty formation. At the same time, the status of the Global Fund as an international organization has been elaborated through a gradual process of legal recognition by national governments. For example, both Switzerland and the United States have formally recognized the Global Fund as an international organization (sic)...." (Newton, 2014).

Granting privileges and immunity to the Global Fund: The story so far... The Global Fund received a lukewarm response to its demand for privileges and immunity on par with UN agencies. In September 2010, the Republic of Moldova was the first to sign the P&I Agreement on the condition that the agreement would come into effect only when a total of ten countries adhere to it[25]. Until 2014, eight countries had signed the P&I Agreement: Ethiopia, Georgia, Ghana, Moldova, Montenegro, Rwanda, Swaziland and Uganda[26]. In 2014, a series of measures were taken to escalate the ongoing efforts. The States represented on the Board were encouraged to support and facilitate the Secretariat's efforts to secure privileges and immunities[27].

The Global Fund Board endorsed continued engagement with relevant counterparts such as the Ministry of Foreign Affairs. Coercive measure of making the recipient countries sign the P&I Agreement as a precondition to secure funding were applied. Within three years of signing the P&I Agreement, the host-country grantees are required to ensure all measures are taken to accord privileges and immunities to the Global Fund[28].

Between 2014 and 2017, the Global Fund claims seven more countries have signed the P&I Agreement, bringing the total number to 15. However, only 13 names are available in public domain. In March 2017, the Republic of Senegal was the latest to sign the P&I Agreement[29].

Privileges and immunity to PPPs: the case against the Global Fund

THE GLOBAL FUND IS NOT AN INTER-GOVERNMENTAL ORGANIZATION Granting of privileges and immunities to public private partnerships in general and to the Global Fund in particular will further jeopardize democratic global health governance. If this is not addressed in time, other global public-private partnerships – such as the GAVI Alliance will demand the same concessions (Aziz, 2009). The Global Fund does not qualify for privileges and immunities in because it is not an inter-governmental organization as it is not established by an international treaty (ILO, 2008).

Non-state participation in the global public–private partnership structure creates legitimacy and accountability issues that are only compounded by the blanket application of P&I regimes. Global public–private partnerships lack such legitimacy because they differ from formal intergovernmental organizations in at least two ways: they are not constituted by a multilateral treaty based on State consent, and they permit the equal participation of non-state actors in decision-making processes. Both features apply in the case of the Global Fund (Aziz, 2009).

Although, the Global Fund argues that the absence of blanket privileges and immunities exposes its resources, staff and mission to serious risks and challenges (The Global Fund Observer, 2014), yet it provides no valid examples. The Global Fund does not implement programmes directly. With 700 staff based in Geneva, the Global Fund describes itself as a lean and efficient organization that does not have country offices[30].

CONFLICTS OF INTEREST: GLOBAL FUND'S ENGAGEMENT WITH PRIVATE AC-TORS The Bill & Melinda Gates Foundation (BMGF), Global Fund's key partner, funds 'Friends of the Global Fund' and other organizations in both developing and developed countries to carry out advocacy for Global Fund worldwide[31]. The five regional 'Friends of the Global Fund', erroneously described as 'independent', are entrusted with developing contacts and garnering political and financial support for the Global Fund[32].

The Global Fund, offers business opportunities and lucrative contracts to the private sector. International management and auditing firms such as PriceWaterhouseCoopers (PwC), KPMG, Cardno EM, etc. are given lucrative contracts to operate as the Local Fund Agents (LFAs), Fiscal Agents and external auditors.

Evidence shows international management and auditing firms promote policies that favour private sector to the detriment of public health (see Chapter D3). The Local Fund Agents (LFAs) oversee, verify and report on grant performance[33]. The Global Fund describes LFAs as its 'eyes and ears' within recipient countries during pre-grant phase, grant implementation period and grant renewal process. Currently, there are a total of 141 LFA's in 150 countries[34]. LFAs are entrusted with important oversight roles for technical health issues in which they hold negligible or limited expertise. LFAs are expensive and of questionable quality (McCoy, 2013). A revolving door between LFAs, the Global Fund and the grant recipients gives rise to conflicts of interest. LFAs are expected to interact closely with grant recipients and can attend Country Coordinating Mechanism (CCM) meetings[35]. The CCM meetings provide LFA's opportunity to interact with other development partners and legitimize their role in public health interventions in which these hold no expertise.

In addition to the LFAs the Global Fund has also appointed fiscal agents in 23 countries for tighter financial control and building the financial management capacity of grant-recipients[36]. Fiscal agents are also private contractors (for profit agencies, e.g. GFA Group, Cardno consulting, etc.). The Fiscal Agent reviews, pre-approves and verifies all transactions related to grant activities and utilization[37]. LFAs and Fiscal Agents come at a high financial cost and administrative burden to the programmes as these are 'for profit' private consulting or audit agencies. Exact costs are not available. However, the 2017 Audit Report on Global Fund Grant Management in High Risk Environments mentioned costs for 23 countries: Fiscal agents cost an estimated US\$ 10 million a year; Local Fund Agents come at an annual cost of US\$ 14 million; and External Auditors at an estimated cost of US\$ 3 million. The report also points out that despite spending significant resources for mitigating fiduciary risks in high risk countries, the gaps in financial management remained[38].

DEBT2HEALTH INITIATIVE: GLOBAL FUND'S INVOLVEMENT IN SOVEREIGN DEBT In 2007, with assistance from BMGF, the Global Fund launched the 'Debt2Health' initiative[39] while it was still under the Administrative Services Agreement with the WHO – thus, providing it the legitimacy of a multilateral organization. Curiously, this was done just before the Global Fund was set to terminate its agreement with the WHO and launch itself as an independent financing organization. Very little about the initiative is in public domain. What is known is that under these Global Fund facilitated agreements creditors (States) forgo repayment of a portion of their sovereign debts (development aid credits) on the condition that the beneficiary countries (States) invest an agreed upon counterpart amount in health through the Global Fund (part of it going the Fund's overhead costs and part to be paid to private contractors). The Global fund calls this an 'innovative financing initiative' when in fact it is a sovereign debt swap involving a public private partnership.

The pilot phase 2007–2009 involved: Indonesia, Peru, Pakistan and Kenya. With this initiative the Global Fund clearly steps out of its remit as a public private partnership and raises the larger issue of the ethics of private sector involvement in sovereign debts.

Conclusion

GAVI is extolled for massive increase in resources for immunization. What is however not often discussed is the fact that this has come at the cost of promoting the 'Gates approach' to health governance that places emphasis on technological solutions to achieve quantifiable, quick, short-term results (Birn, 2005). It places great emphasis on new and novel vaccines rather than ensuring universal access to known and effective traditional vaccines (Heaton et al., 2002). GAVI promotes a market driven vision that includes protection of IPRs and market based pricing mechanisms. In spite of claims to the contrary GAVI does not promote Health System Strengthening, nor does it promote national manufacture of vaccines. Key to these deficiencies is GAVI's governance structure, which includes private entities, though the bulk of GAVI's funding is public.

Another mega PPP, the Global Fund, seeks formalization of its status as a global organization that rivals inter-governmental organizations in power and privileges. Since 2009 it has been demanding blanket immunities and privileges from the grant recipient countries. Immunities and privileges to global public private partnerships in general and to the Global Fund in particular would further undermine democratic governance in health.

The unfettered power of both PPPs represent a threat to the hitherto nation state driven system of global governance for health. They clearly represent instances of private sector influence on activities which are public funded and which essentially take place in the public sphere.

Notes

1 See GAVI website: http://www.gavi.org/support/sustainability/countries-eligible-for-support/

2 Global Alliance for Vaccines and Immunization 1999, First Board Meeting, UNICEF House, New York, October 28.

3 GAVI, Governance, www.gavi.org/about/governance/gavi-board/composition/independent-individuals/

4 GAVI, Partners, www.gavi.org/about/partners/bmgf/

5 GAVI, Governance, http://www.gavialliance.org/about/governance/gavi-board/composition/

6 GAVI, the Vaccine Alliance, Supply and Procurement Strategy 2016-20.

7 Hurvitz, J A 2008, Covington & Burling – Biography, http://www.cov.com/jhurvitz/

8 Other terms used for tiered pricing are: "differential", "preferential", "discounted pricing", and "market segmentation".

9 Pan American Health Organization 1977, Resolution CD25.R27, 25th Directing Council, Washington, D.C.

10 PAHO, 52nd Directing Council, Principles of the Pan American Health Organization Revolving Fund for Vaccine Procurement, CD52/17, http://www.paho.org/hq/index.php?option=com_content&view=article&id=8833&Itemid=40033&lang=en#resolutions

11 ibid.

12 GAVI, HSS Support, www.gavi.org/support/hss/

13 GAVI, Health systems goal indicators. http://www.gavi.org/results/goal-level-indicators/health-systems-goal-indicators/. Published 2017. Accessed 22 March, 2017.

14 The Global Fund, *Government Donors: Overview*, https://www.theglobalfund.org/en/government/

15 ibid.

16 The Global Fund, *Governance*, http://www.theglobalfund.org/en/documents/governance/

17 1) Implementing Country governments (7 Seats); 2)donor Country governments (8 Seats); 3) Foundations interested in providing financial and intellectual support to the Global Fund; 4 Private sector); 5) Civil Society, developed Countries ; 6) Civil Society, developing Countries; 7) Communities; 8) Non-voting Seats (8 seats) Includes the United Nations Joint Programme on HIV/AIDS (UNAIDS); WHO, Partners (Roll Back Malaria, Stop TB, UNITAID), World Bank, host Country, Chair, Vice-Chair, Executive Director, http://www.theglobalfund.org/en/documents/governance/

18 The Global Fund, *Governance*, http://www.theglobalfund.org/en/documents/governance/

19 The Global Fund, *Government Donors: Overview*, https://www.theglobalfund.org/en/government/

20 The Global Fund 2008, The Global Fund becomes an administratively autonomous institution as of 2009, 19 Decemberhttp://www.theglobalfund.org/en/mediacenter/newsreleases/2008-12-The_Global_Fund_becomes_an_administratively_autonomous_institution_as_of_2009/

21 The Global Fund 2010, *Moldova signs agreement to grant privileges and immunities to the Global Fund*, 28 September, https://www.theglobalfund.org/en/news/2010-09-28-moldova-signs-agreement-to-grant-privileges-and-immunities-to-the-global-fund/

22 Global Fund 2014, Thirty-Second Board Meeting, GF/B32/19 Montreux, Switzerland, 20–21 November.

23 ibid.

24 The Global Fund 2010, *Moldova signs agreement to grant privileges and immunities to the Global Fund*, 28 September, https://www.theglobalfund.org/en/news/2010-09-28-moldova-signs-agreement-to-grant-privileges-and-immunities-to-the-global-fund

25 The Global Fund 2010, *Moldova signs agreement to grant privileges and immunities to the Global Fund*, 28 September, https://www.theglobalfund.org/en/news/2010-09-28-moldova-signs-agreement-to-grant-privileges-and-immunities-to-the-global-fund/

26 The Global Fund 2014, Thirty-Second Board Meeting, GF/B32/19 Montreux, Switzerland, 20-21 November.

27 ibid.

28 ibid.

29 The Global Fund 2017, *Senegal and the Global Fund Extend Their Partnership*, 21 March, https://www.theglobalfund.org/en/news/2017-03-21-senegal-and-the-global-fund-extend-their-partnership/

30 The Global Fund, *Staff*, <https://www.theglobalfund.org/en/staff/>.

31 The Global Fund, *Bill and Melinda Gates Foundation*, https://www.theglobalfund.org/en/private-ngo-partners/bill-melinda-gates-foundation/

32 The Global Fund, *Friends*, https://www.theglobalfund.org/en/friends/

33 The Global Fund, *LFA*, http://www.theglobalfund.org/en/lfa/

34 ibid.

35 The Global Fund, *CCM*, http://www.theglobalfund.org/en/ccm/

36 The Global Fund 2017, *Audit Report: Global Fund Grant Management in High Risk Environments*, Geneva, Switzerland,GF-OIG-17-002,23 January.

37 ibid.

38 ibid.

39 The Global Fund 2007, *Q&A Debt2Health*, August.

References

Arie, S 2011, How should GAVI build on its success?, *BMJ*.343:d5182, 8 September.

Aziz, D A 2009, *Privileges and Immunities of Global Public-Private Partnerships: A Case Study of the Global Fund to Fight AIDS, Tuberculosis and Malaria*, Institute for International Law and Justice Emerging Scholars Papers IILJ, Emerging Scholars Paper 14 (A Sub series of IILJ Working Papers) ISSN: 1552-6275

Balasubramaniam K 2001, 'Equitable Pricing, Affordability and Access to Essential Drugs in Developing Countries: Consumers Perspective', Workshop on Differential Pricing and Financing of Essential Drug held in Høsbjør, Norway April 2001.

Balasubramaniam, K V, &Sita, V 2014, 'Access to Vaccines and the Vaccine Industry – An Analysis', *J Vaccines Vaccine*, 5, 218, doi: 10.4172/2157-7560.1000218.

Benedict Cooper, How the "free market" in vaccines is neither free nor fair, 3 March 2016, http://www.newstatesman.com/politics/health/2016/03/how-free-market-vaccines-neither-free-nor-fair

Birn, A E 2005, 'Gates's grandest challenge: Transcending technology as public health ideology', Lancet, 514–519.

Birn, A E 2014, 'Philanthrocapitalism, Past and Present: The Rockefeller Foundation, the Gates Foundation, and the Setting(s) of the International/ Global Health Agenda', *Hypothesis,* vol. 12, no. 1.

Castro, A, Cinà, M, Helmer-Smith, M, Vlček, C, Oghor, C, Cazabon, D 2017, 'A case study of Gavi's human papillomavirus vaccine support programme', *J Health Spec*, 5, 2-7.

Cooper, B 2016, 'How the "free market" in vaccines is neither free nor fair', 3 March, http://www.newstatesman.com/politics/health/2016/03/how-free-market-vaccines-neither-free-nor-fair

Farlow, A 2004, 'Over the rainbow: the pot of gold for neglected diseases', *Lancet*, 364(9450), 2011-12.

GAVI 2008, GAVI Implementation Working Group. Advance Market Commitment for Pneumococcal Vaccines, Geneva, July.

GAVI Alliance, 'GAVI Alliance Support for Access to Appropriate Pricing for GAVI Graduates and Other Lower Middle Income Countries', www.gavi.org/library,cited in Médecins Sans Frontières 2015, *The Right Shot: Bringing Down Barriers to Affordable and Adapted Vaccines*, 2nd Edition, January.

Gjerde, R 2008, 'Vaccine money right out of the window (in Norwegian)', *Aftenposten*, 3-4 March Sect. A1-3.

Government of Honduras 2013, 'Honduras GAVI Alliance Annual Progress Report 2012', Honduras; May,<http://www.gavi.org>, cited in Médecins Sans Frontières 2015, *The Right Shot: Bringing Down Barriers to Affordable and Adapted Vaccines*, 2nd Edition, January.

Hamblin, J 2016, *Is the Gates Foundation always a force for good? Why Doctors Without Borders Refused a Million Free Vaccines*, October 14, https://www.theatlantic.com/health/archive/2016/10/doctors-with-borders/503786/.

Heaton, A, & Keith, R 2002, 'A long way to go: a critique of GAVI's initial impact', Save the Children, cited in Birn, A E 2014, 'Philanthrocapitalism, Past and Present: The Rockefeller Foundation, the Gates Foundation, and the Setting(s) of the International/ Global Health.

International Labour Office 2008, *Matters relating to the Administrative Tribunal of the ILO Recognition of the Tribunal's jurisdiction by the Global Fund to Fight AIDS, Tuberculosis and Malaria*, Fifteenth Item on the Agenda, GB.303/PFA/15/2 303rd Session, Governing Body, Geneva, November.

Johns Hopkins Bloomberg School of Public Health 2006, *GAVI pneumoADIP. GAVI Alliance Investment Case: Accelerating the Introduction of Pneumococcal Vaccines into GAVI-Eligible Countries*, Baltimore, www.gavialliance.org/resources/Pneumo_Investment_Case_Oct06.pdf

Light, D W 2006, 'Basic Research Funds to Discover Important New Drugs: Who Contributes How Much?', in Burke, MA (ed.), *Monitoring the Financial Flows for Health Research Behind the Global Numbers*, Global Forum for Health Research, Geneva, pp. 27-43.

Light, D W 2007, 'Misleading Congress about drug development', *Journal of Health Politics, Policy and Law*, 32, 895-913, http://bioethics.upenn.edu/people/?last=Light&first=Donald

Light, D W 2009, *Current Realities and Alternate Approaches*, A HAI Europe/ Medico International Publication, Health Action International (HAI) Europe, Paper Series Reference 03-2009/01.

Martens, J & Seitz, K 2015, *Philanthropic Power and Development: Who shapes the agenda?*, November, Bischöfliches Hilfswerk MISEREOR.

Mccoy, D 2013, *BBC Panorama – The Global Fund and Corruption.*

Médecins Sans Frontières 2015, *The Right Shot: Bringing Down Barriers to Affordable and Adapted Vaccines*, 2nd Edition, January.

ModiPandav, S 2014, *Presentation on Tiered Pricing and Access to Medicines*, Seminar on Making Medicines Affordable: Role of Pricing Policies, OSF Access to Medicines Initiative, Istanbul, Turkey, October 13, 2014.

Newton, G A 2014, *The Global Fund Enlarges Efforts to Secure Privileges and Immunities*, Press Release, 30 July, http://en.sgdl.ch/news/the-global-fund-enlarges-efforts-to-secure-privileges-and-immunitiesnal-labour-organisation.aspx

PAHO 2013, *Recent Developments of the PAHO Revolving Fund for Vaccine Procurement*, November, http://scm.oas.org/pdfs/2013/CP32037E.pdf

Ryckman T, Cornejo, S 2014, 'Overcoming challenges to sustainable immunization financing: early experiences from GAVI graduating countries',*Health Policy Plan*, Feb 8, http://www.heapol.oxfordjournals.org/cgi/doi/10.1093/heapol/czu003, cited in Médecins Sans Frontières 2015, *The Right Shot: Bringing Down Barriers to Affordable and Adapted Vaccines*, 2nd Edition, January.

Schoen-Angerer 2008, 'Questioning the 1.5 billion vaccine deal', *Development Today*, April 28, http://www.accessmed-msf.org/

no_cache/resources/press-clips/ddt-tvsa-editorial-on-a

Schoofs, M & Phillips, M M 2002,'Global disease fund to be strict for better change to get results', *The Wall Street Journal*, Feb 13, http://online.wsj.com/news/articles/SB1013554027358224600

Sell, S K 1998, *Power and Ideas: North-South Politics of Intellectual Property,* University of New York Press, Albany, NY State.

Storeng, K T 2014, 'The GAVI Alliance and the 'Gates approach' to health system strengthening', *Glob Public Health,* Sep 14, 9, 8, 865–879 doi: 10.1080/17441692.2014.940362 PMCID: PMC4166931.

Strategic Advisory Group of Experts on Immunization (SAGE) 2016, *Midterm review of the Global Vaccine Action Plan*, http://www.who.int/ immunization/global_vaccine_ action_plan/SAGE_GVAP_Assessment_Report_2016_EN.pdf?ua=1

The Economist 2001, 'Aid and AIDS: gambling with lives', May 31, http://www.economist.com/node/639326

The Global Fund, Observer Newsletter 2014, 'Privileges and immunities', Issue 256, 24 November.

Wirgau, J S, Kathryn, W F, K,W & Jensen, C 2010, 'Is Business Discourse Colonizing Philanthropy? A Critical Discourse Analysis of (PRODUCT) RED', Voluntas, 21:611–630 cited in *Philanthropic Foundations and the Public Health Agenda* 2011, August 3, http://www.corporationsandhealth.org/2011/08/03/philanthropic-foundations-and-the-public-health-agenda/

World Health Organization (WHO) 2007 Everybody's business: strengthening health systems to improve health outcomes: WHO's framework for action. 2007:1-56. http://www.who.int/healthsystems/strategy/everybodys_business.pdf

Yamey, G 2002, 'WHO 's management: struggling to transform a — fossilised bureaucracy', *BMJ*, 325:1170, http://dx.doi.org/10.1136/bmj.325.7373.1170

D5 | INVESTMENT TREATIES: HOLDING GOVERNMENTS TO RANSOM

Introduction

As the WHO pushes for the implementation of the Framework Convention on Tobacco Control (FCTC), the tobacco industry has, in the words of outgoing WHO Director General Margaret Chan, "made it absolutely clear that it has no intention of abandoning a business model that depends on enticing millions of new users – especially young people – to its deadly products"[1]. For the multinational tobacco industry, the weapon of choice in thwarting the adoption and implementation of the FCTC has been the use of provisions in investment treaties that allow investors to initiate binding arbitration against governments in international forums.

Nearly all developing countries have signed bilateral investment treaties (BITs) with developed countries. Increasingly, free trade agreements (FTAs) also feature investment protection chapters. There are 3268 treaties with investment protection provisions, of which 2923 are BITs (Reid Smith and Allas Portilo, 2016). BITs were originally aimed at protecting foreign investors from nationalization of their investments. However over time, both the provisions in BITs and their interpretation have expanded the meaning and scope of protections available to investors. Protection to 'investors' is now interpreted to include scrutiny of social, environmental and health policies of sovereign governments. Such policies are now being challenged by foreign investors on the plea that they put their investments at risk. Such challenges can involve the Investor-State Dispute Settlement (ISDS) mechanisms that are embedded in trade and investment treaties.

Understanding investment treaties and ISDS

Investment treaties incorporate provisions which protect investments by private entities from being expropriated by a foreign government. They also grant 'fair and equitable' treatment to foreign investors as is enjoyed by national investors. Such protection is often in conflict with public interest.

These treaties generally have a very broad definition of property that goes well beyond the commonly understood definition of property, to include intellectual property rights, licences and permits, debt securities and loans and profits and future/expected profits. They also define investors very broadly and in several treaties simply having a branch office is sufficient to recognize a company as an investor. Under the now shelved Trans Pacific Partnership

(TPP) for instance, the mere act of 'channelling resources or capital in order to set up a business' or 'applying for permits and licences' would have been sufficient to qualify as an investor[2].

'Investors' are then entitled to various protections under these treaties. The first being 'national treatment' which requires that national policies and laws must apply equally to foreign investors as they do to local firms. Further, 'most favoured nation' (MFN) clauses in these agreements require that if a country is party to one investment treaty, it must provide investors covered by other investment treaties with the same protection and privileges as available in the former case.

Investors are also entitled to 'fair and equitable treatment'. There is a wide range of interpretations of 'fair and equitable treatment' which governments have found difficult to comply with. This can be seen in the statistics for disputes under US trade or investment treaties where 74 per cent of the time when investors win, there has been a violation of fair and equitable treatment (FET); for instance tribunals have found that laws or policies that differed from investors' 'reasonable expectations' have amounted to FET violations[3]. Broad interpretations of this provision in tribunal decisions can lead companies to claim reasonable expectations about future profits arising from intellectual property filings. Thus changes to IP laws that impact their expectations of profits could be interpreted as a FET violation.

Another entitlement is protection from expropriation without compensation. Typically in these treaties expropriation is only permissible if it is for a public purpose and carried out in a non-discriminatory manner. Further any expropriation requires the prompt payment of adequate and effective compensation, even in cases where expropriation is done for a public purpose. The quantum of compensation is required to be equivalent to the fair market value of the investment before expropriation. Expropriation is traditionally understood to mean nationalization and the taking of physical property but these treaties also protect from 'indirect expropriation'. This has been interpreted to mean reduction in the value of a foreign investment due to regulations and other government actions (Kelsey and Wallach, 2012). Thus, for example, issuing compulsory licences by governments to allow production of cheaper generic versions of patented medicines could be interpreted as 'indirect expropriation'.

When investors claim violation of their rights, as laid down in these treaties, they can initiate arbitration proceedings against governments claiming compensation in specialized tribunals. Such tribunals include the World Bank's International Centre for the Settlement of Investment Disputes (ICSID), the UN Commission on International Trade Law (UNCITRAL), the Permanent Court of Arbitration at the Hague or in chambers of commerce. Thus, foreign investors pursue claims against the host country outside the country's judicial system. If they are successful, arbitration tribunals may make awards both in the form of monetary damages, including applicable interest, and/or in the form of property restitution.

The ISDS system enables foreign investors and corporations to directly sue governments. It may be recalled that the BITs or Free Trade agreements (FTAs) themselves are signed between countries. Typically, if there is a dispute over the implementation of these international agreements, the signatories to the agreement – the governments – file disputes against each other. The ISDS mechanism allows investors, who were never signatories to the agreements, to bring disputes against governments. Disputes between governments often may not be pursued or may be settled out of diplomatic considerations. However private businesses face no such diplomatic constraints as evidenced by the cases described below.

Philipp Morris sues Uruguay and Australia

The cases filed by US cigarette manufacturer, Philipp Morris, against Uruguay (Porterfield and Byrnes, 2011) and later Australia (BBC, 2011) illustrate the implications of ISDS for public health. In these disputes, Philipp Morris alleged that tobacco warnings on cigarettes or rules for plain packaging amounted to infringements of their trademarks which are considered to be 'investments'.

The case against Australia[4] originated with the Tobacco Plain Packaging Act, 2011 which required removal of brands from cigarette packs. Under the Hong Kong–Australia BIT, Philip Morris Asia Limited (PMA) initiated arbitration

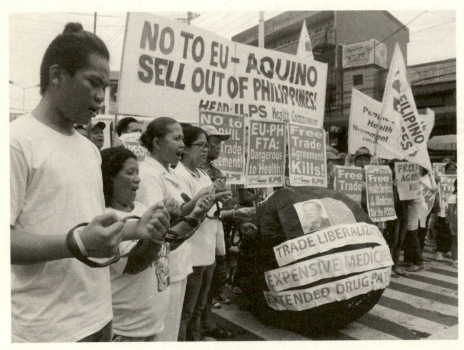

Image D5.1 Protest against EU Philippines FTA, 26 May2016 (M3M)

against Australia for the expropriation of its IP due to this legislation. The IP in question were trademarks held by an Australian subsidiary of PMA. In December 2015, the arbitration tribunal established for this dispute at the Permanent Court of Arbitration (PCA) held that the case could not be heard on a jurisdictional issue; specifically that Philip Morris Asia changed its corporate structure to take advantage of the provisions of the Hong Kong-Australia BIT. It was only in February 2011 that PM Asia acquired all shares of PM Australia and became the direct owner of Philipp Morris's investment in the country. The tribunal held that whether such a restructuring was indeed an abuse depended on whether there was a foreseeable dispute and since by February it was evident that Australia would be introducing plain packaging rules, a dispute was indeed foreseeable.

In Philipp Morris' case against Uruguay[5] in 2010 the claim was brought by two Swiss companies and one Uruguayan company from the Philip Morris Group under the Switzerland-Uruguay BIT. The measures challenged by these companies were Ordinance 514 of August 18, 2008 which required tobacco warnings on cigarette packs and prohibited variants of brands such as *Light*, *Blue* and *Fresh Mint* in the case of Philip Morris. Also challenged was Presidential Decree 287/009 of 15 June, 2009 which increased the size of the warnings from 50 to 80 per cent (Brauch M D 2016). These measures, according to Philip Morris amounted to an expropriation of its investment and a violation of the requirement of fair and equitable treatment among other things.

In July 2016, a tribunal at ICSID dismissed Philip Morris's case, ordered it to bear the entire costs of the arbitration and partially reimburse Uruguay's legal expenses to the tune of US$ 7 million. The tribunal found that trademarks do not confer an absolute right of use which is free of state regulation but only the right to exclude others from using it. They also held that the limitation of space for Philip Morris to display its brand on the cigarette pack to 20 per cent did not substantially deprive the value of their investment and so held that the claims of expropriation were invalid. Rejecting claims of violation of fair and equitable treatment, the tribunal found that Uruguay's actions were based on the WHO's FCTC process which was supported by scientific evidence and were adopted in good faith to protect public health and were not discriminatory or arbitrary.

Pharmaceutical companies in the fray

The tobacco disputes have not been the only ones involving the ISDS mechanisms. The implications of ISDS on access to generic medicines became evident in the dispute between the pharmaceutical company Eli Lilly and the Government of Canada filed under the North American Free Trade Agreement (NAFTA). In Canada, Eli Lilly's patents on two drugs – atomoxetine and olanzapine – were revoked on grounds of failure to prove the 'utility' of the patented drug, as required under Canada's patent law. Eli Lilly filed its intention to initiate formal proceedings under NAFTA in 2012 and then filed an arbitration notice in 2013.

Eli Lilly claimed that the patent revocation violated the minimum standard of treatment and fair and equitable treatment guaranteed to foreign investors under NAFTA which obliged signatories to accord to another party "treatment in accordance with international law, including fair and equitable treatment and full protection and security". Eli Lilly further claimed that the patent revocation discriminated against Eli Lilly in favour of generic firms, in violation of Canada's national treatment obligations under NAFTA. Eli Lilly also alleged that the patent revocation amounted to an expropriation of property rights, alleging violation of the WTO TRIPS Agreement, NAFTA's intellectual property rules, the Patent Cooperation Treaty and the Paris Convention for the Protection of Intellectual Property. Eli Lilly demanded a compensation of 500 million Canadian dollars for these violations.

In 2017, the tribunal established under ICSID dismissed all of Eli Lilly's claims against Canada and directed it to pay all of Canada's arbitration costs and 75 per cent of their costs of legal representation and assistance.

Energy and environment sector

Several cases have been filed by investors in a number of countries, both developd and developing, in response to government regulations in the environment and energy sector. Table D5.1 summarizes some of the important cases.

TABLE D5.1: Cases related to investor state disputes in the environment and energy sector

Policy being challenged	Bans on mining due to environmental concerns	Regulations to fight for energy transition and against climate change	Other environmental protection measures
Case	Pacific Rim v. El Salvador	Vattenfall v. Germany I (environmental restrictions on coal)	Methanex v. United States (chemical and groundwater contamination)
	Renco v. Peru	Vattenfall v. Germany II (phasing out nuclear energy)	
	Gabriel Resources v. Romania	Lone Pine Resources v. Canada (fracking moratoria)	
	Infinito Gold v. Costa Rica	Perenco/Burlington v. Ecuador (oil taxes)	Ethyl v. Canada (ban of environmentally damaging gasoline additive)
	Bilcon v. Canada	TransCanada v. United States (cancellation of pipeline due to environmental concerns)	
	Glamis v. United States		

Source: TNI, Friends of the Earth International and CEO, 2017, Winning the debate against pro-ISDS voices: An activist's argumentation guide, https://www.tni.org/files/9837452346812786.pdf

Limited victories

Supporters of ISDS have characterize cases, where tribunals ruled against corporations, as evidence that the ISDS system works and is not arbitrary or stacked in favour of investors. However, experience has shown, that the threat of private international arbitration and the exorbitant compensation awarded to investors has had a chilling effect on government regulations and often governments opt for settlements that favour foreign investors. It is important to note that investment treaties can have different provisions, so success for a government in one investment treatment dispute does not guarantee success in a dispute brought under a different investment treaty. There is also no real system of precedent followed in investment disputes and across the multiple dispute settlement forums. In some cases, the mere filing of a dispute is sufficient to achieve a change in laws and policies.

In January 2017, Ukraine settled a dispute filed by Gilead Sciences Inc. in which Gilead reportedly claimed US$ 800 million in relation to its Hepatitis C drug sofosbuvir. This particular dispute highlights another key concern with the ISDS system, i.e. information about the disputes are at times dependent on both parties consenting to make it public. Information about this dispute has been pieced together from some Ukraine government documents with the actual settlement not being made public. The dispute likely related to the registration of a generic version of sofosbuvir. Gilead objected to this in local courts seeking an injunction based on the fact that the Ukraine has data exclusivity laws that prevent the registration of a subsequent generic for five years after Gilead's version was registered. Gilead obtained registration in mid-2015 and in November 2015, a state registry of medicines listed Grateziano, a generic version of the drug produced by Egyptian owned manufacturer Europharma International.

It needs to be noted that Gilead has specifically excluded the Ukraine from voluntary licences given to Indian companies that would have allowed access to cheaper generic versions of sofosbuvir for the millions of people living with Hepatitis C in the Ukraine. Nor does Gilead have a patent on this drug yet. Even as it challenged the generic registration in the local courts, Gilead initiated an investment dispute under the US-Ukraine BIT. It is unclear what arguments and claims Gilead was relying on. An interagency working group set up by the government of Ukraine recommended settling the dispute and a settlement, which remains secret was reached and approved in January 2017. A public statement issued by the Ministry of Justice implied that a discounted price offered by Gilead was also part of the settlement. The Ministry of Health later announced that it was de-registering the Egyptian company's version to comply with this settlement.

Although Australia and Uruguay eventually won the arbitration cases filed against them, it is of note that several countries received warnings from the tobacco industry of similar actions against them and Costa Rica, for instance, dropped plans to implement tobacco control measures in light of the ISDS cases[6]. Recently, leaked documents revealed by Swiss NGO Public Eye showed that Novartis threatened Columbia with an investment dispute under the Swiss-Columbian BIT over the government ordered reduction in prices of its drug imatinib (Public Eye, 2017).

The fear of adverse findings and huge awards apart, simply the costs involved in defending an investment arbitration are sufficient for several countries to avoid such disputes. Although Philip Morris and Eli Lilly were ordered to cover 75 per cent of the legal costs of the states they were suing, that still left a substantial amount for the States to pay themselves. In the Philip Morris-Uruguay case, the costs claimed by the parties exceeded the claim of US$ 25 million made by Philip Morris.

IP safeguard proposals

Several countries have now started considering introducing safeguards in new BITs and FTAs to prevent a repeat of cases described above. For instance, the India-Japan Comprehensive Economic Partnership Agreement (CEPA) contains an investment chapter which includes intellectual property in the definition of investment. Article 92(5) of the investment chapter states that the provisions would not be applicable to compulsory licences issued in accordance with the TRIPS agreement. This, however, means that companies can still challenge compulsory licences by claiming that they violate the TRIPS agreement. This introduces another layer of complexity as under the TRIPS agreement only another government can challenge non-compliance with the TRIPS agreement before the WTO Dispute Settlement Body.

Expanded versions of this exception now appear in recent BITs and FTA negotiations in which the USA is involved. These provisions exempt revocation of patents and compulsory licensing from the definition of expropriation. However it is of note that there is no exemption of these measures from claims of violation of fair and equitable treatment. In the case of the tobacco disputes, an exception to ISDS for tobacco control was agreed in Art 29.5 of the TPP [7].

Not just intellectual property rights

Several public interest groups and academics recommend that intellectual property (IP) be removed entirely from the definition of investments. While this may remedy a serious area of concern, it should be noted that IP is not the only basis of ISDS challenges to health policies. Investment provisions have also been used to challenge Poland's attempts to prevent the privatization of its public health insurance company[8] and the ability of Canada to regulate chemicals that can cause health problems (Public Citizen, 2000).

In addition BITs and investment provisions in FTAs have provisions related to 'market access'. Typically they restrict the ability of governments to impose barriers to free flow of goods and services. Barriers imposed by countries can be tariff barriers (duties on imports for example) or non-tariff barriers (not allowing certain goods into the market on health grounds, for example). The loss of flexibility to impose barriers to market access, can pose problems. Traditionally countries (especially developing countries) have used market access restrictions to promote domestic industry. In areas such as medicine production, this may be a vital tool, as it could allow the development of a local pharmaceutical industry.

While developed countries press for market access in trade and investment agreements, they oppose provisions related to 'performance requirements' (PRs). PRs are conditions imposed on foreign investors and can be used to channelize foreign investments in a manner that supports development of local industry, research, etc. Thus a PR that could help local industry, for example, is the requirement of 'technology transfer'. There is a trend towards barring PRs in trade and investment treaties.

A key concern with including investment provisions in FTAs as opposed to stand alone BITs is the link this creates between trade and investment. Where a developing country finds that the abuse of investor protections in these BITs is significant enough to warrant that they be revoked, they would be unable to revoke investment provisions in an FTA as that would involve the revocation of the entire FTA.

Reform, reject, repeal

It is evident that the rights given to investors in BITs and FTAs can significantly restrict a government's ability to regulate how companies operate

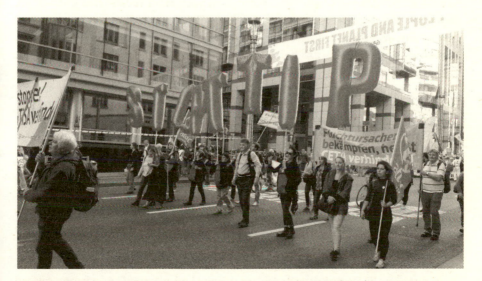

Image D5.2 Demonstration in Europe against the Transatlantic Trade and Investment Partnership (third world health aid)

within its national borders. Investment treaties or provisions are increasingly being questioned even as the manner in which these provisions have been used by multinational companies to challenge health, environment and other laws and policies have come to light (Oxfam, 2011).

There are now increasing calls for the rejection or the overhaul of the global investment treaty framework. In South Korea, judges have openly objected to investor-state dispute mechanisms highlighting its impact on the sovereignty of the country and on the judiciary[9]. At the height of the tobacco disputes, Australia declared that the government would no longer sign any trade agreement which include investor-state dispute mechanisms[10]. Eventually they did agree to ISDS in the TPP but after having tobacco excluded from the scope of any disputes. South Africa and Indonesia are withdrawing from existing BITs in favour of domestic investor protection laws while others like India are adding safeguards to their model BITs/FTA investment chapters and requesting renegotiations of existing BITs. The US push for ISDS played a significant role in the 2014 suspension of FTA talks between the USA and EU. The EU is now pushing for a permanent, multilateral investment court to address many of the criticisms of the current system. In early 2017, Canada and the EU made an informal proposal for such a multilateral ISDS mechanism to come within the WTO; a proposal that was rejected by India, Brazil, Japan and Argentina.

Even as states grapple with attempts to reform the global investment treaty framework, UN agencies and experts have expressed grave concern over the interplay between BITs and ISDS with human rights treaties. In June 2015, a joint statement by 10 UN experts and special rapporteurs stated that there was "a legitimate concern that both bilateral and multilateral investment treaties might aggravate the problem of extreme poverty, jeopardize fair and efficient foreign debt renegotiation, and affect the rights of indigenous peoples, minorities, persons with disabilities, older persons, and other persons leaving in vulnerable situations[11]." They made key recommendations calling for transparency and public consultation in current trade and investment agreement negotiations, human rights impact assessments of BITs and FTAs and robust safeguards embedded in current BITS and FTAs to ensure full protection and enjoyment of human rights (Reid Smith, 2015).

In his testimony to the European Parliament in 2016, the UN Independent Expert on the promotion of a democratic and equitable international order was more direct, challenging claims that investors need protection, stating: "It is States, particularly developing States, and their populations that need protection from predatory investors, speculators and transnational corporations, who do not hesitate to engage in frivolous and vexatious litigation, which are extremely expensive and have resulted in awards in the billions of dollars and millions in legal costs.' As he noted, 'the time has come to abolish ISDS...and to ensure that henceforth, trade works for human rights and not against them[12]."

Notes

1 See speech by Margaret Chan 'Every tobacco death is an avoidable tragedy. The epidemic must stop here': http://www.who.int/mediacentre/commentaries/early-tobacco-death/en/

2 See TPP text available at website of Analysis and Policy Observatory: http://apo.org.au/system/files/58399/apo-nid58399-98391.pdf Chapter 9, P. 4

3 See note by Public Citizen on this issue: http://www.citizen.org/documents/MST-Memo.pdf

4 Morris Asia Limited v. The Commonwealth of Australia, PCA Case No. 2012-12 http://www.italaw.com/sites/default/files/case-documents/italaw7303_0.pdf

5 Philip Morris Brands Sàrl, Philip Morris Products S.A. and Abal Hermanos S.A. v. Oriental Republic of Uruguay, ICSID Case No. ARB/10/7http://www.italaw.com/sites/default/files/case-documents/italaw7417.pdf

6 See: ' Tobacco Companies Bully Countries: https://sites.psu.edu/stopthetobaccoindustry/tobacco-companies-bully-people-into-purchasing-their-products/

7 See TPP Text here: https://www.tpp.mfat.govt.nz/text

8 Marinn Carlson (Partner) and Peter Kasperowicz, Sidley Austin LL,Dutch insurer Eureko, Polish government settle investment dispute, setting up IPO for Poland's state-owned insurer, available at http://arbitration.practicallaw.com/6-500-6640

8 See: 'Judges debate KORUS FTA task force', The Hankyoreh, 3 December 2011.

10 Public Statement on the International Investment Regime, 31 August 2010 available at http://www.osgoode.yorku.ca/public-statement/documents/Public%20Statement%20%28June%202011%29.pdf

11 See: http://www.ohchr.org/EN/NewsEvents/Pages/DisplayNews.aspx?NewsID=16031

12 See" ' Investor-State dispute settlement undermines rule of law and democracy, UN expert tells Council of Europe'http://www.ohchr.org/EN/NewsEvents/Pages/DisplayNews.aspx?NewsID=19839&LangID=E#sthash.TkSKjpD6.dpuf

References

BBC 2011, 'Philip Morris sues Australia over cigarette packaging', BBC News Asia, 21 November 2011 http://www.bbc.co.uk/news/world-asia-15815311

Brauch M D 2016, 'Philip Morris v. Uruguay: all claims dismissed; Uruguay to receive US$7 million reimbursement' Investment Treaty News, August 10 2016 https://www.iisd.org/itn/2016/08/10/philip-morris-brands-sarl-philip-morris-products-s-a-and-abal-hermanos-s-a-v-oriental-republic-of-uruguay-icsid-case-no-arb-10-7/

Kelsey J, Wallach L, 2012, '"Investor-State" Disputes in Trade Pacts Threaten Fundamental Principles of National Judicial Systems' April 2012. https://www.citizen.org/documents/isds-domestic-legal-process-background-brief.pdf

Oxfam 2011, 'Sleeping Lions: International investment treaties, state – investor disputes and access to food, land and water', Oxfam Discussion Paper, Oxfam, May 2011 available at http://www.oxfam.org/sites/www.oxfam.org/files/dp-sleeping-lions-260511-en.pdf

Porterfield M C and Byrnes C R, 2011, 'Philip Morris v. Uruguay: Will investor-State arbitration send restrictions on tobacco marketing up in smoke?' Investment Treaty News, International Institute for Sustainable Development, 12 July 2011, http://www.iisd.org/itn/2011/07/12/philip-morris-v-uruguay-will-investor-state-arbitration-send-restrictions-on-tobacco-marketing-up-in-smoke/

Public Citizen, 2000, 'Another Broken NAFTA Promise: Challenge by U.S. Corporation Leads Canada to Repeal Public Health Law' 2000 available at http://www.citizen.org/trade/article_redirect.cfm?ID=5479

Public Eye, 2017, 'Compulsory licensing in Colombia: Leaked documents show aggressive lobbying by Novartis' 12. April 2017 https://www.publiceye.ch/en/media/press-release/compulsory_licensing_in_colombia_leaked_documents_show_aggressive_lobbying_by_novartis/

Reid Smith S 2015, 'Potential human rights impacts of the TPP' Third World Network, 2015 http://www.twn.my/title2/FTAs/General/TPPHumanRights.pdf

Reid Smith S, Allas Portilo M, 2016, ' Impact of trade and investment agreements on access to affordable medicines' submission by Third World Network to UN Secretary general's High level Panel on Access to Medicines, February 28, 2016. http://www.unsgaccessmeds.org/inbox/2016/2/28/third-world-network

D6 | FRAMING OF HEALTH AS A SECURITY ISSUE

Introduction

In the last couple of decades, political actors' perceptions of what constitutes a threat to international security has broadened. Health issues, particularly those related to infectious diseases, have increasingly been presented as security threats. The framing of health as a security issue, or 'health securitization', is often a successful strategy for generating interest in, and resources for, a specific health issue. Nevertheless, it is also problematic in several respects. This chapter describes the evolution of health securitization and critically analyses the impact that it has on global health. We first introduce the concept of securitization and follow it up with an exploration of how health issues have been securitized over the last two decades, with particular attention to the manner in which the outbreak of Ebola in West Africa in 2014 was presented primarily as a security threat. Finally we examine the problems associated with the increased tendency to securitize health issues.

What is securitization?

The notion of securitization has been conceptualized by the Copenhagen School of Security Studies (Buzan, Wæver and De Wilde, 1998). The argument is that a security threat is not an objective condition that exists independently of the person or organization that is representing it as such. Securitization refers to the discursive process by which an issue is socially constructed as a security threat through the speech and representations of relevant political actors. The central issue for securitization studies is not how much of a security threat a particular issue poses. Rather, it aims to understand who defines the threat to security and whose interests are being served by securitization.

Securitization occurs when an actor claims that the referent object faces an existential threat, demands that urgent and extraordinary countermeasures be taken to deal with the threat and persuades an audience that such action is necessary. Buzan, Wæver and De Wilde (1998) point out that there is no universal definition of an existential threat. Existential threats are problems that, if not tackled, will render "everything else…irrelevant (because we will not be here or will not be free to deal with it in our own way)" (ibid., p. 24). What constitutes a threat can only be understood with reference to the particular character of the referent object, but the nature of the referent object varies between sectors.

The Copenhagen School argues that security is invoked in a variety of different arenas: that is, it does not just refer to military threats to the state. It identifies four other sectors: political, societal, economic and environmental. In the military sector, the referent object will usually be the state and it can be subject to threats to its sovereignty from either external aggressors or internal dissidents. But in the environmental sector, for example, the referent objects can be anything from individual species (including humans) to planet Earth, and these are subject to threats to their survival from human activity of various sorts.

The Copenhagen School argues that framing an issue in terms of security is the most effective strategy for bringing about a large-scale response (Buzan, Wæver and De Wilde, 1998). It is, nevertheless, troubled by securitization as a mode of dealing with problems. One reason is that securitization legitimates the bypassing of normal political rules of the game: for example, public debate, democracy, legal-rational decision-making procedures and respect for another countries' sovereignty. Thus, securitization allows the state to take extraordinary measures in order to deal with perceived existential threats. In the most extreme cases, security might be invoked to legitimize the use of force, as in a declaration of a state of emergency or an attack on another country. Another reason that the Copenhagen School is concerned with securitization is that it can result in a misallocation of resources. An issue that has been successfully securitized will garner disproportionate attention and resources as compared to one that has not, even when the latter actually poses a greater threat.

Securitizing health

The end of the Cold War, the War on Terror and the increasing focus on domestic security in developed countries have led to a broadening of the perception of what constitutes a threat to security (ibid.). Since the 1990s, health issues have increasingly been framed as security threats, and health has become one of the most important non-traditional security issues (Heymann et al., 2015). The securitization of health has occurred in two distinct ways, which are often conflated and confused with each other.

In one, the referent object is individual human beings and the health issue is a presented as a threat to their well-being and lives. This is apparent in a report published by the United Nations Development Programme (UNDP) in 1994 entitled *New Dimensions of Human Security*, which identifies seven categories of threat to human security, including health. It distinguishes between the idea of human security, an individual, people-centred concept and the more traditional state-centred concept of security. The report argues that, irrespective of the threat, people rather than borders, international relations or economics should be the primary concern of politicians and policymakers. In the field of health policy, this has been referred to as "individual health security", which is defined as "security that comes from access to safe and effective health services, products, and technologies" (ibid., p. 1884).

In the second, the referent object is the state and the health issue is presented as a threat to international peace. Heymann et al. (2015) refer to this as collective health security. This is the dominant way in which health security is conceptualized, for example in the International Health Regulations. It has its roots in the efforts to stop the spread of bubonic plague in the fourteenth century. The increased securitization of health in the past couple of decades has been driven by the concern that infectious diseases have the potential to cause problems far beyond public health. In large part, this has been the result of fears about the HIV/AIDS epidemic, as well as the outbreak of SARS in 2003 and fears about avian flu. In 2000, HIV/AIDS was the first health issue to be recognized by the UN Security Council as a threat to international security, when it passed Resolution 1308, pertaining to the impact of HIV/AIDS on peacekeeping operations in Africa. The securitization of health has also been a result of the perceived threat of 'bioterrorism' in the wake of the sarin gas attack in the Tokyo subway system in 1995 and the mailing of anthrax spores to US senators and the media in 2001 (Calain and Sa'Da, 2015, p. 29).

Securitizing Ebola The securitization of infectious diseases reached its apogee in the (delayed) reaction to the 2014 Ebola outbreak in West Africa (Burci, 2014, pp. 27–39). Concern for the people of West Africa was not what motivated the concerted international reaction to Ebola in West Africa. Rather, it was fear that the epidemic could spread out of Africa and cause harm to Western societies (Calain and Sa'Da, 2015, p. 29). Three political decisions taken in September 2014 followed this reasoning. First, the UN Security Council adopted Resolution 2177, which stated that the Ebola outbreak constituted a threat to international peace and security. Second, the USA deployed 3,000

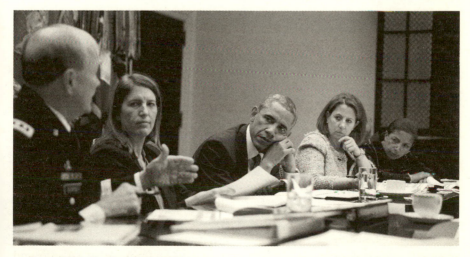

Image D6.1 President Barack Obama convenes a meeting on the Ebola virus at the Center for Disease Control (Official White House Photo by Pete Souza)

military personnel to work on outbreak-control measures in Liberia. While this is generally seen to have had a positive effect on controlling the outbreak, it has also been viewed as an example of the militarization of humanitarian aid (De Waal, 2014). Third, the secretary-general of the United Nations created the first-ever emergency health mission, the United Nations Mission for Ebola Emergency Response (UNMEER).

Depicting Ebola as a threat to international security helped to increase the amount and speed of aid to affected countries. But this was also problematic in several respects. It reinforced the suspicion that global health security priorities are determined by Western conceptions of risk. As Rushton (2011, p. 781) points out, "the result has been the prioritization of measures designed to contain disease within the developing world rather than measures designed to address the root causes of disease". The 'root causes' of the outbreak are not hard to identify. It is widely acknowledged that the extent of the Ebola outbreak was a consequence of dysfunctional national health systems combined with a delayed and fragmented response from global health actors (Moon et al., 2015, pp. 2204–21; Panel of Independent Experts, 2015). Nevertheless, the human insecurity dimension of this failure of health systems (failures both at the national and international levels and played out in multiple countries, and therefore global) has been all but ignored in the literature.

The challenges facing the three Western African countries most affected by Ebola – Liberia, Sierra Leone and Guinea – in rebuilding their health systems are substantial. Internationally, the World Health Organization has convened two high-level meetings on Ebola: the first held in Cape Town in July 2015, followed a year later by a meeting in Bali. Box D6.1 lists the urgent requirements agreed upon amongst participants at the latter meeting (WHO, 2016, p. 12):

Reviewing these requirements, it is easy to see how they might present an additional burden on health systems barely recovering from the Ebola pandemic. The promise of financial assistance has been forthcoming, with two funding mechanisms available for member states: the WHO's first-line Contingency Fund for Emergencies and a longer-term option available through the World Bank's Pandemic Emergency Facility. The latter has approved US$ 110 million in International Development Association financing to help build a disease surveillance system in West Africa. In 2015, Ban Ki-Moon held an International Ebola Recovery Conference, raising US$ 3.4 billion to support West African countries' recovery plans. While the support is welcome, the question remains: How will these countries process such large amounts of money? In an overview of post-Ebola recovery plans in *The Lancet*, Andrew Green recalls an interview with Sjoerd Postma, the chief of party in Liberia for Management Sciences for Health (MSH): "However, that influx of cash created new problems, Postma said, because the countries were not necessarily equipped to absorb it" (Green 2016, p. 2465).

Box D6.1: Recommendations for implementing national preparedness plans to advance global health security

- Country preparedness plans must be urgently developed or updated, taking into consideration 'One Health', 'whole of society' and 'whole of government' approaches.
- Legislative frameworks are required for working together across ministries/sectors.
- Technical guides and controls should be used or designed where necessary, to help ministries work together on zoonoses and shore up the legislative framework. These should be underpinned with training.
- Coordination mechanisms should be established between sectors and guided by a multisectoral steerage committee chaired by a political authority of the highest level.
- Clear definitions should be used for common goals and areas of interest – for example, 'One Health' approach to address, among other problems, antimicrobial resistance (AMR) – underpinned by common frameworks or approaches to anchor collaboration.
- Exercises and simulations should be conducted to strengthen collaboration.

For those with experience of the problems that recipient countries' health systems faced during the early 2000s from large sums of money raised through global health partnerships, these concerns will sound very familiar. So too will Green's further observation, "Now that systems are starting to develop, international interest has been diverted to other hotspots, including the Zika virus response and the ongoing refugee crisis" (ibid.). In the 'rush to implement' post-Ebola security plans, there is the very real risk that: i) recipients of aid will not be able to absorb the levels of external financial assistance either at all or quickly enough; ii) funds will not be spent on reforms to ensure long-term health system strengthening, such as health worker retention and public works such as road building; and iii) donors will not continue to give these funds for long.

Problems with the securitization of health

The notion that collective health security is dominant in global health is underpinned by the assumption that states, specifically Western states, are the referent object under threat. As Rushton (2011, p. 781) summarizes, "[T]he focus tends to be overwhelmingly (albeit implicitly) on securing states against the ingress of disease." As such, collective health security is concerned with preventing potential threats to developed countries – to health, to the economy, or as a matter of non-proliferation of biological weapons and counter-terrorism. This is problematic for several reasons.

One problem is that there is no real empirical basis for the argument that infectious diseases have the potential to cause political instability, especially in the developed world (Burci 2014, pp. 27–39). There are some historical examples of infectious diseases having grave effects on international peace and security. The Plague of Justinian is said to have contributed to the decline of the Eastern Roman Empire in the sixth century CE (Rosen, 2007). The intentional and unintentional introduction of smallpox and other infectious diseases to the Americas had a devastating effect on the local population and facilitated the European colonial conquests (Diamond, 1988). The Black Death, which killed about one-third of the population of Europe, radically changed the relationship between feudal lords and their chattels, resulting in a series of peasant rebellions in Europe and ultimately being a contingent factor in the transition to capitalism (Brenner 1977, p. 25). Nevertheless, there are no recent examples and even the biggest infectious disease outbreaks of modern history – for example, Spanish influenza and HIV/AIDS – have not had a significant negative effect on international peace and security (De Waal, 2010).

Another problem with the dominant form of health securitization is the presumption that disease is the primary source of risk. This constructs a dynamic in which global health actors are focused on the biological determinants of disease. They become focused on developing surveillance systems and 'fighting wars' against outbreaks when and where they occur. This means that the underlying structural causes of epidemics, which are rooted in the lack of access to healthcare and the underlying social, economic and political determinants of health, are overlooked. But unlike states, humans are not immune to the health insecurity that comes with poverty, discrimination or migration. It is apparent, therefore, that collective health security overlooks humans and the idea of human or individual security.

One possible alternative to the dominant view would be to advocate a more people-centred approach to health security. Such an approach would be positive because it would prioritize human life over the interests of the state and society. Nevertheless, it could be argued that individual health security is problematic because it invokes fear in order to legitimize a reaction to health issues. Andrew Lakoff (2010) suggests 'humanitarian biomedicine' as an alternative to the security vision of global health. The former is motivated by a concern for the suffering of others, whereas the latter is implicitly motivated by fear and selfishness (Hofman and Au, 2017). Thus, humanitarian biomedicine aims to alleviate the suffering of individuals in developing countries for its own sake by, for example, taking a long-term approach and building up health systems.

What is more, securitization creates problems that go beyond securitization itself. As public health is increasingly seen as a tool of domestic politics and foreign policy, global health actors become entangled in a wider set of political disputes than would be the case if focus had been solely on public health issues (Elbe, 2006, pp. 119–144). In Syria, for example, the Assad regime has severely restricted access to organizations providing medical aid to rebel-controlled areas (Kennedy and Michailidou, 2017, pp. 690–98). This has exacerbated the health crisis in these areas. In the most extreme examples, global health programmes are used as a cover for political interventions in foreign states.

Perhaps the most notorious case is that of the Central Intelligence Agency (CIA) of the USA using a fake Hepatitis B campaign in Abbottabad, Pakistan, in a failed attempt to obtain DNA from Osama bin Laden's children prior to his assassination (Kennedy, forthcoming). This led to a boycott of vaccination campaigns in militant-controlled areas of northwestern Pakistan, which was a setback for the global efforts to eradicate polio. After a public outcry, the Obama administration pledged that vaccination schemes would never again be used to collect intelligence (Gambino, 2014). Nevertheless, it is clear that this was not an isolated incident. For example, in 2014 it was revealed that the United States Agency for International Development (USAID) had used HIV prevention workshops in Cuba as a cover for attempts to encourage political opposition (Associated Press, 2014). Such activities undermine trust between health workers and local populations, which is especially problematic in postcolonial countries where a great deal of work has been done to counter mistrust that resulted from the colonial encounter.

Conclusions

Although the securitization of health can be a useful tactic for generating interest and resources, there are a variety of problems associated with it. There is no real empirical basis for securitization. It operates by encouraging feelings of selfishness and fear rather than compassion. It can result in the misallocation of scarce resources in a manner that undermines efforts to extend universal health coverage and improve the social determinants of health. And it can, more generally, lead to the dangerous entanglement of politics and health. As such, the securitization of health should be treated with scepticism by global health activists and academics.

References

Associated Press 2014, *USAID programme used young Latin Americans to incite Cuba rebellion*, https://www.theguardian.com/world/2014/aug/04/usaid-latin-americans-cuba-rebellion-hiv-workshops

Brenner, R 1977, 'The origins of capitalist development: a critique of neo-Smithian Marxism', *New Left Review*, vol. 104, p. 25.

Burci, GL 2014, 'Ebola, the Security Council and the securitization of public health', *Questions of International Law*, vol. 10, pp. 27–39.

Buzan, B, Wæver, O & De Wilde, J 1998, *Security: a new framework for analysis*, Lynne Rienner Publishers, Boulder, CO.

Calain, P & Sa'Da, CA 2015, 'Coincident polio and Ebola crises expose similar fault lines in the current global health regime', *Conflict and Health*, vol. 9, no.1, p. 29.

De Waal, A 2010, 'Reframing governance, security and conflict in the light of HIV/AIDS: a synthesis of findings from the AIDS, Security and Conflict Initiative',

Social Science & Medicine, vol. 70, no. 1, pp. 114–20.

De Waal, A 2014,'Militarizing global health' https://www.bostonreview.net/world/alex-de-waal-militarizing-global-health-ebola

Diamond, J M 1998 *Guns, germs and steel: a short history of everybody for the last 13,000 years*, Random House, London.

Elbe, S 2006, 'Should HIV/AIDS be securitized? The ethical dilemmas of linking HIV/ AIDS and security', *International Studies Quarterly*, vol. 50, no. 1, pp. 119–144.

Gambino, L 2014, 'CIA will not use vaccination schemes for spying, says White House official' https://www.theguardian.com/world/2014/may/20/cia-vaccination-programmes-counterterrorism

Green, A 2016, 'West African countries focus on post-Ebola recovery plans', *The Lancet*, vol. 388, no. 10059, pp. 2463–65.

Heymann, D L, Chen, L, Takemi, K, Fidler, D P, et al. 2015, 'Global health security: the wider lessons from the West African Ebola virus disease epidemic', *The Lancet*, vol. 385, no. 9980, pp. 1884–901.

Hofman, M & Au, S (eds) 2017, *The politics of fear: Médecins Sans Frontières and the West African Ebola epidemic*, Oxford University Press, Oxford.

Kennedy, J forthcoming, 'How drone strikes and a fake vaccination program have inhibited polio eradication in Pakistan', *International Journal of Health Services*.

Kennedy, J & Michailidou, D 2017, 'Civil war,

contested sovereignty and the limits of global health partnerships: a case study of the Syrian polio outbreak in 2013', *Health Policy and Planning*, vol. 32, no. 5, pp. 690–98.

Lakoff, A 2010, 'Two regimes of global health', *Humanity: An International Journal of Human Rights, Humanitarianism, and Development*, vol. 1, no. 1, pp. 59–79.

Moon, S, Sridhar, D, Pate, MA, Jha, A K, Clinton, C, Delaunay, S, Edwin, V, Fallah, M, Fidler, D P, Garrett, L, Goosby, E, Gostin, L O, Heymann, DL, Lee, K, Leung, G M, Morrison, J S, Saavedra, J, Tanner, M, Leigh, J A, Hawkins, B, Woskie, L R & Pio, P 2015, 'Will Ebola change the game? Ten essential reforms before the next pandemic. The report of the Harvard-LSHTM Independent Panel on the Global Response to Ebola', *The Lancet*, vol. 386, no. 10009, pp. 2204–21.

Panel of Independent Experts 2015, 'Report of the Ebola Interim Assessment Panel – July 2015', http://www.who.int/csr/resources/publications/ebola/ebola-panel-report/en/

Rosen, W 2007, *Justinian's flea: The first Great Plague and the end of the Roman Empire*. Penguin.

Rushton, S 2011, 'Global health security: security for whom? Security from what?'*Political Studies*, vol. 59, pp. 779–96.

WHO 2016, *Advancing global health security: from commitments to action*, http://apps.who.int/iris/bitstream/10665/251417/1/WHO-HSE-GCR-2016.15-eng.pdf?ua=1

D7 | POLITICS OF DATA, INFORMATION AND KNOWLEDGE

Introduction

Data, information and knowledge are core resources for policy, practice and activism in relation to healthcare and population health. However, they do not stand apart from the struggle for health equity. They are not simple representations of an objective reality 'out there'. They are produced in social practice and bear the imprint of power. This chapter works towards a set of understandings regarding the politics of data, information and knowledge in the struggle for health.

Data, information and knowledge are abstract categories that do not map closely to the institutions and practices through which they are generated and used. We use a hybrid framework in this chapter, structuring our discussion around:

- creating, storing and accessing data
- processing data, generating and accessing information
- learning from practice,
- clinical information and exposure/risk information
- health statistics
- research
- programme evaluation
- knowledge: generation, authorization, communication and management.

Creating, storing and accessing data

Of all the institutions involved in the creation, storing and accessing of health-related data, vital registration is perhaps the oldest, in particular the registration of births and deaths. Vital registration is supplemented by population surveys, including the demographic and health surveys used in many low-income countries where vital registration is incomplete. Administrative data, derived in the context of programme administration, is a major source of data, which includes the utilization and servicing of data, data about health sector resources and health financing data. Two further sets of data are from research projects and project/programme evaluations. We will return to them later.

In reflecting on some of the political issues associated with data collection we will highlight:

- data that is not collected
- data that over-claims what it measures, and
- data which is restricted through price or secrecy.

A notorious example of data that is not collected involves vital registration data in some low-income countries. Insofar as health programmes and schools are planned on the basis of a known population of children, those who are not registered at birth stand at risk of being further ignored in vaccination programmes and educational infrastructure. Insofar as preventive programmes are based on estimates of prevalence and incidence, shortfalls in death registrations, for example maternal deaths, may lead to further failures in prevention.

While shortfalls in vital registration are generally due to resource constraints in some cases, the failure to collect data reflects the power of corporate players seeking to avoid public accountability. Tax avoidance is the outstanding example, but in the health sector we can point to the widespread failure of government agencies to collect data regarding prescription and sale of pharmaceuticals, including, in particular, data regarding the clinical indications for prescribed drugs.

A different issue is where the data that is collected bears only a loose relationship to the concept it claims to represent. A well-known example of this concerns the concept of 'social capital', which in some cases is measured by arbitrary and culturally rooted questions, such as how many organizations the respondent belongs to.

Equally troubling is data that is restricted through price or secrecy. An example of the latter is access to doctor-specific prescribing patterns. Such data is commonly collected by agents of the pharmaceutical industry to evaluate and target their marketing strategies. This data is either not available to public-interest regulators or available at a very high price. Similar secrecy shrouds data about food retailing, which is commonly collected on behalf of the supermarket chains and which provides detailed data about shopping choices, sometimes down to identified families.

Processing data, generating and accessing information

The political forces operating on the transformation of health data into health-related information may be traced in a number of different settings:

- learning from practice
- clinical information and exposure/risk information
- health statistics
- research reports, and
- programme evaluation.

Learning from practice We start with 'learning from practice' because this is commonly overlooked. Vast amounts of 'data' are generated in the ordinary practice of families, healthcare practitioners and, importantly, patients and people living with disabilities. This data constitutes observations about 'What happens when I do such and such thing?'

The data is 'processed' through reflection and discussion where it is converted into information and knowledge, which is then carried and transmitted in culture. The learning from professional practice in the clinic finds its way into conventional wisdom through teaching and into formal expression in books and journals. The learning from the practice of patients and families is shared in communities of interest and sometimes finds its way into literature and film.

In political terms, the key issue here concerns the discounting of learning from practice by the knowledge establishment and the potential significance of systematic reflection and discussion, and the capturing and sharing of such knowledge. This is particularly true in relation to the learning from the practice of social movements, including the 'Health for All' movement.

Clinical information and exposure/risk information The focus under this heading is, first, information about patients' clinical situation – diagnosis, prognosis, treatment options and so on; and, second, information about exposure and health risk.

Information asymmetry in the clinic is well recognized but poorly managed. Proselytizers for private healthcare would suggest that market pressures should encourage clinicians to develop communication skills and provide the information patients want. But they don't. The US Institute of Medicine (1999, 2001), which has published several important reports on the quality of healthcare, states that good communication is an issue of clinical culture and argues that the institutions of healthcare should cultivate the attitudes, skills and practices that will ensure such communication in the clinic. And they should. However, it is also important to recognize the incentive pressures (economic and administrative) that arise in the clinical environment and which militate against the development of such a culture.

The primary healthcare approach envisages working not only to encourage a culture of respect and communication but also to change the institutional relationships and accountabilities that frame clinical practice. In Australia, Aboriginal Community Controlled Health Organizations (ACCHOs) are governed by community representatives and staffed by a mix of Aboriginal and non-Aboriginal practitioners. There are challenges in implementing this model, especially since it runs counter to so much in conventional healthcare. However, the ACCHOs are working deliberately and consciously to implement this approach. (See Chapter B2.)

A different issue under the politics of health information concerns occupational and environmental health exposures. The role of the mining industry in deliberately concealing what it knew about asbestosis (Peacock, 2009) and black lung disease (Berman 1977, pp. 63–87) has been documented in detail. A comparable case concerns tobacco and the role of the tobacco industry in concealing the knowledge (Malone and Balbach, 2000)of the health dangers of tobacco smoking.

One of the most egregious cases of risk concealment was the Tuskegee syphilis experiment between 1932 and 1972 involving black farm workers in Alabama, around half of whom had syphilis (Reverby, 2011). It appears that the government-sponsored study commenced as a study of the natural history of the disease but after penicillin became available the study continued as before, simply observing clinical progress. Not only did the researchers fail to organize treatment for the study participants, they discouraged them from seeking treatment elsewhere.

The Tuskegee case is not an isolated instance. Since then numerous cases have come to light of drug companies undertaking clinical trials in low-income countries on poor and poorly educated populations without the informed consent provisions that would be required in high-income countries (Illes, Sahakian and Dyke, 2011).

A more systemic case, concerning data that is not collected, deals with the adverse effects of pharmaceuticals. The regulation of the marketing of new drugs takes place in two phases: the first is marketing approval and the second is post-marketing surveillance. In most countries post-marketing surveillance is weak, depending only on clinicians reporting adverse events following exposure. This means that low-incidence side effects, particularly in infrequently used drugs, may remain undetected for many years.

A different set of distortions are evident in the evolving protocols for pre-marketing approval, with the introduction of 'data exclusivity', which defines the period during which generic manufacturers are not allowed to rely on the initial documentation regarding safety and efficacy as part of their application for marketing approval.

Finally, food labelling provides a further instance where risk information is being systemically denied to consumers. An aggressive campaign has been waged over many years by the food and beverage industry in order to prevent regulations that might require them to provide informative and accessible information about the health risks associated with their products.

Health statistics The field of health statistics constitutes another domain where the politics of measurement fogs health policy analysis. The principal reason governments collect and publish health statistics is to inform public policy. Information is power in the sense that if governments know what they are doing they can modify policies to achieve their objectives more effectively. Furthermore, most governments take the view that while integrity and transparency in health statistics can inform protest as well as policy implementation, there are significant costs related to dishonest data and secrecy. Accordingly, for health activists seeking to engage in policy dialogue the various data repositories and, particularly, visualizations can be valuable resources to refer to.

While there is much useful material in national and international health statistics repositories (and observatories) it is also necessary to appreciate how official information systems are cast within, and project, a particular ideology notwithstanding their veneer of objectivity.

DALYs, disability-adjusted life years, were developed in the context of the World Bank's 'Investing in Health' report, published in 1993. DALYs are used as a measure of ongoing disease burden consequent upon disease or injury commencing in the present period (or the disease burden averted by treatments or preventive interventions implemented in the present period). Disability-adjusted life years comprise two components: years of life lost and years lived with disability. Years of life lost compares the estimated survival following the onset of the illness or injury with estimated life expectancy at the same age without the onset of illness or injury. The value of years of life lost well into the future is discounted compared with the years immediately following the onset on the grounds that immediate years are worth more than distant years. The estimate of years lived with disability is based on estimated survival, weighted for the degree of disability. The weighting is expressed in a figure from 0 to 1 and has the effect of reducing the survival estimate in accordance with the level of disability. Thus a disability weight of 0.95 will not alter the survival estimate greatly. However, a disability weighting of 0.2 will reduce by five-fold the estimate of years lived with disability. A year of life lived with such a disability is valued at 20 per cent of a year. Finally, DALYs are further adjusted according to the age of onset. Greater value is assigned to DALYs taken from the 'economically productive' ages as compared to infancy, childhood and old age.

DALYs are conceptually attractive because they reduce to one measure the morbidity and mortality consequent upon events occurring in the present period: the onset of disease or injury, or treatments delivered, or preventive interventions. However, the incidence data and the survival data on which they are based are often very rough 'guesstimates' and the transformations involved in discounting future years by applying disability weights and adjusting for age of onset all reflect judgements about the value of human lives, judgements that are not always evident to readers of publications using DALYs. The processes involved in determining disability weightings are particularly dubious.

A second example of hidden value judgements in apparently objective statistics are the health system league tables published in the World Health Report of 2000. This exercise purported to compare national health systems using three measures: health status, responsiveness and fairness in financing. We do not have space here to itemize the weaknesses in the crude data assembled for this exercise or the value judgements incorporated in the selection of evaluative criteria or the flawed logic expressed in the selection of the three principal measures. Suffice it to say that the product of this exercise was completely lacking in credibility and greatly damaged the WHO's reputation.

Research reports Access to research funding through both government-funded research councils and philanthropic bodies is generally dependent on the value of the anticipated knowledge and the technical quality of the research proposal. Both are subject to the gatekeepers' interpretation of both the social value of the anticipated knowledge production and the proposed methodology.

The most striking measure of political bias in research funding is the imbalance between, on the one hand, the funding of basic science and clinical medicine and, on the other, (the lack of) funding for research on the delivery of healthcare and prevention. Notwithstanding shortfalls in access, quality and efficiency in healthcare delivery, the focus of health-related research globally is on the biology of health and disease and technical advances in clinical practice.

Gatekeeping with respect to methodology favours the generalizable over the contingent, the quantitative over the qualitative, and privileges methods that are high in the 'hierarchy of evidence'.

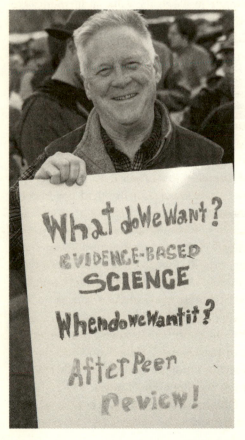

Image D7.1 Support for evidence-based science and peer review (By scattered1 from USA; License: CC BY-SA 2.0, https://commons.wikimedia.org/w/index.php?curid=58260940)

The hierarchy of evidence is a reflection of the reductionism that dominates health research funding and practice. This is epitomized by the double-blind randomized controlled trial (RCT), which is represented as producing the most compelling research. The genius of the RCT is that it controls for variations in context. The inclusion criteria and the nature of the intervention are specified and, through random allocation to treatment or control, all of the contextual factors that might affect the impact of the intervention are controlled. The paradox is that healthcare and health promotion are highly context-dependent, where context includes patient variables and environmental factors. Thus, because the treatment of blood pressure in middle age has been shown to improve outcomes, the need to control blood pressure is taken as mandatory even in the very old, amongst whom very few RCTs have been done.

One of the consequences of the increasing authority of statistics has been an increasing preference for research methodologies that yield quantitative estimates, amenable to statistical testing, over qualitative methods. There is a perception that quantitative methods are more 'objective' or less imbued with value judgements. This is not so. The big difference is that the value judgement goes into the definition of the variables *before* the data is collected in quantitative research, while in qualitative research the value judgements are present in the questions that are asked and the interpretation of the findings.

Social class is an example par excellence of an emergent phenomenon that has properties at the macro level that are not computable on the basis of micro variables and relationships. This is highly relevant to public health both in relation to the social (and political) determinants of health and the political configurations that shape health systems.

Looming over these factors is the academic citation/impact fetish. Increasingly, the research performance (and funding) of universities is being measured in terms of publication in highly cited journals and the citations achieved by individual papers. This has the effect of discounting journals that do not service a large constituency, no matter the social significance of the field covered by that journal. This has the effect of encouraging papers that offer widely applicable generalizations rather than focusing on context-specific questions. The consequence is that academic collaboration with communities, learning from practice, and locally relevant knowledge are discounted in favour of technological research-oriented material useful for the new globalized marketplace.

The drivers of industry research are much more closely tied to market opportunities and treat knowledge as private property. A field of industry research that is of particular relevance to health policy and is particularly influenced by health politics is that of clinical trials, in particular of drugs and vaccines. We have referred to Tuskegee and its modern equivalent, the use of Third World subjects for evaluating safety and efficacy. John le Carré's novel, *The Constant Gardener*, is a beacon in this context. The book was based on a clinical trial conducted by Pfizer in Nigeria on the treatment of meningitis. The trial was carried out without authorization from the Nigerian government and without consent from the children's parents. Eleven children died.

The issues go beyond unethical recruitment and exposures. Of more general concern is the prevalence of fraudulent analyses of clinical trials data and the failure to publish negative studies. As a consequence, proposals for mandatory registration of all clinical trials and for clinical trials data repositories are gaining increasing support. The corrupting influence of corporate sponsorship of clinical trials affects methodology as well as publication. For example, trials that focus on the impact on intermediate endpoints need to be supplemented by further studies that confirm that there is a net benefit in terms of long-term outcomes. This is not always the case.

Programme evaluation How does politics shape the transformation of evaluation data into information and knowledge? We start by noting the tendency to discount formative as opposed to summative evaluation. Formative evaluation follows the implementation of a programme with a view to learning how to do it better. Summative evaluation sums up the outcomes of the programme, often with a view to satisfying funders that their investment has been well spent; the focus is on accountability rather than learning. The distinction is between single loop learning (What am I learning about how to achieve the original goals we established for this programme?) and double loop learning (What am I learning about how to achieve the original goals *and* what am I learning about whether these were the right goals?).

The problem arises sharply when agencies distributing funds are also accountable to original donors who need to be assured that their funds are being productively used. If the funding agency is obligated to report that promised goals are being achieved (perhaps the distribution of insecticide-treated bed nets) they will not be disposed to allow the flexibility of double loop learning to the funding recipients. So if the recipients come around to the view that some of their efforts should be applied to preventing mosquito access through improved window and door fittings and if this leads to fewer insecticide bed nets being distributed, then the funder will be disadvantaged vis-à-vis the donor. Both learning and accountability are important, but in this instance learning on the ground is sacrificed to accountability.

The concept of programme logic is central to this dynamic. Applicants for funding are required to specify the programme logic underpinning their application. This is a useful discipline; it specifies how the strategies to be implemented will contribute to the putative outcomes and suggests performance indicators that enable the project managers to determine how well the strategies are being put in place and if so whether they are working. However if that programme logic is locked into place for accountability purposes there is no space for double loop learning.

Knowledge: generation, authorization, communication and management

Knowledge is generated, transmitted and stored in:

* hard copy (academic research, libraries, books and journals)
* soft copy (the Internet, artificial intelligence, smart phones, digital mode)
* wet copy (teaching/learning, mentoring, culturally embedded knowledge, experiential knowledge, practical knowledge).

With the information explosion, speed of change and global integration, knowledge management (the capture, storage, access and retrieval of previously encoded knowledge) is attracting increased formal attention. At a systemic level we can identify the following institutions of knowledge management: libraries and journals, search engines, knowledge portals, observatories and knowledge brokers. Many large organizations are also exploring at a corporate level how they can better manage 'their' knowledge, including through corporate memory and computers or by developing a culture of recognizing and sharing the 'wet copy' knowledge of experienced workers.

We highlight three important issues involving the politics of knowledge: ideology, marketization, and the embeddedness of knowledge in the workforce (or human resources).

We have referred earlier to the role of hegemonic ideology in shaping how knowledge is generated, authorized, valued, and made available. Among the assumptions that are promoted by neoliberalism are these: that market mechanisms are preferable to administration, planning and regulation; that private enterprise is generally more efficient than government; that society is constituted of a myriad of separate competing consumers; that inequality reflects the necessary discipline of market forces, sorting people according to their worth (Harvey, 2005). The intellectual framework for this ideology is provided by conservative economists and philosophers, but its driving forces are rooted in the transnational capitalist class. These include the financial press and ratings agencies working in tandem with the dispersed forces of 'market discipline', the stock market and the money market speculators who collectively hobble political leaders.

Through neoliberal ideology the transnational capitalist class is able to influence the climate within which knowledge is generated and applied. Thus charity (international development assistance) is a proper and necessary mechanism for supporting healthcare and nutrition in low-income countries (and it would be bad form to harp on the power relations and dynamics of the global economy that perpetuate national poverty).

Hegemonic ideology can be challenged. In the mid-1990s when anti-retroviral drugs became available, there were many voices saying that treating AIDS in low- and middle-income countries was impossible and that the only rational policy was one of 'prevention'. This position reflected an acceptance of high prices and poor governments, an acceptance of the monopoly pricing power provided to Big Pharma through the extended intellectual property provisions of the TRIPS Agreement. However, this status quo position was not accepted by the treatment access movement, which challenged the basic assumptions of the free trade juggernaut. The delegitimation of TRIPS by the treatment access movement was a major factor motivating rich nations and philanthropists to mobilize billions for new global health initiatives and for the Millennium Development Goals.

The privatization and marketization of knowledge is fully consistent with the neoliberal celebration of market forces and the expanded protection and policing of intellectual property. Price barriers to accessing knowledge arise in part from the corporate ownership of academic journals, which restricts electronic access to journals and e-books to employees of large organizations such as universities. One of the active debates in this area is the controversy over the digitization of hard copy libraries. No one argues against the digitization of this legacy but the question is whether it should be done privately (perhaps by Google?) or as a publicly funded open access initiative.

Perhaps the largest pool of usable knowledge, including information on how to access the knowledge, is embedded in the workforce, hence the term 'human resources'. This has implications for the politics of knowledge, including the power relations of communication and of teaching and learning.

The concept of the proletarianization of knowledge workers provides a useful framework for interpreting contemporary movements in knowledge management. Braverman (1974) speaks of the appropriation of shopfloor knowledge by engineers in the 'front office'. As the engineers acquire more detailed knowledge of the production process they are able to redesign the work flow, including a greater division of labour (and reduction in the work span of individual workers), in order to increase efficiency and profit. As the workers on the shop floor are transformed from skilled artisans into assemblyline operatives they are disempowered and increasingly alienated from their work.

The transfer of wet knowledge (held in memories and culture) into soft knowledge (held in computers) is happening in the health sector, although at different rates and in different ways. Perhaps the most dramatic example is the rise in the power of health insurance corporations in the medical arena in the USA.

Conclusion

The struggle for health is complex and difficult. A thoughtful approach to data, information and knowledge is a necessary part of effective engagement. We have reviewed some general ideas and a few specific case studies. This is just the beginning of a discussion towards a set of insights that might usefully inform practice.

References

Berman, D 1977, 'Why work kills: a brief history of occupational safety and health in the United States', *International Journal of Health Services*, vol. 7, no. 1, pp. 63–87, DOI10.2190/8m31-316b-guej-frcw.

Braverman, H 1974, *Labor and monopoly capital: the degradation of work in the twentieth century*,Monthly Review Press, New York.

Institute of Medicine 1999,*To err is human: building a safer health care system*,National Academy Press, Washington, DC, http://www.nap.edu/books/0309068371/html/

Institute of Medicine (US) Committee on Quality of Health Care in America 2001, *Crossing the quality chasm: a new health system for the 21st Century*, National Academies Press, Washington, DC.

Harvey, D 2005, *A brief history of neoliberalism*, Oxford University Press, Oxford.

Illes, J, Sahakian, B J & Dyke, C V 2011,*Ethical perspectives: clinical drug trials in developing countries*, Oxford University Press, Oxford.

Le Carré, J 2001, *The constant gardener*, Scribner, New York.

Malone, R E & Balbach, E D2000, 'Tobacco industry documents: treasure trove or quagmire?'*Tobacco Control*, vol. 9, http://dx.doio.org/10.1136/tc.9.3.334

Peacock, M 2009, *Killer company: James Hardie exposed*, ABC Books.

Reverby, S M 2011, *Examining Tuskegee*, University of North Carolina Press, Chapel Hill.

In 2011, the members of the World Health Organization (WHO) adopted a ground-breaking agreement, the Pandemic Influenza Preparedness Framework (PIP Framework), for the first time linking access to pathogens to fair and equitable sharing of benefits arising from their use.

The right of governments to fair and equitable benefit-sharing was established in 1992, with the adoption of the Convention on Biological Diversity (CBD).[1] This right follows from the CBD's recognition of a state's sovereign right over its natural resources and the recognition that access to and use of genetic resource is subject to prior informed consent and mutually agreed terms.[2] The Nagoya Protocol on Access and Benefit-Sharing, which entered into force in 2014 further elaborates on these elements.[3]

The PIP Framework, adopted by the World Health Assembly Resolution WHA64.5, builds on the legal principles of the CBD and recognizes the sovereign right of states over their biological resources. It also recognizes that the members of the WHO have a commitment to virus-sharing and benefit-sharing on an "equal footing", as they are "equally important parts of the collective action for global public health".[4] Accordingly, the framework sets out international rules governing the access to influenza viruses of pandemic potential (IVPP) and the benefit-sharing obligations of the recipients of IVPP.

Five years of implementation reveals the framework to be a 'success story' in equitable pandemic preparedness and a significant precedent to be followed in relation to the WHO's handling of other pathogens and related epidemics and pandemics (Shashikant 2017).

PIP Framework: theorigins[5]

World attention focused on access and benefit-sharing in early 2007 when Indonesia's minister of health, Siti Fadilah Supari, announced that Indonesia would suspend the sharing of viruses with the WHO Collaborating Centres (WHO CCs) as the then WHO flu virus-sharing scheme, the Global Influenza Surveillance Network (GISN), was 'unfair' (Khor and Shashikant, 2007a, 2007b).

The affected countries would send potentially pandemic avian flu virus samples to certain national laboratories designated as WHO CCs and located in developed countries.[6] These laboratories would characterize the virus, develop candidate vaccine strains and, in violation of the WHO guidelines, send viruses

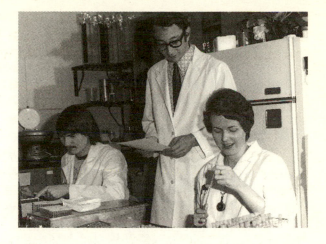
Image D8.1 Viruses shared by countries are used by industry to develop vaccines (https://pixnio.com/)

to the commercial sector for vaccine development, without the consent of the contributing country. Worse still, the vaccines developed by the private sector, using viruses obtained from the GISN, were unavailable and/or not affordable to developing countries (Shashikant, 2010).

Indonesia, severely affected by the highly pathogenic H5N1 virus, found that its viruses shared with WHO CCs were used for vaccine development without its permission, and the same vaccines were being offered to Indonesia by an Australian drug company for US$ 20 a dose. As the country might need to vaccinate its entire population of over 200 million should a pandemic occur, the cost at this price level would be astronomical (Khor and Shashikant, 2007b).

Patent claims were also filed over influenza virus and virus parts, that is, viral gene segments and their sequences, shared in good faith with the GISN by avian influenza-affected countries such as Indonesia, Vietnam, China and Thailand (Hammond, 2009, 2011).

Thus the GISN virus-sharing system had a clear set of winners: the vaccine companies that gained access to flu viruses and developed proprietary flu vaccines to be sold at high prices; developed countries that entered into advance purchase agreements with vaccine manufacturers for the supply and stockpile of (pre) pandemic vaccines; and national laboratories in those countries that gained access to flu vaccines and claimed scientific recognition and patents. On the other hand were the losers: especially, developing countries facing dangerous outbreaks, astronomical bills for the purchase of vaccines and other treatments, and even difficulty in accessing such supplies at all, due to their limited availability. Technologies and know-how used in vaccine development and production (largely based in developed countries) are also protected as intellectual property, potentially creating more obstacles for developing countries seeking to build their own production capacity.

It also soon became apparent that the GISN's operations were inconsistent with the principles and provisions of the CBD, which subjects the access to and use of genetic resources to prior informed consent and fair and equitable benefit-sharing on mutually agreed terms with the country providing the resource.

All of these issues came to a head at the World Health Assembly in 2007 as a number of developing countries led by Indonesia expressed outrage at the inequities and indifference of the then WHO GISN to the needs of developing countries and the lack of adherence to the principles of the CBD and sought to overhaul the system. The 2007 assembly adopted Resolution 60.28 titled 'Pandemic Influenza Preparedness: sharing of influenza viruses and access to vaccines and other benefits', which for the first time linked the sharing of viruses to benefit-sharing and kicked off four years of often tense negotiations that eventually led to the adoption of the PIP Framework.

Achievements and challenges of the PIP Framework

The PIP Framework overhauled the WHO's influenza virus-sharing system and the basis on which potentially pandemic flu viruses are accessed. It replaced the GISN with the Global Influenza Surveillance and Response System (GISRS) and set out the terms of references (TOR) for GISRS laboratories. The WHO GISRS is an international network of influenza laboratories coordinated by the WHO, which comprises 143 National Influenza Centres (NIC), 6 WHO Collaborating Centres (WHO CCs), 13 WHO H5 Reference Laboratories (H5RL) and 4 Essential Regulatory Laboratories (ERLs).

The objective of the PIP Framework is "to improve pandemic influenza preparedness and response, and strengthen protection against pandemic influenza by improving and strengthening WHO GISRS, with the objective of a fair, transparent, equitable, efficient, effective system for, on an *equal footing* [emphasis added]: (i) the sharing of H5N1 and other influenza viruses with human pandemic potential; and (ii) access to vaccines and sharing of other benefits."

The scope of the framework is limited to the IVPP (influenza viruses of pandemic potential) and does not extend to seasonal influenza viruses or any other pathogens. The framework subjects all transfers of IVPP (also known as PIP biological material) among the WHO GISRS laboratories and with entities outside the GISRS system to the Standard Material Transfer Agreements (SMTAs) and commits all recipients of PIP biological material to benefit-sharing. The framework also puts in place a transparent traceability mechanism, the Influenza Virus Tracking Mechanism (IVTM), which tracks in real time the movement of PIP biological material into, within and out of the WHO GISRS (WHO, 2017b).

Under the PIP Framework, WHO member states "should in a rapid, systematic and timely manner" through their NICs, or other authorized laboratories, provide PIP biological materials from "all cases" of IVPP "as feasible" to the WHO CCs or H5RL laboratories of their choice. By providing PIP biological materials "Member States provide their consent for the onward transfer and use of PIP biological materials" to entities outside of the GISRS "subject to provisions in the Standard Material Transfer Agreements [SMTA)]".

It is noteworthy that the framework does not prevent a WHO member state from providing PIP biological material "directly to any other party or body on a bilateral basis provided that the same materials are provided on a priority basis" to the WHO CC or the H5RL.

All transfers of PIP biological material within the WHO GISRS (for example, from an NIC to a WHO CC) are subject to mutually agreed terms contained in SMTA1.[7] This requires, inter alia, the following: the compliance of the recipient with its respective TOR for GISRS laboratories; the recording of any shipments of PIP biological materials to entities inside and outside WHO GISRS, in the IVTM; the active involvement of scientists from the originating laboratories, especially those from developing countries, in scientific projects on clinical specimens or influenza viruses and their active engagement in the preparation of manuscripts for presentation, and the publication and acknowledgement of their contributions. SMTA1 also makes it clear that neither the provider nor the recipient should seek to obtain any intellectual property right on the materials.

Disputes between the provider and the recipient are to be resolved through amicable means, or, if that fails, the matter is to be referred to the director general of the WHO, who may seek the advice of the Advisory Group (established to guide the implementation of the framework), with a view of settling it. The framework further provides the director general with the authority to suspend or revoke the WHO designation of the relevant GISRS laboratory in the event of a serious breach of its TOR.

All transfers of PIP biological material by the WHO GISRS to entities outside of the GISRS network are also subject to legally binding, mutually agreed terms contained in SMTA2.[8] This material transfer agreement is a one-time agreement between the WHO and the entity outside of the GISRS network. SMTA2 lists the different benefit-sharing options for different types of recipients. Box D8.1 shows the different options for different categories of recipients.[9]

As at March 2017, the WHO had signed nine agreements with vaccine and antiviral manufacturers (Table D8.1) providing the WHO real-time access to an estimated 400 million doses of pandemic vaccine during the next pandemic (WHO, 2017a). However none of the agreements commit the manufacturers to technology transfer, as is possible under A5 and A6 benefit-sharing options of the SMTA2.

Box D8.1 Benefit-sharing options

Category A: Manufacturers of vaccines and antivirals are to commit to at least two of the following options:

- A1. Donate at least 10 per cent of real-time pandemic vaccine production to the WHO.
- A2. Reserve for the WHO at least 10 per cent of real-time pandemic vaccine production at affordable prices.
- A3. Donate at least X treatment courses of needed antiviral medicine for the pandemic to the WHO.
- A4. Reserve at least X treatment courses of needed antiviral medicine for the pandemic at affordable prices.
- A5. Grant to manufacturers in developing countries licences on mutually agreed terms that should be fair and reasonable, including in respect of affordable royalties, taking into account the development levels, in the country of end use of the products, of technology, know-how, products and processes for which it holds IPR for the production of (i) influenza vaccines, (ii) adjuvants, (iii) antivirals and/ or (iv) diagnostics.
- A6. Grant royalty-free licences to manufacturers in developing countries or grant to WHO royalty-free, non-exclusive licences on IPR, which can be sublicensed, for the production of pandemic influenza vaccines, adjuvants, antivirals products and diagnostics needed in a pandemic. The WHO may sublicense these licences to manufacturers in developing countries on appropriate terms and conditions and in accordance with sound public health principles.

Category B: Manufacturers of other products relevant to pandemic influenza preparedness and response shall commit to one of the following options: A5, A6, B1, B2, B3 and B4.

- B1. Donate to the WHO at least X2 diagnostic kits needed for pandemics.
- B2. Reserve for WHO at least X2 diagnostic kits needed for pandemics at affordable prices.
- B3. Support, in coordination with the WHO, the strengthening of influenza-specific laboratoryand surveillance capacity in developing countries
- B4. Support, in coordination with the WHO, the transfer of technology, know-how and/or processes for pandemic influenza preparedness and response in developing countries.

Category C: The recipient shall, in addition to the commitments selected under A or B above, consider contributing to the measures listed below, as appropriate:

- donations of vaccines
- donations of pre-pandemic vaccines
- donations of antivirals
- donations of medical devices
- donations of diagnostic kits
- affordable pricing
- transfer of technology and processes
- granting of sublicences to the WHO
- laboratory and surveillance capacity-building.

TABLE D8.1: Agreements with vaccine and antiviral manufacturers

Company	Benefit-sharing commitments of influenza vaccines and antiviral manufacturers under SMTA2			
	Donation of real-time pandemic vaccine to the WHO (%)	Reservation of real-time pandemic vaccine for supply at affordable prices (%)	Antiviral donation	Antiviral reservation
China National Biotech Group (CNBG)	8.0	2.0		
Glaxo Group Limited	7.5	2.0	2 million treatment courses	3 million treatment courses
Kitasato Daiichi Sankyo Vaccine Co., Ltd	8.0	2.0		
MedImmune LLC	9.0	1.0		
The Research Foundation for Microbial Diseases of Osaka University (BIKEN)	8.0	2.0		
Sanofi	7.5	7.5		
Seqirius, UK	10.0	2.5		
Serum Institute of India	8.0	2.0		
Sinovac Biotech Ltd	8.0	2.0		

Source: World Health Organization, 2017, Manufacturers of vaccines & antivirals, current status, http://www.who.int/influenza/pip/benefit_sharing/SMTA2_pieChart_A.pdf?ua=1

The WHO has also concluded 50 SMTA2s with academic and research institutions and received 22 benefit-sharing offers. Most of these institutions have offered to provide laboratory and surveillance capacity-building as a benefit contribution. The WHO has also signed a SMTA2 with a diagnostic company.

In addition to SMTA2 commitments, the framework requires influenza vaccine, diagnostic and pharmaceutical manufacturers "using the WHO GISRS" to make an "annual partnership contribution to the WHO". The sum of annual contributions is set at "50 per cent of the running costs of the WHO GISRS", with the understanding that costs may change over time and the partnership contribution will change accordingly. At the point of the framework's adoption, these running costs were estimated to be US$ 56.5 million.

Thus, companies that access the GISRS are collectively responsible for contributing US$ 28 million annually. How much each company pays is based on a formula agreed among the industry representatives (WHO, 2013). Table D8.2 shows that from the start of 2012 to 31 January 2017, the total partnership contribution collected from 47 contributors stood at US$ 117,758,149 (WHO, 2015b). The use of the partnership contribution is decided by the director general, based on the advice from the Advisory Group, following consultations with manufacturers and other stakeholders.

The first high-level implementation plan approved for the period 2013 to 2016 was based on the allocation of 70 per cent of the contribution for preparedness, that is, for activities in the following categories: (i) laboratory and surveillance capacity, (ii) burden of disease, (iii) regulatory capacity, (iv) risk communications and (v) planning for deployment (WHO, 2015a). Thirty per cent of the contribution has been reserved for response activities in the event of a pandemic.

A five-year review In 2016, following five years of implementation, an Expert Review of the PIP Framework concluded that the framework is a "bold and innovative tool for pandemic influenza preparedness", and "its implementation has led to greater confidence and predictability in the global capacity to respond to an influenza pandemic" (WHO, 2017c). Noteworthy is the review's conclusion that "the principle of the Framework of placing virus-sharing and benefit-sharing on an equal footing remains relevant today".

The review also identified several on-going and new challenges specifically in relation to the PIP Framework and its relevance to other pathogens shared within the WHO. A particularly urgent challenge is the relevance of the framework in view of rapid technological developments. Viruses may be generated in whole or in part from the genetic sequence data (GSD), supplanting the need for the transfer of biological material, including for production of vaccine strains (Dormitzer et al., 2013). This development has brought to the forefront the issue of how the GSD should be handled and the importance

TABLE D8.2: Contributions by companies accessing GISRS (in US$)

Contributors	Total contributions (US$)	Contributors	Total contributions (US$)
GlaxoSmithKline	30,110,587	Scientific Research Institute of Vaccines and Sera	59,812
F.Hoffmann-La Roche AG	26,707,341	Serum Institute of India	33,168
Sanofi Pasteur	22,057,029	Diasorin Molecular LLC	29,692
Novartis Vaccines and Diagnostics, Inc.	15,292,743	China National Biotec Group (CNBG)	20,000
MedImmune, LLC	5,160,754	VABIOTECH	10,300
Seqirus	3,779,042	Cadila Healthcare	10,261
BioCSL Pty. Ltd	2,667,715	Fast-track Diagnostics	8,136
Kaketsuken	2,580,379	Princeton BioMeditech Corporation	8,136
The Research Foundation for Microbial Diseases of Osaka University (BIKEN)	2,369,318	Cepheid	8,130
Denka Seiken Co., Ltd	1,754,659	The Government Pharmaceutical Organization (GPO)	8,130
Kitasato Daiichi Sankyo Vaccine Co., Ltd	1,347,821	Quidel Corporation	8,130
Green Cross Corporation	1,347,781	Takeda	8,113
Sinovac Biotech Ltd	409,323	Institute of Vaccines & Medical Biologicals (IVAC), Vietnam	5,437
Shangai Institute of Biological Products Co., Ltd	409,317	Response Biomedical	5,417
Becton, Dickinson and Company	296,432	Nanotherapeutics	5,337
Baxter International Inc.	209,205	NPO Petrovax Pharm	5,337
Changchun Insitute of Biological Products Co., Ltd	208,231	InDevR, Inc.	4,984
Fluart Innovative Vaccines Kft	160,077	Medicago	4,984
Beijing TiantanBiological Products Co., Ltd	149,518	Nanosphere	4,984
Omninvest Vaccine Manufacturing, Researching and Trading Ltd.	149,443	PT Bio Farma	4,984
Alere Inc.	117,153	Protein Sciences Corporation	4,944
Focus Diagnostics, Inc.	83,844	UMN PharmaInc.	2,799
Adimmune Corporation	65,543	Lanzhou Institute of Biological Products Co., Ltd	2,173
Qiagen	61,506	Total receipts	117,758,149

Source: World Health Organization, 2017, Partnership Contribution Implementation Portal, https://extranet.who.int/pip-pc-implementation/budget.aspx?year=2012

of treating it in a manner equivalent to viral isolates, with access to the PIP GSD contingent on acceptance of benefit-sharing and other obligations of the framework.[10]

On the latter subject, the review also concluded that the framework 'is a foundational model of reciprocity for global public health that could be applied to other pathogens'.

An access and benefit-sharing model for other pathogens

In 2003, following the outbreak of SARS coronavirus, a major controversy broke out. Teams of scientists in Canada, Hong Kong and the USA, brought together by the WHO to address the outbreak, filed patent applications on all or part of the SARS virus genome and on the virus itself, which were reported to be sufficiently broad to allow their holders to claim rights in most diagnostic tests, drugs or vaccines that had been or would be developed to cope with the outbreak (NBCNEWS. com 2003; Simon et al., 2005, pp. 707–10).

In 2014, another dispute erupted, this time over the Middle East respiratory syndrome (MERS) virus. It emerged that Erasmus University in the Netherlands had filed patent applications over the MERS virus, which was sent to the Netherlands without permission from the country of origin, Saudi Arabia (Hammond, 2014).

These controversies are symptomatic of the inequities and bias prevailing in global health governance. The 2007 avian flu controversy led to a multilateral access and benefit-sharing with equity at the core of the arrangement, with the WHO financially and otherwise resourced to facilitate pandemic preparedness at the national and international levels. However a similar benefit-sharing arrangement does not exist for seasonal influenza viruses (although annually 28,000 such viruses are shared with the GISRS network and relevant strains with vaccine manufacturers) and other pathogens shared in situations of emergencies.

Even in the devastating outbreak of Ebola, the Review Committee on the Role of the International Health Regulations (2005) in the Ebola Outbreak and Response found that a number of states parties expressed concern that data-sharing was not be balanced by benefit-sharing (WHO, 2016). The same committee has recommended that the WHO Secretariat and member states consider using the PIP Framework or similar existing agreements as a template for creating new agreements for other infectious agents that have caused, or may potentially cause, a Public Health Emergency of International Concern (PHEIC), based on the principle of balancing the sharing of samples and data with benefit- sharing on an equal footing (ibid.).

Following the Ebola outbreak, the WHO is engaged in developing a blueprint for research and development preparedness and rapid research response covering 11 pathogens, which are likely to cause public health emergencies. The WHO's documentation suggests that it is involved in ad hoc activities with multiple actors – such as the Wellcome Trust, Chatham House, Institut

Pasteur and the Coalition for Epidemic Preparedness Innovation (CEPI), which includes initiatives linked to biological samples, such as developing global norms for sharing data and results, the development of bio-banks and capacity building on material transfer agreement. However, absent from the various activities of the blueprint is a transparent process engaging all the WHO members in the establishment of clear, equitable rules governing the use of pathogens or related GSD, and especially establishing fair and equitable benefit-sharing consistent with the objectives and provisions of the CBD and the Nagoya Protocol.

The lack of international rules governing access to pathogens and fair and equitable benefit-sharing is a major deficiency and risks the re-occurrence of controversies as seen in SARS, MERS and avian flu, with the consequence of erosion of trust and the weakening of pandemic preparedness and response.

Notes

1 The CBD has 196 parties.

2 See the Preamble and Article 15 of the CBD (United Nations 1992).

3 For the text of the Nagoya Protocol, see Secretariat of the Convention on Biological Diversity (2011).

4 For the Preamble (paras 3, 11 and 14) as well as the objectives of the PIP Framework, see WHO (2011).

5 See Shashikant (2010).

6 From 2003 to April 2007, 291 confirmed human cases (including 172 deaths) of avian influenza A(H5N1) were reported to the WHO. The most affected countries were Vietnam (93 confirmed human cases and 42 deaths in 2003–2005), Indonesia (81 cases, 63 deaths in 2005–2007), Egypt (34 cases, 14 deaths in 2006–2007), Thailand (25 cases, 17 deaths in 2004–2006), China (24 cases, 15 deaths in 2005–2007), Turkey (12 cases, 4 deaths in 2006), Azerbaijan (8 cases, 5 deaths in 2006), Cambodia (7 deaths in 2005–2007), Iraq (3 cases, 2 deaths in 2006), Laos (2 deaths in 2007), Nigeria (1 death in 2007) and Djibouti (1 case in 2006).

7 See Annex 1 of the PIP Framework (WHO 2011).

8 See Annex 2 of the PIP Framework (ibid.)

9 See ibid.

10 It is noteworthy that the Expert Review has recommended that the definition of PIP biological material in the PIP Framework be amended to explicitly include the genetic sequence data. The Advisory Group set up to monitor implementation of the PIP Framework is investigating the handling of the GSD.

References

Dormitzer, P R, Suphaphiphat, P, Gibson, D G, Wentworth, D E et al., 2013, 'Synthetic generation of influenza vaccine viruses for rapid response to pandemics', *Science Translational Medicine*, vol. 5, no. 185.

Hammond, E 2009, *Some intellectual property issues related to H5N1 influenza viruses, research and vaccines*, TWN Intellectual Property Series 12, http://www.twn.my/title2/IPR/pdf/ipr12.pdf

Hammond, E 2011, *An update on intellectual property claims related to global pandemic influenza preparedness*, TWN Intellectual Property Series 15, http://www.twn.my/title2/IPR/pdf/ipr15.pdf

Hammond, E 2014, *MERS virus claimed in Dutch University's international patent application*, TWN Info Service on Intellectual Property Issues, 6 June, http://www.twn.my/title2/intellectual_property/info.service/2014/ip140601.htm

Khor, M & Shashikant, S 2007a, *Health: winners and losers in the sharing of avian flu viruses*, TWN Info Service on Intellectual Property Issues, 11 May, http://www.twn.my/title2/health.info/twninfohealth089.htm

Khor, M & Shashikant, S 2007b, *'Sharing' of avian flu virus to be a major issue at WHA,*

TWN Info Service on Intellectual Property Issues,8 May, http://www.twn.my/title2/intellectual_property/info.service/twn.ipr.info.050704.htm>

NBCNEWS. com 2003, *Scientists race to patent SARS virus: efforts to claim property rights spark ethical debate*, http://www.nbcnews.com/id/3076748/ns/health-infectious_diseases/t/scientists-race-patent-sars-virus/#.V45S6q7hWWA>

Secretariat of the Convention on Biological Diversity 2011, *Nagoya Protocol on access to genetic resources and the fair and equitable sharing of benefits arising from their utilization to the Convention on Biological Diversity: text and annex*, Secretariat of the Convention on Biological Diversity, United Nations Environmental Programme, Montreal, https://www.cbd.int/abs/doc/protocol/nagoya-protocol-en.pdf

Shashikant, S 2010, *Pandemic preparedness: creating a fair and equitable influenza virus and benefit sharing system*, Third World Network, http://www.twn.my/title2/books/Pandemic.Preparedness.htm

Shashikant, S 2017,*Pandemic flu framework a 'success story' with challenges*, TWN Info Service on Intellectual Property Issues, 7 February, http://www.twn.my/title2/intellectual_property/info.service/2017/ip170206.htm

Simon, J H M, Claassen, E, Correa, CE & Osterhaus ADME 2005, 'Managing severe acute respiratory syndrome (SARS) intellectual property rights: the possible role of patent pooling', *Bulletin of the World Health Organization*, vol. 83, pp. 707–10, http://www.who.int/bulletin/volumes/83/9/707.pdf

United Nations 1992, *Convention on biological diversity*, https://www.cbd.int/convention/text/

WHO 2011, *Pandemic influenza preparedness framework for the sharing of influenza viruses and access to vaccines and other benefits*, http://apps.who.int/iris/bitstream/10665/44796/1/9789241503082_eng.pdf

WHO 2013, *Pandemic influenza preparedness framework: distribution of partnership contribution among companies*, 8 May, http://www.who.int/influenza/pip/pc_distribution.pdf

WHO 2015a, *Partnership contribution implementation plan, 2013–2016*, http://www.who.int/influenza/pip/pip_pcimpplan_update_31jan2015.pdf

WHO 2015b, *PC budget. Budget 2012–2016*, https://extranet.who.int/pip-pc-implementation/budget.aspx?year=2012

WHO 2016, *Implementation of the International Health Regulations 2005: report of the Review Committee on the role of the International Health Regulations 2005 in the Ebola outbreak and response*, Doc. A69/21, http://apps.who.int/gb/ebwha/pdf_files/WHA69/A69_21-en.pdf?ua=1

WHO 2017a, *Influenza SMTA2: signed agreements and benefits*, http://www.who.int/influenza/pip/benefit_sharing/smta2_signed/en/

WHO 2017b, *Infuenza virus traceability mechanism*, https://extranet.who.int/ivtm/

WHO 2017c, *Review of the pandemic influenza preparedness framework*, Doc. A70/17, http://apps.who.int/gb/ebwha/pdf_files/WHA70/A70_17-en.pdf

D9 | TOTAL SANITATION PROGRAMS AT THE COST OF HUMAN DIGNITY

In Global Health Watch 4 we critically interrogated the currently dominant approach to sanitation termed 'Community Led Total Sanitation' (CLTS). CLTS is now being adopted in the rural areas of many Asian and African countries and is being promoted by the World Bank's Water and Sanitation Programme, the Water Supply and Sanitation Collaborative Council, UNICEF, WaterAid, PLAN International and other international NGOs. By 2012 at least 20 countries had designated CLTS as their national sanitation approach in rural areas. The starting point for CLTS is the contention that communities should control their own development and that 'outsiders' should play the role of 'triggering' community responses. The 'community' ensures that households build their own toilets using their own resources. CLTS facilitators 'trigger' communities to recognize the link between open defecation and disease. The community then formulates its own plan for each household to build a latrine, so eradication of open defecation is 'total'. A distinctive feature of CLTS is that it forces participants to confront their 'shit' by using this word, and by identifying and visiting places where people openly defecate.

We pressed for a critical examination of CLTS within a broader socio-political and economic context. CLTS arguably exemplifies several features of a neoliberal approach to development – one which individualizes problems and their solutions and frees governments from promoting the welfare of their citizens. CLTS, we argued, needs also to be seen in terms of individual human rights versus the health of the 'community', as well as the balance between a person's right to dignity and their right of access to sanitation as well as the right of the 'community' to a faecal-free environment. The chapter concluded that: "There is a need for systematic monitoring and analysis to move past anecdotes about the sustainability and impact of CLTS. What is missing is a basis on which to assess local change in the context of broader impacts of the approach, which may be negative (People's Health Movement et al 2014)".

To explore further the issue of coercion that is innate to the CLTS approach, presented below are case studies from the Chhattisgarh state of India – one of the poorest Indian states.

Toilet Tyranny: case studies from Chhattisgarh in India

Kuwar Bai,now a well-known name in the Indian media and government, is a 104-year-old lady from Dhamtari district of Chhattisgarh who sold her ten goats to build two toilets in her house. According to news reports, she wanted to highlight the importance of sanitation and toilets and got these toilets built for the use of the women family members and neighbours. The media extolled her efforts, the government celebrated her more than once, with the Prime Minister touching her feet as a sign of respect (Drolia, 2016a). However, no one questioned why this lady had to sell her precious livestock to build toilets, when the government was in fact supposed to give her funds for constructing them[1].

Swachh Bharat Abhiyan (SBA) or Clean India Campaign is one of the flagship programmes of the current Indian Government. Previous governments had implemented similar programmes, like the Total Sanitation Campaign and the Nirmal Bharat Abhiyan. The National Democratic Alliance (NDA) government launched the Swachh Bharat Abhiyan (SBA) immediately after coming to power in 2014 with the aim to "accelerate the efforts to achieve universal sanitation coverage and to put focus on sanitation"[2]. All these programmes, past and present, follow the CLTS model, albeit with some modifications (for example unlike in the 'pure' CLTS model, the government subsidizes money spent by the poor on latrine construction).

Subsequently, states like Chhattisgarh have gone all out to make this programme a 'success'. The aim of SBA in the state is to make all villages 'open defecation free' (ODF). Chhattisgarh, with 5.6 million households, aims to construct 2.6 million toilets by 2019 (Business Standard, 2015).

Access to proper sanitation and clean drinking water is a serious problem in India and in Chhattisgarh, especially for the poor. However, the manner in which this stand-alone 'toilet construction' programme is being implemented has been problematic. This programme also does not take into consideration, the dimensions of water availability, community choice, affordability, caste, gender and other issues.

The coercive and mandatory nature of this programme has led to a number of infringements of people's legal entitlements, privacy, financial security and human rights (see the statement by People's Health Movement-India on the public lynching of a social activist protesting the shaming of women while defecating, by municipal workers in the state of Rajasthan, Box D9.1). This impact is being felt more by the poorer and vulnerable sections of society. The following cases in Chhattisgarh illustrate this.

Withholding legal entitlement of subsidised grain unless toilets are built Chhattisgarh has been highly praised for its government's Public Distribution System (PDS) which is a programme that entitles families to receive subsidised grain (ration) every month. It was one of the first states to enshrine this provision in law through the state legislation on Food Security and Nutrition. However, there have been numerous instances in which the subsidized PDS grain has been withheld because families have not constructed toilets. Such instances

Box D9.1: Lynching in the name of Total Sanitation Campaign[3]

The Jan Swasthya Abhiyan (JSA) expresses deep shock at the murder of Zafar Hussain, a 55 year old social worker of Pratapgarh in Rajasthan. Zafar Hussain was publicly lynched in a frenzy by Municipal employees linked to the government's 'Swachh Bharat Abhiyan' (SBA), led, according to Press reports, by Nagar Parishad Commissioner Ashok Jain. Zafar Hussain's only crime was that he objected to the photographing of women defecating in the open. Those being photographed included the victim's wife and 14 year old daughter. Reports suggest that a massive cover up of the incident is being attempted and the perpetrators are yet to be apprehended.

Zafar had in the past submitted a memorandum against the harassment of women by civic officials, which included bullying and shaming of women blamed of defecating in the open, taking their photographs, running after women, seizing their water mugs and abusing them while they defecated.

Vigilantism is rampant in the SBA

The above is not an isolated incident but a consequence of the SBA's 'name and shame strategy' where personnel linked to the program organize vigilante squads that hound individuals they find violating the program's objectives. Instances of such vigilante actions are being reported from many parts of the country. As the bulk of people who do not have domestic latrines or access to community latrines are the poor, this strategy has become an excuse for victimizing the poor for their appalling living conditions.

In Pratapgarh, reports clearly indicate that the people being victimized were obliged to defecate in open fields because latrines had not been provided. In fact only days before the murder the victim himself had petitioned authorities demanding latrines and other sanitary facilities in the colony. A recent report indicates that data on open defecation free (ODF) villages is being fudged extensively and at least 25% of villages declared ODF in the country do not have functioning toilet facilities accessible to all households.

Blaming the poor for their conditions of living

As a health coalition JSA believes that access to latrines and good sanitation is a basic human right and the poor stand to benefit the most from such access. However, the manner in which the poor are being victimized in the course of the campaign smacks of extreme insensitivity to the conditions in which they live and an attitude of contempt towards their situation. People do not choose to survive amid squalor and dirt, but are forced to do so because the country's developmental processes have continued to ignore their needs. The stark reality of 21st century India is that in many states vigilantism linked to the campaign prevents the poor accessing the public distribution system and other government benefits.

Put an Immediate Stop to this heinous practice of 'name and shame'
The Jan Swasthya Abhiyan demands that a high level inquiry be instituted into the lynching in Pratapgarh so that the perpetrators are arrested and justice is served.

The JSA demands that the strategy of 'name and shame' linked to the SBA be stopped forthwith and all vigilante squads be disbanded. Victimization of those unable to construct or access latrines should be stopped immediately.

The JSA is very concerned at theassault on privacy of individuals (especially of women) through photographing or videography that has been legitimised by the government as part of Swachh Bharat Abhiyan strategies. We demand that all states must put an immediate stop to all such practices. Such acts should be viewed as gender based violence and viewed as a crime related to sexual harassment of women.

The JSA supports any sensitive and participatory process that aims to ensure universal access to sanitation facilities. The design of the Swachh Bharat Abhiyan's that relies on vigilantism and coercion and promotes 'victim blaming'can neither ensure equitable access to sanitation nor promote human rights.

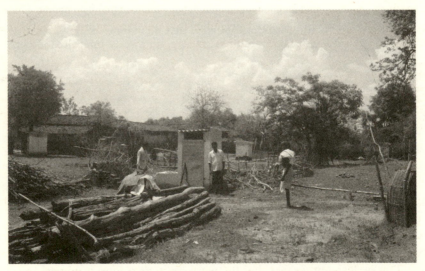

Image D9.1 Building a toilet in India in a rural setting (Sulakshana Nandi)

have become so widespread that the Chief Secretary of the state had to issue an order to all districts that rations entitled under law should not be withheld for people not constructing toilets. Despite this order, due to the immense pressure on the district administration and structures at a lower level to declare villages as ODF, officials in many districts have resorted to denying rations to pressurise people to build toilets (Krishna Das, 2015). For instance in village Karji, the block officer threatened the villagers that their monthly PDS ration will be withheld unless they construct toilets. The villagers complained and the media took up the case, after which they received their entitled grain.

The entitlement to grain is critical for the poorer and more vulnerable groups like the particularly vulnerable tribal groups (PVTGs) who are the most impoverished of tribal groups, having extremely high malnutrition levels. However, there have been cases in which whole villages of PVTGs have been denied grain as they have not managed to build toilets. Rice was given only after complaints were made to the food department. In another instance, families from the Baiga PVTG community were unable to build toilets as a few years previously they had invested in constructing toilets and the promised money from the government never came. They hence lacked money to re-build the toilets and neither could they take loan. Their PDS ration was withheld and it was only allocated after they organised a sit-in at the PDS shop.

Secret ballot to identify people who are not using toilets The Jashpur district administration ordered a secret ballot, using school children, to find out who in their village was not using toilets (Times of India, 2017b). Nearly 49,000 students from 1987 primary and secondary schools submitted names of people in their village, obtained through a secret ballot, who still practise open defecation. This is to be repeated periodically. This authoritarian practice has features of fascism, and using children in this manner is unethical.

CCTVs installed in the village In Balod district the district administration head has motivated the villagers to install closed-circuit TV (CCTV) cameras in the lanes to capture images of anyone going outside their home to defecate[4], totally disregarding the privacy of the villagers.

Financial distress and its consequences Even though the government is meant to provide some of the funds for constructing toilets, the money never arrives in time. People have to construct the toilets with their own money. Often the village heads are forced to advance money for toilet construction.

There has been a long delay in the release of funds from the central government to the state and consequently, from the state to the districts and below. This is despite that fact that the whole administration is engaged in this project and Employment Guarantee Scheme funds that were previously used to build critical infrastructure like roads, ponds and improvement of farming land has been diverted for building toilets (Sharma, 2017).

The delays in the arrival of funds have caused great financial hardship for families and village heads who have been forced to construct the toilets with money they have arranged through borrowing or selling assets, resulting in a rise in rural indebtedness.

In one instance in Kanker district, 11 village heads became so indebted as a result of advancing money for toilets that they wrote to the government in desperation, threatening to commit suicide (Drolia, 2016b) unless the funds were released immediately.

There are media reports of families having been forced to migrate or become bonded labour in order to pay off the debts incurred through toilet construction (Ghose, 2017). A lady whose family had migrated in order to pay off the debts but were now being abused and harassed by the employer, told a reporter: "Tell me, do officials not care about us when they make their plans? What do these words sarkar (government), palayan (migration), Swachh Bharat mean if we die?" (ibid.).

One strategy that the government has employed in order to ensure universal toilet construction is to withhold funds unless all families in the village build toilets and the village is declared ODF. This is done in order to build peer pressure within the community. In Rajnangadon district it resulted in villagers beating their neighbour to death as he had been unable to construct a toilet due to lack of money. He had asked for some more time to arrange money to build his toilet. However, the Diwali festival was approaching and others in the village wanted to receive their funds in time for the festival. He became a scapegoat for their not receiving the funds on time, and was consequently beaten to death (Drolia, 2016c).

Restrictions on participation in local panchayat elections Chhattisgarh (among other states) modified the Panchayat Act (local self government Act) to make possessing a toilet a mandatory qualification for standing for the local panchayat elections (Jaiswal, 2015). This has been implemented in retrospect, with the existing elected panchayat members under threat of losing their seats if they did not construct toilets (Times of India, 2017a). Such a rule is bound to affect the participation of those from poorer and marginalised communities, including tribal and dalits, as often they are the ones without household toilets.

Other concerns While communities and families grapple with these problems, there are many other reasons to be concerned about the SBA. The first big issue concerns availability of water for the toilets and safe potable water. While on the one hand, toilets are being promoted, the situation with respect to water availability for the toilets remains bleak and that has implications for the women, already burdened with numerous other household tasks. Women now have to fill and carry water for servicing the toilet, in addition to arranging water for cooking, drinking, washing, etc.

Another issue concerns cleaning of the toilets. This has been a caste-based role, with Dalits being forced to undertake this work. They have suffered centuries of indignity and discrimination as a result of this. The SBA does not acknowledge this as an issue nor try to address it (The Hindu, 2016).

There are also technical issues concerning the siting and construction of toilets such as contamination of drinking and underground water during monsoons where toilets and pits are sited inappropriately in terms of their drainage. Moreover, with proliferation of toilets in a village, it is no longer possible to maintain the recommended distance between toilets and the source of drinking water. This has serious public health implications. The past two years have seen a rise in cholera outbreaks in Chhattisgarh: the possible relationship with the current toilet building programme merits urgent investigation.

It is patently clear that there is an urgent need for the Indian government to review the way the sanitation programme is being rolled-out. An emphasis on dignity and respect for people must inform this programme and its perverse effects, especially on equity, must be recognised and eliminated.

'Victim blaming' is a constant feature of CLTS programs

The stories related in the preceding sections do not represent a new trend in India, though it is likely that the coercive elements of the sanitation campaign have intensified recently. A 2011 report pointed to very similar coercive tactics being employed in the state of Karnataka. The report describes "squads of teachers and youths, who patrolled the fields and blew whistles when they spotted people defecating". School children whose families did not have toilets were humiliated in the classroom. Men followed women – and vice versa – all day, denying people the opportunity even to urinate. Squads threw stones at people defecating. Women were photographed and their pictures displayed publicly. The local government institution, the gram panchayat, threatened to cut off households' water and electricity supplies until their owners had signed contracts promising to build latrines (Chatterjee, 2011).

Neither is the phenomenon peculiar to India. A 2014 paper argued that the CLTS approach in Indonesia, was not only "inadequate" but also "echoes coercive, race-based colonial public health practices" (Engel and Susilo, 2014). A disturbing report from Bangladesh described how arbitration in rural Bangladesh was denied to young women and girls who were raped while openly defecating (Mahbub, 2009).

CLTS practitioners claim that the 'shame' spoken of in CLTS comes from self-critique and not from "externally imposed humiliation (to shame), and certainly not by the facilitators" (Musembi and Musyoki 2016). However, in practice, CLTS programmes in many countries appear to thrive on coercive practices that often lead to gross violation of the rights of poor people. Clearly a course correction in the model of the CLTS programme is overdue.

Notes

1 In a modification of the CLTS model, the government in India subsidizes the cost of toilet construction.

2 See Guidelines: http://www.mdws.gov.in/sites/default/files/SwachBharatGuidlines.pdf

3 Excerpts from Press Release by People's Health Movement-India on 19th June, 2017, full text available here: http://phmindia.org/2017/06/19/press-release-jsa-demands-an-end-to-vigilantism-in-the-name-of-the-swachh-bharat-abhiyan/

4 See: https://factordaily.com/cctv-cameras-open-defecation-swachh-bharat

References

Business Standard, 2015, Chhattisgarh to construct 2.6 million toilet blocks, February 15, 2015 http://www.business-standard.com/article/current-affairs/chhattisgarh-to-construct-2-6-million-toilet-blocks-115021600020_1.html

Chatterjee L 2011, Time to acknowledge the dirty truth behind community-led sanitation, the Guardian, 9 June 2011 https://www.theguardian.com/global-development/poverty-matters/2011/jun/09/dirty-truth-behind-community-sanitation

Drolia R, 2016a, Modi felicitates 104-yr-old woman for building toilets, Times of India, Feb 21, 2016 http://timesofindia.indiatimes.com/city/raipur/Modi-felicitates-104-yr-old-woman-for-building-toilets/articleshow/51078507.cms

Drolia R 2016b Swachh Bharat: 11 village sarpanches threaten suicide, Times of India, Sep 4, 2016, http://timesofindia.indiatimes.com/city/raipur/Swachh-Bharat-11-village-sarpanches-threaten-suicide/articleshow/54003026.cms

Drolia R 2016c, Man killed for buying time to build toilet, Times of India, Oct 8, 2016, http://timesofindia.indiatimes.com/city/raipur/Man-killed-for-buying-time-to-build-toilet/articleshow/54742845.cms

Engel S. and Susilo A 2014, 'Shaming and sanitation in Indonesia: a return to colonial public health practices?', Development and Change, 45(1): 157–78, doi: 10.1111/dech.12075.

Ghose D 2017, Money for toilets they built never came, now they are trapped, The Indian Express, February 17, 2017 http://indianexpress.com/article/india/money-for-toilets-they-built-never-came-now-they-are-trapped-uttar-pradesh-chhattisgarh-swachh-bharat-abhiyan-4529164/

Jaiswal A 2015, Toilets at homes must for contesting panchayat polls in Chhattisgarh, Times of India, Nov 19, 2015 http://timesofindia.indiatimes.com/city/raipur/Toilets-at-homes-must-for-contesting-panchayat-polls-in-Chhattisgarh/articleshow/49847932.cms

Krishna Das R 2015, In a Chhattisgarh town, no PDS rations if toilet not built, October 20, 2015 http://www.business-standard.com/article/current-affairs/in-a-chhattisgarh-town-no-pds-rations-if-toilet-not-built-115102000703_1.html

Mahbub, A 2009, 'Social dynamics of CLTS: inclusion of children, women and vulnerable', CLTS Conference, 16–18 December, Brighton.

Musembi, C and Musyoki, S 2016, 'CLTS and the Right to Sanitation', Frontiers of CLTS issue 8, Brighton: IDS https://opendocs.ids.ac.uk/opendocs/bitstream/handle/123456789/10133/Issue8_Human_Rights_FINAL.pdf?sequence=1

People's Health Movement, ALAMES, Third World Network, Medicos International and Health Action International, 2014, 'Talking Shit: Is Community Led Total sanitation Empowering or Divisive?' in Global Health watch 4, Zed Books, London, 2014 http://www.ghwatch.org/sites/www.ghwatch.org/files/C5_0.pdf

Sharma S 2017, Chhattisgarh report: How Modi government's new approach is undermining a decade of gains in rural India, July 9th 2017, scroll.in https://scroll.in/article/727633/chhattisgarh-report-how-modi-governments-new-approach-is-undermining-a-decade-of-gains-in-rural-india

The Hindu, 2016, Who will clean the Swachh Bharat toilets, asks Wilson, October 18, 2016 http://www.thehindu.com/news/cities/Delhi/Who-will-clean-the-Swachh-Bharat-toilets-asks-Wilson/article14585219.ece

Times of India, 2017a, No toilet at home: Notices to panchayat representatives, January 24, 2017, http://timesofindia.indiatimes.com/city/raipur/no-toilet-at-home-notices-to-panchayat-representatives/articleshow/56752298.cms

Times of India, 2017b, 'Swachhata' ballot to validate ODF status, March 16, 2017 http://timesofindia.indiatimes.com/city/raipur/swachhata-ballot-to-validate-odf-status/articleshow/57661244.cms

RESISTANCE, ACTIONS AND CHANGE

E1 | SOCIAL MOVEMENTS DEFEND PROGRESSIVE HEALTH REFORMS IN EL SALVADOR

Introduction

Since the implementation of comprehensive health reforms in 2009, health outcomes in El Salvador have shown significant improvements. The last decade has witnessed a substantial decline in maternal and child mortality rates, at 38 per 100,000 and 8 per 1,000 live births, respectively, in 2013 as compared to 66 per 100,000 and 16 per 1,000, respectively, in 2006.[1] The share of the health budget increased from 9 per cent to 16 per cent of the total government budget between 2008 and 2010 and in the following five years, it has maintained an average share of 15.4 per cent.

In the initial phase of the health reforms, foreign loans played a significant role, accounting for close to a quarter of the health budget. But this was clearly unsustainable in the long term, in a country that already spends more than a quarter of its government budget on debt repayment. Gradually, general taxation has become the major source of financing for the health budget. However constraints exist in expanding the tax base in an economy that has limited productive capacity.

The design and implementation of the health reforms have been jointly conceived by the government and social movements for the right to health. A novel component of the Salvadoran health reforms is the institutionalization of social participation, and the design and implementation monitoring of services. The National Health Forum (Foro National para la Salud or FNS) has taken on the role of a pressure group to influence key political actors. As the struggle for health expands into the political and economic arenas of the country, the role of social movements as a political force will be a decisive factor for the reforms to proceed.

Health reforms: key interventions

The government of the left-wing Frente Farabundo Marti para la Liberacion Nacional (FMLN), which came to power in June 2009, inherited a fragmented health system focused on curative care. Different institutions provided care of varying quality to specific populations. An underfunded network of facilities under the Ministry of Health (MINSAL), partly financed by co-payments, provided care to the general population. An insurance based system, funded by contributions from employers, employees and government, covered around 20 per cent of the population. These were supplemented by a small charitable sector and a few private tertiary care hospitals for the elite, which had emerged in the 1990s.[2]

In the 1990s, public hospitals and specialty care services faced the threat of privatization. By the 2000s, this threat extended to the social insurance system and primary care facilities. However, a wave of public protests stalled these attempts. It is in this backdrop that Mauricio Funes came to power. The new government initiated discussions on a new health policy by issuing a proposal for reform titled *Construyendo la Esperanza* or 'Building Hope' (People's Health Movement et al., 2014). The proposal was based on the recognition that health is a public good and a fundamental human right guaranteed by the state. Eight core areas of action were defined in the document:

i. comprehensive, integrated health services network
ii. national medical emergency system
iii. accessibility of essential drugs and vaccines, including through curbing the power of pharmaceutical companies
iv. addressing determinants of health and inequities among population groups
v. national health forums for organizing local community participation
vi. national institute of health for institutional research policies;
vii. unified health information system
viii. creation of human resources for health development.

Advances in health reform

Towards a stronger, primary care-based health system During the eight years of the FMLN government, bold policy decisions were taken and implemented, which aimed at restructuring the health system and build a robust system that emphasized primary care. Within 100 days of installation of the Funes administration, fees for treatment were abolished in facilities under the Ministry of Health, leading to a 25 per cent increase in demand for services from 2009 to 2010 (Menjivar, 2012).

In 2010, community health teams were rolled out in the country's poorest 125 municipalities and this number increased to 575 in 2016 (MINSAL, 2011, 2016b). Fifty more are planned for 2017. In these eight years, 402 health facilities were added, most of them community clinics. In addition to expanding the capacity of primary care through community clinics and community health teams, the area-wise division of the population has ensured that each person is under the responsibility of a specific health facility and team. These teams are connected to the rest of the health system through referral and reverse referral (from the tertiary and secondary levels to the primary level) mechanisms.

The efforts at restructuring the health system (MINSAL, 2015a. p. 38) are visible in the budgetary allocation that shifted the priority from secondary

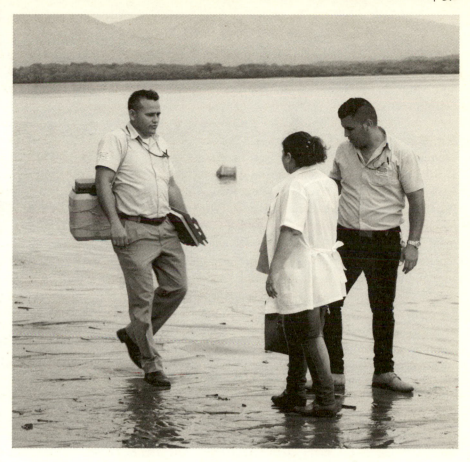

Image E1.1 Health workers on the Pacific coast in El Salvador (Boris Flores)

hospitals to primary level of care, leading to proportionally more consultations in the latter (Table E1.1).

TABLE E1.1: Number of consultations at different levels of care (2008–2015)

	Primary	Secondary	Tertiary
2008	1,908,950	121,878	
2010	2,139,428	141,964	3,073
2011	2,258,607	116,864	3,257
2012	2,443,413	79,715	4,765
2013	2,637,754	74,548	8,200
2014	2,953,343	80,168	11,900
2015	2,983,990	88,691	9,218

Source: MINSAL 2015a

Overall, the capacity of the public health system has been consolidated. Of the estimated 8,800 human resources required, 7,100 had been hired by 2015. Across the board, infrastructure was repaired and expanded, and equipment was acquired at an estimated cost of US$ 225 million for hospitals and USD 80 million for primary care facilities in the period between 2009 and 2014 (MINSAL, 2015b).

Curtailing the power of 'big pharma' Despite open hostility from the pharmaceutical industry, the Medicines Act was passed in 2012. The 2012 Act ensures a unified regulatory system. It has removed pharmaceutical manufacturers from the Medicines Regulatory Board and made a new body, the National Administration of Medicines, in charge of medicines-related policy as well as purchase and procurement. Further, the Medicines Act has instituted a price regulation system and quality control mechanisms. This has resulted in an increase in the availability of medicines in public facilities and has contributed to reducing the out-of-pocket expenditure of patients.

Increased health budget The share of health in the government budget has increased from 9 per cent in 2008 to 16 per cent in 2016. In the initial period significant resources were sourced as loans from international institutions such as the Inter-American Development Bank (US$ 60 million over five years) and the World Bank (US$ 80 million over four years).[3] In the period between 2009 and 2015, cumulative foreign loans amounted to US$ 306.5 million. However, as the loans contributed to the overall indebtedness of the country, there has been a steady trend towards reducing the reliance on loans. Foreign loans' share in the MINSAL budget has declined from 23 per cent to 5.1 per cent between 2008 and 2015 and is projected to further decline to 3.6 per cent in 2016. Thus, the largest source of resources for MINSAL is general taxation and the share of general taxation in MINSAL's budget has

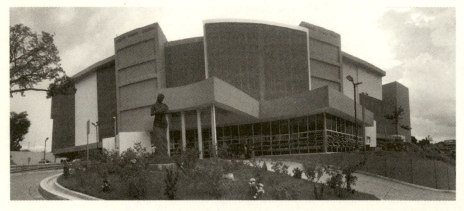

Image E1.2 New infrastructure of the National Women's Hospital in El Salvador (Boris Flores)

increased steadily, from 72 per cent in 2009 to 89.2 per cent in 2015, with projections of an increase to 90.8 per cent in 2016 (MINSAL, 2016a, p. 41).

Positive change in indicators Various indicators reflect the sector wide effects of the reforms (Minsal, 2013; Orellana, 2012; Pan American Health Organization & MINSAL, 2013):

- El Salvador has met the target for MDG 5 on maternal mortality in 2011.
- The private-to-public spending ratio has changed from 50 per cent private and 50 per cent public in 2004 to 34 per cent private and 66 per cent public in 2015 (MINSAL 2016a).
- Prenatal care coverage has gone up to 88.1 per cent and institutional delivery coverage is at 99.6 per cent (ibid.).
- Hospital beds increased from 0.7 per 1,000 population in 2009 to 1.14 in 2013.
- Institutional child and infant mortality dropped by 20 per cent between 2007 and 2012.
- Drug shortages in the public network reduced from 60 per cent to 20 per cent between 2008 and 2013.

Challenges to the health reforms

Not yet a unified system Although it had been envisaged that the health sector reforms would lead to a unified system, progress has been slow and the sector remains fragmented. The Salvadoran public health sector includes MINSAL-run facilities, as well as a series of networked autonomous health facilities financed through co-payments of workers and employers. The latter includes the Instituto Salvadoreno de Seguridad Social (ISSS), which covers most workers in formal employment; Instituto Salvadoreño de Bienestar Magisterial (ISBM), which covers the teaching profession; and Comando de Sanidad Militar (COSAM), which covers the military.

The fragmentation leads to a resource drain on MINSAL, which subsidizes the other facilities through different routes, such as purchase of medicines and public health initiatives. In addition, when patients insured in other entities come to the public system, they access healthcare without paying for treatment. However, when non-insured patients go to other facilities, treatment is charged to MINSAL. The ISBM has subcontracted services to private facilities and private practitioners and, in consequence, its per capita cost is much higher than other institutions (see Figure E1.1).

Medicine costs remain high Despite the effect of the Medicines Act on out-of-pocket expenditure, the expected effect on medicine cost to MINSAL has not materialized. It is becoming clear that the supplier base needs to be broadened. New initiatives are required which would support the expansion of production capacity for medicines in the country. The government is set to propose a soft loan for medicine manufacturers interested in increasing production capacity and improving quality of locally manufactured medicines.[4]

Per capita expenditure remains low Among the different public health institutions, MINSAL is in charge of providing healthcare to about 72 per cent of the population, or around 4.4 million persons. MINSAL's modified budget (which includes allocated budget and additional or extraordinary allocations) has increased by 51.8 per cent, from US$ 399.3 million in 2008 to US$ 606.2 million in 2015 (MINSAL, 2014, p. 40 and 2016a, p. 37) . This has allowed the per capita expenditure of MINSAL to increase from US$ 87 to US$ 130 between 2008 and 2015, a 49 per cent increase (MINSAL, 2014, p. 53 and 2016a, p. 38). Despite this, per capita expenditure by the Ministry of Health (MINSAL) is still low as compared to other public health institutions (social insurance based) in the country (See Figure E1.1), or to other countries in the Central American region. While the per capita expenditure on health in El Salvador is higher than in Guatemala, Honduras and Nicaragua, it is still much below the levels of Mexico, Costa Rica and Panama (Datosmacro.com, n.d.).

Uncertainty regarding financial sustainability According to Violeta Menjivar, the minister for health, if health is to be a right and not a commodity or a gesture of altruism, general taxation has to be the base of its financing.[5] It is estimated that MINSAL requires at least 6 per cent of the GDP for it to be adequately resourced. Yet, in the absence of sufficient resources, MINSAL

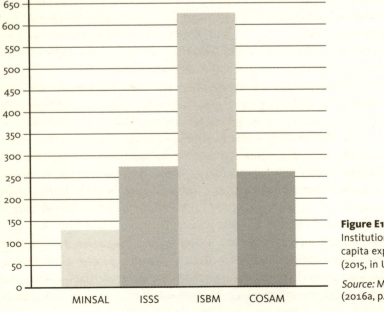

Figure E1.1:
Institution-wise per capita expenditure (2015, in US$)

Source: MINSAL (2016a, p. 38).

has only received between 2.2 per cent and 2.4 per cent of the GDP in the past decade.[6]

Under pressure to control the fiscal deficit, the government instituted austerity measures in the public sector starting 2011, which were reaffirmed in September 2014 (Public Sector Austerity and Savings Policy 2014). Five per cent has been cut from the approved budget, which means that all the allocated resources that have not been used as planned cannot be diverted to other activities. Medicines have not been affected as the Medicines Act provides for the allocation of a fixed percentage of the budget.

Economists have pointed out that the government will soon have exhausted its capacity to increase the health budget without increasing its overall budget.[7] In fact, the 2014 health budget was slightly lower than that of the previous year, and the year on year increase from 2014 to 2015 and from 2015 to 2016 was marginal – 1.8 per cent and 2.2 per cent, respectively (MINSAL 2016, p. 43). For the health reforms to be effective, fiscal reforms that can boost government revenues and spending, as well as the sustained development of the productive economy, are clearly necessary.

Economic landscape and government revenues

The budgetary constraints that limit the ability of the government to expand public health infrastructure and healthcare delivery need to be seen in a broader context, which is discussed below.

Structural challenges El Salvador faces structural challenges, such as indebtedness, a large trade deficit and a low, though increasing, tax to GDP ratio. Its economy is dominated by a large services sector and export-oriented agriculture and manufacturing, led by monoculture plantations and *maquiladoras* (foreign-owned, export-oriented factories). The country depends on imports to fulfil its requirements in primary goods and food. As a consequence, import houses and their owners are very powerful in the political landscape.

The lack of employment opportunities, persecution during the civil war and high crime rates have driven a large proportion of the population to migrate out of the country. It is estimated that a fourth of Salvadorans live and work outside the country, sending back remittances that account for 16 per cent to 17 per cent of the GDP (Gammage, 2007). In the absence of a productive economy, oriented towards the domestic market, remittance inflows are largely spent on imported consumer goods and fuel the large trade deficit, which was more than 18 per cent of the GDP in 2015 (Index Mundi, 2016).

The Economic Stabilization Programmes and Structural Adjustment Programmes (ESPs/SAPs) of the 1990s had a deep impact on government finances (SAPRIN, n.d.). The ESPs/SAPs led to the privatization of financially healthy public banks, state-owned companies and public services (pension system, and electricity and telephone companies). This resulted in a loss of government revenues and an explosion of its internal debt. By 2015, the public debt stood at 64.2 per cent of the GDP, with debt repayment absorbing between a quarter and a third of the government budget every year (projected at 35 per cent for 2017) (Carta Economica, n.d. b).

Yet, despite the drain on government resources, El Salvador has one of the lowest tax rates in the American continent. The tax to GDP ratio stood at 12.6 per cent in 2009. Tax evasion (illegal non-payment of taxes) and tax avoidance (legal rebates and sops) represent significant losses to the exchequer, estimated at more than US\$ 2,600 million in 2015, or 10 per cent of the GDP. The quantum of tax evasion is 3.2 times the public health budget.

Further, the fiscal structure is deeply unfair. Fiscal reforms were undertaken by the earlier administrations led by the right-wing Alianza Republicana Nacionalista (ARENA),[8] to change the fiscal structure of the economy in a way that the overwhelming burden of taxes fell on households (82 per cent in 2012), rather than on corporations and those in the high income bracket.

Government response and governance The FMLN government marks a political shift from the earlier government of ARENA. It recognizes the need to address the limitations of the current economic structure. In certain areas, concrete measures have been promoted, such as a substantial increase in minimum wages across sectors – between 20 per cent and 40 per cent, depending on the sectors (Carta Economica, n.d. e), legislative amendments to curtail tax avoidance, proactive measures to curtail tax evasion and the introduction of laws for progressive taxation.

However, ARENA remains dominant in the legislative assembly, with 35 deputies out of a total of 84 (the FMLN has 31 deputies) and the judiciary is under the control of the country's elite. In consequence, progressive measures have been systematically stalled. In 2013, in an attempt by the government to address the practice of private companies to declare bankruptcy in order to avoid paying taxes, the government had introduced a tax of 1 per cent on gross sales of companies declaring bankruptcy but not closing within two years. The constitutional bench had struck it down and the government later introduced a 1 per cent tax on assets of companies that did not otherwise pay taxes. In 2015, this measure was also struck down by the same bench, the argument being that it would amount to double taxation.[9] In 2014, when the government, in another attempt to curb tax evasion, published the names of companies that were not paying their taxes, the constitutional bench intervened *suo moto* and ruled that the list should be removed from public domain.

Since 2010, the government has taken several measures to move to a more progressive fiscal system, with the result that the contribution from indirect taxation has decreased from 64 per cent to 60 per cent. Yet, in the absence of deeper measures, the impacts remain insignificant.[10] Due to the lack of financing options, government arrears have accumulated and resulted in a liquidity crunch

(Central America Data, 2017). As a consequence, austerity measures have been in place since 2014. Observers speak of a systematic blockage of government finances by ARENA in Parliament[11] and by the constitutional bench of the Supreme Court, backed by right-wing think tanks (such as FUSADES and FUNDE) and the media owned by the corporate lobby ANEP.[12]

International commitments In the face of the liquidity crisis, the government turned to the International Monetary Fund (IMF). In its July 2016 report (IMF 2016), the IMF criticized the "distortionary" taxation measures of the government, proposed further regressive reforms of the pension system and a further contraction of the fiscal deficit. These conditionalities will add to the existing political pressure on the government to hold back progressive measures in these areas.

El Salvador's international commitments pose further challenges. El Salvador is signatory to the World Trade Organization and several free trade agreements which provide for the gradual elimination of a number of import duties. This reduces the ability of the government to protect domestic enterprises from competition.

Role of social movements In such a politically adverse environment, social movements have played a key role in pressing for progressive measures.

In November 2012, a loan of US$ 60 million for health reforms had to be approved by a two-third majority in Parliament (56 out of the 84 members). However, ARENA and its allies blocked the decision. The National Health Forum (FNS) mounted a campaign, 'I am the 56th MP'. Through mobilizations and road blocks, the FNS put pressure on parliamentarians. The loan was finally approved.

In another instance in October 2013, health professional unions supported by ARENA had called for a march to Parliament protesting MINSAL's inability to increase salaries of health professionals in breach of dearness allowance provisions. Two organizations of health professionals (Movimiento Salvador Allende and Asociación de Estudiantes Formados en Cuba) supported by the FNS called for a parallel march to the ANEP office, asking for the latter's constituents to pay their taxes so as to enable the government to pay health workers the dearness allowance. This was an important initiative that shifted the focus on the structural issue of who pays taxes and who does not.[13]

Despite leading the executive, the FMLN does not enjoy the support of the judiciary or the legislative branches of the state. The support of independent and vibrant social movements is therefore critical. Street mobilizations have already shown how the balance of power in Parliament, where the government currently has a minority of the seats, can be shifted. The challenge will be to convince people why fiscal reforms are necessary and to develop joint actions and campaigns.

Popular mobilization in defence of progressive reforms

Foro Nacional de la Salud (FNS) The guiding document on health reforms in El Salvador, 'Building Hope', recognizes the need for a mechanism for people's participation in policymaking and implementation.[14] This led to the creation of the FNS. According to its coordinator, Margarita Posada, the FNS is an autonomous entity separate from political parties and economically independent, which fulfils the role of social auditing of the health system and providing information to the public and the Ministry of Health.[15] The FNS is a formal institution, but it is not legally registered. It does not have infrastructure, paid staff or its own funds.

The FNS is organized thematically and territorially, that is, in thematic working groups and provincial (*departamentos*) and district (*municipios*) chapters. By 2015, there were six thematic working groups and five provincial chapters covering one hundred and fifty districts (MINSAL, 2015, p. 23). Each chapter has one or two point persons (*referentes*) who are responsible for addressing specific issues and closely interacting with the primary care facility and hospital administration in their areas. In addition, the FNS creates social alliances that link health issues with other social issues and with the broader economic and political structure.

District chapters are made up of community-based leaders. NGOs, especially those involved with service delivery, are the outreach arm of the FNS in the communities where they have worked and created trust. However, NGO professionals do not represent the community in the FNS local structure.[16]

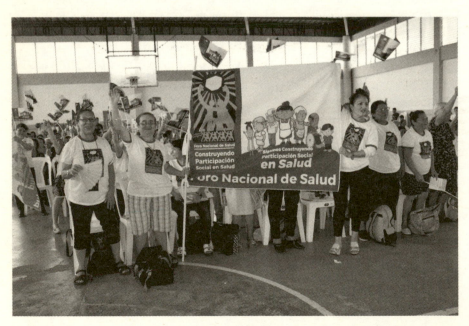

Image E1.3 Seventh anniversary of the National Health Forum, El Salvador (Boris Flores)

Box E1.1: Allied but independent

Since 2002, there had been several proposals for a legislation that would address the price of medicines, which was extremely high in the country. Members of the FNS have been in the forefront of pushing for this demand. Under the aegis of Isabel Rodriguez, minister of health, and Eduardo Espinoza, vice-minister for health policies, a comprehensive law was drafted to address the issues related to the commercialization, quality and prices of medicines. The Medicines Bill was place before Parliament in February 2012. Though the FMLN had supported the move, its committee-in-charge did not reach a clear decision to support the bill.[18] In its response, the FNS mobilized widely, organized marches to Parliament and engaged in road blockades in the capital city, calling for the support of the bill. It also decided to make public the names of the parliamentarians who pronounced themselves in favour of the bill, in a move to push all parties to take a stand.[19] The FMLN raised an objection, but the FNS went ahead. The law was approved unanimously, with 80 out of 84 votes (Anonymous, 2012).

The FNS is independent of MINSAL and does not receive financial or in-kind support from the latter. However, the formalization of each new chapter is attended by the vice-minister for health policies, which gives the institution a strong legitimacy. In addition, there are established channels of communication, consultation and negotiation between the two institutions (monthly meetings with key functionaries of MINSAL, such as the vice-ministers, directors of hospitals and directors of primary care networks). Each side shares their perspective and disagreements are identified and discussed.[17] On the other hand, the FNS has maintained close links with the FMLN to ensure that important legislations are enacted, while also maintaining its role of an independent pressure group (Box E1.1).

The FNS has developed a methodology which allows it to leverage on its political influence. This includes disseminating information through workshops and seminars attended by FNS constituents. This is followed by training workshop in the different departments where the FNS has a presence. In parallel with this the perspectives of the FNS are communicated through press conferences and gatherings (*concentraciones*) and by creating social alliances with like-minded organizations. After the passing of new decisions, laws or policies, the FNS monitors the implementation by ensuring that structures for implementation are created and by developing systems to check the implementation on the ground (see Box E1.2).

Box E1.2: Intervention by FNS to ensure access to care

Alejandro, a six-year-old, broke his foot on October 2015 near his house in Sensuntepeque, in the province of Cabanas. When brought to the Sensuntepeque regional hospital, a public facility, on that same day, his mother, Sara, was asked to pay US$ 400 for his treatment. Alejandro's uncle, Nelson, a driver in one of the FNS member organizations reported the case to Ernesto, the FNS point person in the district, and requested him to take up the matter.

Ernesto requested a meeting with Vicente Robira, director of the Sensuntepeque hospital, which took place at Vicente's private clinic on 31 October. The meeting was attended by Ernesto, Nelson and Boris (family doctor and FNS member) and Susana (author of this report). The doctor justified himself by saying that he was not charging for treatment but only providing an opportunity for the patient to be treated closer to his place of residence. He explained that as the needed equipment was not available in the Sensuntepeque hospital, the family would have had to go to another city to seek treatment and his intention was to facilitate buying the required medical supplies and equipment.

After the meeting, the team went to the hospital to meet Sara and Alejandro. The guards were unfriendly despite the written permission from the director of the hospital, but backed off when the team mentioned its link with the FNS.

Sara clarified that she had not been given any option for free treatment in another hospital, but that her son was offered a cast or an operation for the cost of US$ 400. She was also not aware that there was no urgency to conduct the operation. The team felt that the doctors had kept her in the dark intentionally. Sara is a self-employed vendor, with an income of around US$ 100 a month.

The team established that the hospital was in error, and that there was no reason to not bring in the necessary equipment from another hospital, and, further, that this had been done previously for similar operations. Transfer of supplies and equipment was part of the routine functioning of the hospital network and could have been done on request by the hospital director.

Alejandro's family decided against getting him operated in Sensuntepeque hospital to avoid possible lack of support by the senior staff. Ernesto facilitated the child's transfer and care to another hospital close by with help from the hospital director. The FNS followed up the case with the vice-minister for health services, responsible for overseeing hospital directors.

FNS interventions to implement health reforms The FNS has played a key role in monitoring the implementation of the health reforms. At the level of facilities, there has been unwillingness by the administration and health professionals to change their way of working or be accountable to patients and their families, especially when the latter are less wealthy or less educated. Representatives of FNS intervene on behalf of the latter (see Box E1.2).

Furthering reforms through tax justice In 2012, news reports referred to statements by the minister of finance that budgetary constraints would make it difficult to fulfill the expectations of different sectors, among them the health sector. In response, the FNS decided to deepen its understanding of government finances and to mobilize public opinion to demand fiscal reforms to further health reforms.[20] To this end, it launched a two-year campaign to bring clarity on fiscal issues and their link with the health reforms.

FNS was successful in making tax reforms an issue of public debate[21] and, in early 2013, FNS developed a fiscal reform proposal, as a precursor to the introduction of a Bill in Parliament. However, in the parliamentary election of 2015, ARENA gained more seats than the FMLN, creating an unfavourable situation in Parliament for such a reform to be passed.[22] In the light of this new situation, it is evident that it is now even more important to broaden the social alliance for comprehensive tax reforms.

Reversal of privatization of pension funds Pensions constitute a large part of the internal debt. This is linked to pension reforms implemented by the previous government. As a result of the reform any employee below 35 years was compulsorily shifted to the private system, while employees above 35 were given the choice to stay with the government pensions fund or leave (most stayed). As a result, the government pension fund has a large number of members receiving pension and a smaller number of members paying a contribution, creating a large financial burden on the government exchequer. The FNS launched a campaign to strengthen public opinion in favour of reversing the privatization of pension funds and linked this demand to the need for tax reforms in order to increase the government budget.[23]

Conclusion

Low- and middle-income countries face challenges to adequately resource their health systems. The structure of a country's health system is linked to policy choices that governments make. In many countries, the challenge for people's movements is the lack of political will to opt for a model that is truly fair and effective and avoids wastages created by private interests and private sector participation in healthcare delivery.

In El Salvador the government has the political will to propose and advance reforms that will deliver better health outcomes. Yet, this is not sufficient, as even a well-structured system needs to be adequately financed. This case study has shown that a transformation of economic and fiscal structures is required in order to achieve adequate financing. Further, as the case study highlights, private interests and local elites can take democratic institutions hostage and sabotage reforms that benefit the majority. In such a situation, strong and independent people's movements and organizations have a key role to play to protect and further progressive reforms.

The dilemma faced by the progressive government in El Salvador is typical of what other progressive governments face. In a globalized world where the global economy is integrated through myriad mechanisms, countries find it extremely difficult to create fiscal space for welfare. This calls for international mobilization designed to break the power of the international financial institutions, the international trade regime and multinational corporations. Countries such as El Salvador just cannot conduct a lone battle, and progressive initiatives such as in El Salvador will flounder in the absence of international solidarity.

Notes

1 From mid-2014, the base data of both indicators was changed; thus 2013 data is used for consistency. For maternal mortality, see MINSAL 2015a, p. 58; for child mortality, MINSAL 2010, pp. 143, 175.

2 For an analysis of the evolution of the Salvadorean health system, see Chapter E2, 'Social change in El Salvador and the health sector' (Global Health Watch, 2014).

3 See MINSAL (2012, p. 156).

4 Eduardo Espinoza, vice-minister for health policy (2015), interview, 27 October.

5 Menjivar (2015), interview.

6 Author's own calculation based on GDP figures. See Trading Economics (2017) and MINSAL (2016a, p. 37).

7 Cesar Villalona, economist (2015), interview, 28 October.

8 ARENA, founded in 1981, is socially conservative and economically liberal. ARENA controlled the National Assembly until 1985 and controlled the presidency from 1989 until 2009.

9 Villalona (2015), interview.

10 Villalona (2015), interview.

11 Margarita Posada, convenor of Foro Nacional para la Salud (2015), interview, 23 October.

12 FUSADES is the Fundación Salvadoreña para el Desarrollo Económico y Social (FUSADES n.d.); FUNDE is the Fundación Nacional para el Desarrollo (FUNDE n.d.); and ANEP is the Asociación Nacional de la Empresa Privada (ANEP 2016)

13 Hernandez (2015), interview.

14 The document states, '[I]n continuity with the participatory process already begun, a National Health Forum will be created immediately, which will formulate the elements for the new system and contribute to making fundamental decisions about its development.' See Rodriguez (2009, p. 5).

15 Posada (2015), interview.

16 Roxana Rodriguez, independent consultant and member of FNS (2015), interview, 27 October.

17 Rodriguez (2015), interview; Magdalena Cortes, executive director of NGO Fundación Maquilishuatl (FUMA) and member of FNS (2015), interview, 28 October.

18 Giovani Guevara, director for medicines (2015), interview, 28 November.

19 Rodriguez (2015), interview.

20 Rodriguez (2015), interview.

21 Ibid.

22 While the introduction of new taxes only requires a simple majority of votes in Parliament, a comprehensive fiscal reform would require a 2/3rd majority.

23 Rodriguez (2015), interview.

References

ANEP 2016, http://www.anep.org.sv/

Anonymous 2012, 'Diputados aprueban Ley de Medcamentos', *La Prensa Grafica*, 22 February, http://www.laprensagrafica.com/el- salvador/politica/249983-diputados-aprueban-ley-de-medicamentos.html

Carta Economica n.d. a, *Análisis económico en El Salvador 2016–2017, Cuadro 1*, http://cartaeconomica.com/analisis-economico-en-el-salvador-2016-2017/

Carta Economica n.d. b, *El presupuesto recesivo del 2017 garantiza pagar la deuda pero no cumple con la obligación del Estado: proteger los intereses de la población*, http://www.cartaeconomica.com/el-presupuesto-recesivo-del-2017-garantiza-pagar-la-deuda-pero-no-cumple-con-la-obligacion-del-estado-proteger-los-intereses-de-la-poblacion

Carta Economica n.d. c, *En El Salvador los hogares –el pueblo– pagan 25.9 ctvs. x dólar recibido y las empresas sólo 4.7 ctvs. x dólar de utilidades ¡Ya no más impuestos al pueblo!*, http://cartaeconomica.com/en-el-salvador-los-hogares-el-pueblo-pagan-25-9-ctvs-x-dolar-recibido-y-las-empresas-solo-4-7-ctvs-x-dolar-de-utilidades-ya-no-mas-impuestos-al-pueblo/

Carta Economica n.d. d, *Reforma fiscal y declaración de suspensión del pago de la deuda financiera*, http://cartaeconomica.com/reforma-fiscal-y-declaracion-de-suspension-del-pago-de-la-deuda-financiera/

Carta Economica n.d. e, *Un llamado a los trabajadores para que defiendan los nuevos salarios mínimos aprobados: con huelgas y tomas de calle si es necesario*, http://cartaeconomica.com/un-llamado-a-los-trabajadores-para-que-defiendan-los-nuevos-salarios-minimos-aprobados-con-huelgas-y-tomas-de-calle-si-es-necesario/

Central America Data 2017, *El Salvador's debt rating downgraded again*, 2 February, http://www.centralamericadata.com/en/article/home/El_Salvadors_Debt_Rating_Down_Graded_Again

Datosmacro.com n.d., *Gasto público salud*, http://www.datosmacro.com/estado/gasto/salud

FUNDE n.d., http://www.funde.org/

FUSADES n.d. http://fusades.org/

Gammage, S 2007, *El Salvador: despite end to civil war, emigration continues*, Migration Policy Institute, http://www.migrationpolicy.org/article/el-salvador-despite-end-civil-war-emigration-continues

People's Health Movement, Medact, ALAMES et al 2014, 'Social change in El Salvador and the health sector,' in *Global Health Watch 4*, 2014, Zed Books, London

Index Mundi 2016, *El Salvador economy profile 2016*, http://www.indexmundi.com/el_salvador/economy_profile.html

IMF 2016, *IMF executive board concludes 2016 Article IV consultation with El Salvador*, http://www.imf.org/external/pubs/ft/scr/2016/cr16208.pdf

Menjivar, V 2012, 'Redes integrales e integradas de servicios de salud: Avances y desafíos', presentation at International Forum Logros de la reforma de salud en El Salvador y desafíos para su consolidación, 30 August, San Salvador.

MINSAL 2010, *Informe de labores 2009–2010*, Government of El Salvador, San Salvador.

MINSAL 2011, *Lineamientos operativos para el desarrollo de actividades en los Ecos familiares y Ecos especializados*, Government of El Salvador, San Salvador.

MINSAL 2012, *Informe de labores 2011–2012*, Government of El Salvador, San Salvador.

MINSAL 2013, *Informe de labores 2012–2013*, Government of El Salvador, San Salvador.

MINSAL 2014, *Informe de labores 2013–2014*, Government of El Salvador, San Salvador.

MINSAL 2015a, *Informe de labores 2014–2015*, Government of El Salvador, San Salvador.

MINSAL 2015b, *Rendicion de cuentas 2009–2014*, Government of El Salvador, San Salvador.

MINSAL 2016a *Informe de labores 2015–2016*, Government of El Salvador, San Salvador.

MINSAL 2016b, *Rendicion de cuentas 2015–16*, Government of El Salvador, San Salvador.

Orellana, G S 2012, 'MINSAL cumplió el objetivo 5 del Desarrollo del Milenio', *Diario Co Latino*, 14 June, http://www.diariocolatino.com/

Pan American Health Organization & MINSAL 2013, *El Salvador: aportes de la reforma de salud en El Salvador al desarrollo del sistema de salud y los objetivos de cobertura universal y dialogo político para la sostenibilidad de los logros*, PAHO, Washington, DC.

Public Sector Austerity and Savings Policy 2014, *Diario oficial*, http://www.diariooficial.gob.sv/diarios/do-2014/09-septiembre/02-09-2014.pdf

Rodriguez, M I 2009, *Building hope: strategies and recommendations in health, 2009–14*, MINSAL, San Salvador.

SAPRIN n.d., *The impact of economic stabilization and structural adjustment programs in El Salvador – executive summary*, http://www.saprin.org/elsalvador/research/els_exec_summ.pdf

Trading Economics 2017, *El Salvador GDP 1960–2017*, http://www.tradingeconomics.com/el-salvador/gdp

Introduction

An estimated 800 million people suffer from hunger every year in the world, mostly in the developing countries of the South (United Nations, 2015). Hunger adversely and disproportionately impacts those who live on the margins of society. It is estimated that it would require an average US$ 267 billion per year to end hunger in the world by 2030 (ibid.). More importantly, it will require commitment, determination and an enhanced political will on the part of governments, with increased focus on policies of social protection.

In this chapter we use the term malnutrition to refer to 'undernutrition', though 'overnutrition', i.e. overweight and obesity (usually primarily as a result of excess intake of sugars and fats), which is a growing phenomenon in many parts of the world, would also be termed malnutrition. A quarter of all children in the world, mostly in the global South, are undernourished, which increases their chance of death and undermines their potential to learn.

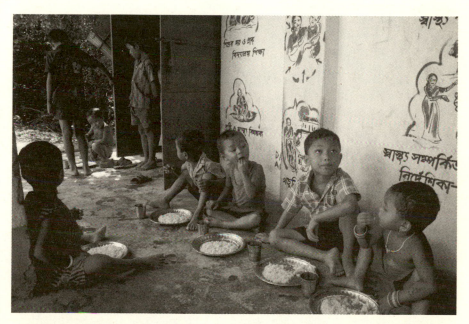

Image E2.1 Mid-day meal programme in a school in India. Such programmes miss the most vulnerable 0–3 age group (Sulakshana Nandi)

Undernutrition is directly linked to poor outcomes in infant and young child health, and is associated with an increased risk of later development of obesity, diabetes and heart disease.

While the Indian economy has been one of the fastest growing economies in the world, with an average growth rate in excess of 6 per cent between 2001 and 2016, the country is also home to the largest number of malnourished children in the world. The Global Hunger Index (GHI) report of 2016 placed India in the 97th position, six notches below Rwanda, which was ravaged by a bloody civil war in the 1990s (Von Grember, 2016). India is among the 20 countries worst affected by hunger in the world, part of a list that includes so-called 'failed states' like Afghanistan, Sierra Leone, etc. (ibid.). The India State Hunger Index (ISHI) shows considerable variations in severity of hunger among various states. Recent data indicate that 32 per cent of children under the age of five are stunted (low height for age, reflecting chronic undernutrition) and 29 per cent are underweight (low weight for height reflecting acute undernutrition) (National Family Health Survey 2015–2016, 2016). While the state of Punjab recently had a hunger index of 13.6, the state of Madhya Pradesh had an index of 30.9 (Menon, Deolalikar and Bhaskar, 2009). Even the best performing state, Punjab, if considered to be a country would be ranked 34th in the GHI 2008 rankings (ibid.). In the worst performing states such as Bihar, Madhya Pradesh and Meghalaya more than 40 per cent of children are stunted.

Tackling malnutrition: the Indian experience

There are two (often contending) streams of thought regarding malnutrition in India:

1. Malnutrition is a medical emergency, which may result in fatality, and which therefore requires specialized treatment under expert care. Treatment of 'uncomplicated' cases is provided through specially designed products called 'Ready to Use Therapeutic Foods' (RUTF), which are standardized in their composition and include essential micronutrients. This is a view that is promoted largely by experts in clinical management of malnutrition.
2. Malnutrition is the outcome of socioeconomic and political inequities. Malnutrition has to be managed in all its stages and manifestations, with a strong focus on the 'root causes'. The processes and products used to address malnutrition need to reflect this overall approach. This view is largely promoted by public health experts.

However, the first approach has come to be regarded as the principal strategy in managing malnutrition. The alarming situation of malnutrition in India demands a comprehensive approach that addresses the needs both of those children who are malnourished and require treatment, as well as preventing much larger numbers with moderate malnutrition from deteriorating further (Prasad and Sinha, 2015). Unfortunately, the approach followed has been informed by a biomedical rather than public health perspective, where malnutrition is often treated without considering its broader social determinants, amongst which household food insecurity dominates.

Efforts to mitigate food insecurity for children in India are primarily channelled through the Integrated Child Development Scheme (ICDS), under the Ministry of Women and Child Development. As part of the scheme, an *'Anganwadi'* or child care centre is established for every 1,000 children between the age of 0 and 3 years. The *'Anganwadi'* provides nutritional supplements and pre-school education. However, the programme has been unable to reach children under the age of 2 years, even though it is widely recognized that this is the age group most critical for intervention (Prasad and Sinha, 2015).

Nutritional Rehabilitation Centres (NRCs) have been established after the rolling out of the National Rural Health Mission (NRHM, 2005) to treat children with Severe Acute Malnutrition (SAM). Experience, however, has shown that NRCs are unable to cope with the large numbers of children suffering from malnutrition and are largely ineffective in addressing the problem. There are serious discrepancies in protocols in the management of SAM between NRCs and ICDS (Prasad, Sinha and Sridhar, 2012) creating operational problems. Families are also unwilling to admit children in the NRCs (often situated far from their homes) for prolonged periods of time. The NRCs treat the children as medical emergencies and do not offer any comprehensive system of prevention or continuity of care(ibid).

RUTFs and conflicting commercial interests

Over the recent past interventions promoted by international agencies such as UNICEF and MSF to address malnutrition have centred on specialized products termed Ready to Use Therapeutic Foods (RUTF). In some settings RUTFs have greatly increased the survival of children aged 6 months to 5 years suffering from severe acute malnutrition (SAM), especially during emergencies (Bazzano, Potts, Bazzano and Mason, 2017). RUTFs are easier to prepare and distribute during nutritional emergencies. They do not require water for preparation, are shelf-stable for 2 years and are generally palatable for children with an appetite (Bazzano, Potts, Bazzano and Mason, 2017). All these factors have led to a surge in the demand for RUTFs in low and middle income countries (LMICs). Production facilities have sprung up across the developing world. These production facilities have emerged not only to meet emergencies, but, increasingly, for supplementation of pregnant women and young children who are not severely malnourished. This increased use of manufactured, commercial products for the treatment and prevention of undernutrition is of great concern since there is a lack of evidence for their long-term health impacts. UNICEF itself has stated that care should be taken to ensure that the

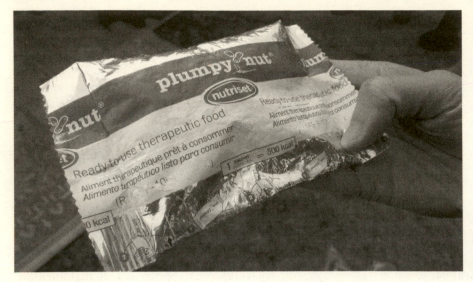

Image E2.2 Plumpy'nut (By Flickr user mastermaq - Flickr image 2874479122; License: CC BY-SA 2.0, https://commons.wikimedia.org/w/index.php?curid=7050129)

RUTFs do not replace nutritional best practices and consumption of normal household foods (UNICEF, Position Paper: Ready-To-Use Therapeutic Food for Children with Severe Acute Malnutrition in UNICEF, 2013).

RUTFs were first commercially produced by the French manufacturer Nutriset and were marketed as 'Plumpy'Nut'. It can be used in places where large numbers have to be fed and health resources are strained. Nutriset patented the product and founded 'Plumpy'Field', a network of Plumpy'Nut manufacturers established through a franchise model. Subsequently many 'Plumpy'Field' factories have been established in countries where the product is needed and locally sourced foods are often employed in its production. After a prolonged advocacy campaign, Nutriset made its patent available in the developing countries, so that generic variants of 'Plumpy'Nut' could be produced. Often, however, the RUTFs do not use locally sourced ingredients, nor does production occur in the end user countries. (Bazzano, Potts, Bazzano and Mason, 2017)

The entry of the private sector has resulted in commercial interests coming into conflict with the public health challenges that RUTFs were originally supposed to address. Edesia, which has the franchise rights for the production of Plumpy'Nut in the USA was set up by a person who has no background in nutrition or public health. It ostensibly operates as a 'Not for Profit' but its website mentions "strategies" to achieve "profit objectives, secure 'new business opportunities" and "penetrate" new markets (EdesiaNutrition, 2017). Similarly, Abbott Nutritionals, makers of infant milk formulas have built a production facility as a 'donation' to Partners in Health to produce 'Norimanba', a RUTF in Haiti (Partners In Health, 2017). The increase in producers of RUTF has coincided with a parallel expansion in the development of RUTFs for consumption by populations that do not suffer from SAM. Nutriset itself has expanded and diversified its range to products like 'Plumpy'Sup' (Supplementary nutrition for stunted children), Plumpy'Mum' (Supplementary food for pregnant and lactating women), 'Plumpy'Doz' (Micronutrient enriched supplementary food), etc. (PlumpyField, 2017).

Another example of conflict of interest is Valid Nutrition, a company based in Ireland. Valid calls itself a 'not for profit' enterprise, while counting former Unilever executives on its board of directors. The company has a factory in Malawi producing RUTFs. Now it has plans to tie up with Amul, India's largest milk brand, to produce RUTFs and also expand its product lines beyond RUTFs to complementary and supplementary foods. The company clearly states that it seeks to profit from selling "low cost nutritional products" (Valid Nutrition, 2017). These product-based 'solutions' being offered to combat undernutrition fail to address issues regarding prevention of malnutrition, continuity of care, sustainability, impact on local food systems and economies or even efficacy (Sachdeva et al., 2016).

Lack of support to caregivers, women in particular, is a primary determinant of child malnutrition. Gender-based discrimination in Indian society contributes significantly to incidence of ill health and malnutrition in women (NFHS 4). It is these women that not only go on to bear children, often with low birth weight, but are also charged with rearing them, often single-handedly and, in particular, feeding them. While acknowledged in various frameworks for managing malnutrition, such societal issues have not been problematized or prioritized for intervention. Although "UNICEF supports community-based management of acute malnutrition with ready-to-use therapeutic foods (RUTF)...and sees it as one part of a medical protocol that should only be used as part of the community-based management of acute malnutrition in children, in accordance with international standards for such care"(UNICEF, Ready-to-use Therapeutic Food for Children with Severe Acute Malnutrition, 2013) in reality, UNICEF's practice of Community based Management of Acute Malnutrition (CMAM), tends to medicalize its management and minimizes the importance of community participation and ownership:

Addressing malnutrition in the Indian context

It has been argued that the type and context of malnutrition in India is substantially different from that seen in humanitarian emergencies in Africa, from where strategies involving use of RUTFs have largely been drawn. (Dasgupta, 2014). Direct evidence is rapidly accumulating to substantiate this contention. Recent data, based on the National Family Health Survey (NFHS 4) confirms the fact that the quality of diets in India is abysmally

Box E2.1: Community-based nutrition programme: an alternative

Practitioners have been attempting to create models of community-based management of malnutrition that take into account the elements of prevention, care, treatment and community participation; and use local resources and food sources. One such attempt incorporates a comprehensive community-based programme involving child care services, participatory learning and action, mobilization of women and social audit. The programme, Action Against Malnutrition (AAM), is designed and implemented by a consortium of organizations: the Public Health Resource Network (PHRN), Ekjut, Child In Need Institute (CINI), Chaupal and IDEA. The programme is being implemented in seven blocks covering four states of India: Jharkhand, Odisha, Bihar and Chhattisgarh. The three key components of the programme are: Creches for child care services, Participatory Learning and Action (PLA) for community mobilization and action, and systems strengthening (Prasad and Sinha, 2015).

1. Creches: It is well known that women from marginalized and deprived communities face a triple burden: child care, household chores and wage work. This compromises a mother's ability to attend to the child, increasing the risk of undernutrition. Therefore, the creche component of the programme addresses this challenge and provides a framework for overall child care with emphasis on prevention of malnutrition. The creches provide safety, learning through play, appropriate feeding, growth monitoring and access to health and referral care. The programme is available to every child in the village irrespective of the level of malnutrition, thus adhering to the principle of universality of care. Within this, special attention is given to those children who exhibit growth faltering so that they do not deteriorate further and become severely malnourished. The programme ensures continuity of care by enabling referral to government institutions. It lays equal stress on community processes and participation while maintaining technical rigour in the identification of cases of malnutrition and their management.

2. Participatory Learning and Action (PLA): Under this, regular meetings are held in the community, primarily with women. At the same time the meetings also involve the participation of men, community leaders and elected representatives. The meetings discuss issues of child malnutrition, child care, government schemes and programmes, etc. The motive is to build community consensus for the programme, find local solutions to tackle the problem of malnutrition and use collective pressure to improve services.

3. Systems Strengthening: This component aims to identify critical gaps in the implementation of government interventions to address malnutrition. AAM works in close coordination with the frontline workers of public health programmes, and district and block level government officials, to ensure that services provided by the government reach the intended beneficiaries.

The outcomes from the programme have shown that, while a medicalized approach may yield short term results in tackling malnutrition, a comprehensive participatory approach provides better access, sustainability and continuity of care at lower costs, with fair outcomes (Prasad and Sinha, 2015). A study was conducted to analyse the outcomes of the intervention among tribal children (Prasad and Sinha, 2015). A cohort of 587 children was taken and was studied for the change in the status of stunting and wasting for a period of four to six months from May 2013 to November 2013. It was seen that there was an increase in the proportion of children in the non-wasted category from 72 per cent to 80 per cent. There was a significant reduction in the percentage of children with Severe Acute Malnutrition (SAM / severe wasting) from 8 per cent to 4 Per cent. It was also observed that there was a significant increase in the proportion of children in the non-underweight category from 43 per cent to 49 per cent and reduction in the severely underweight from 24 per cent to 17 per cent.

66.6 per cent of children saw an improvement in their Z score (Z score is the measure of deviation from normal), with over 80 per cent being classified as normal or improving grades. The average Weight for Height Z-score (WHZ) – an index of wasting or excessive thinness – of the children improved from –1.41 to 1.13 during the 4–6 month period. Over 80 per cent of children with SAM improved with approximately 40 per cent achieving normalcy (cure) (Prasad V. e., 2014) and the rest shifting to moderately acute malnutrition. In another series with a larger number of children with SAM followed for a longer period, similar gains were found to be sustained and even enhanced over time (Under review for publication). A formal evaluation of the project has also shown fair results that await publication. Further, cost-benefit analyses suggest that such programmes are highly cost effective by WHO standards (Under review for publication).

There have been other potential positive spin-offs from the programme such as an increase in women's earnings due to the availability of child care, increased awareness about nutritional practices and hygiene, emergence of a micro market for foodstuffs like eggs and a prevention of the "food-drug" confusion, which may have arisen had the intervention been based on commercially produced RUTF. (Prasad e., 2014).

poor for a large majority, and is largely related to poverty and food insecurity, while there may be some elements of lack of information (National Family Health Survey 2015–2016, 2016). Lack of protein is significant along with lack of micronutrients which are also present in many sources of protein, specially eggs and meat. Simultaneously, even as many poorer communities are culturally inclined to be non-vegetarian there is a political and social push to declare India as a largely vegetarian state – even though over 70 per cent of the country population consumes foods of animal origin such as meat and fish (NFHS 4). The push for 'vegetarianism' has gained traction following the installation of a socially conservative government in 2014. In recent years '*Gaurakshaks*' (cow protectors) have wreaked havoc across North India, specifically targeting Dalits (so called 'lower caste' communities in India who traditionally consume meat) and Muslim communities, who often rely on relatively cheap sources of protein obtained from beef and buffalo meat (compared to poultry or goat meat).

A randomized controlled trial has been conducted by research agencies in India which compares the relative efficacy of three different nutritional products: commercial RUTF, locally produced RUTF and augmented home foods, all mandated by the Government (Bhandari, 2017). The trial showed that the use of commercial RUTF has an impact equivalent to that of augmented home foods. However, locally produced RUTF (identical in composition to commercial RUTF) is seen to be superior for inexplicable reasons. It also shows that even in the best-case scenario of local RUTF, over 40 per cent children fail to recover even after a 4-month period of intervention. Recovery rates across all arms fell to 15 per cent within the next four months after the intervention stopped. The study also noted that satisfactory results could not be achieved without the additional intervention of providing for a paid worker to supervise feeding at household level eight times a day. Paradoxically, the study goes on to advocate the use of RUTF, which seems to go against its own evidence. (Prasad, Reading between the lines of RUTF trials, 2017).

Conclusion

As a result of pressure from civil society organizations such as the International Baby Food Action Network (IBFAN) and People's Health Movement (PHM), UNICEF has reluctantly acknowledged that in 'certain contexts' other strategies may also be tried. This is reflected in the following statement:

"In specific settings where there is provision of adequate resources, the treatment of SAM is based on a therapeutic diet using locally available nutrient-dense foods prepared by the carer at home, without the use of commercially produced products such as RUTF. UNICEF acknowledges that some regions adopt this approach to managing SAM as they believe it be more sustainable and better suited to the country" (Revised UNICEF document for Codex Committee on Nutrition and Foods for Special Dietary Uses – CCNFSDU)

However, it is a matter of concern that UNICEF has announced 13 pilots across 13 states of India, most of which, it is understood, intend to or are already using commercial RUTF. It appears that the push for evidence-based policy making and programming only holds if the evidence is convenient to a particular view – that of reducing food insecurity and malnutrition to a technical issue and seeing it as a medical problem requiring a nutraceutical solutions. Compelling evidence, nonetheless, points to the efficacy and sustainability of comprehensive community based nutrition programmes that incorporate the use of locally devised solutions.

References

Bazzano, A, Potts, K, Bazzano, L, & Mason, J 2017, The Life Course Implications of Ready to Use Therapeutic Food for Children in Low-Income Countries. *International Journal of Environmental Research and Public Health.* http://www.mdpi.com/1660-4601/14/4/403/htm

Bhandari, N 2017, Efficacy of three feeding regimens for home-based management of children with uncomplicated severe acute malnutrion: a randomised control trial in india. *British Medical Journal.*

Dasgupta, R 2014, Can Nutrition Rehabilitation Centers Address Severe Malnutrition in India? *Indian Paediatrics.*

EdesiaNutrition 2017, 1 May. Retrieved from www.edesianutrition.org: http://www.edesianutrition.org/wp-content/uploads/2016/05/busdevmanager052316.pdf

Menon, P, Deolalikar, A, & Bhaskar, A 2009, *India State Hunger: Comparison of Hunger across the states.* Bonn, Riverside, Washington D.C.: International Food Policy Research Institute.

2016, *NATIONAL FAMILY HEALTH SURVEY 2015–2016.* Mumbai: International Institute Of Population Sciences.

Partners In Health 2017, 1 May. Retrieved from www.pih.org: http://www.pih.org/blog/nourimanba-malnutrition-haiti-poverty

PlumpyField 2017, 1 May. Retrieved from www.plumpyfield.com: http://www.plumpyfield.com/about/key-data

Prasad, V e. 2014, *Combating malnutrition: A process document of Action Against Malnutrition(AAM), a multi-strategy intervention in seven blocks of four*

states. New Delhi: Public Health Resource Network.

Prasad, V & Sinha, D 2015, Potentials, Experiences and Outcomes of a Comprehensive Community Based Programme to Address Malnutrition in Tribal. *International Journal of Child Health and Nutrition,* 151-162.

Prasad, V, Sinha, D, & Sridhar, S 2012, Falling between two stools:Operational inconsistencies between ICDS and NRHM in the management of severe malnutrition. *Indian Paediatrics,* 181-185.

Sachdeva H P S, Kapil U, Gupta A, Prasad V, "Sustainable developmental solutions or product- based illusions for addressing severe acute malnutrition?" Paper submitted to the World Nutrition Conference2016, held in Cape Town, South Africa from 30th August to 2nd September 2016.

UNICEF 2013, *Position Paper: Ready-To-Use Therapeutic Food for Children with Severe Acute Malnutrition in UNICEF.* New York: UNICEF.

UNICEF 2013, *READY-TO-USE THERAPEUTIC FOOD FOR CHILDREN WITH SEVERE ACUTE MALNUTRITION.* UNICEF. Retrieved from www.unicef.org: http://www.unicef.org/media/files/Current_Issues_Paper_-_Ready_To_Use_Therapeutic_Food.pdf

United Nations 2015, Retrieved from www.un.org: http://www.un.org/sustainabledevelopment/hunger/

Von Grember, K e. 2016, *2016 Global hunger index: Getting to zero hunger.* Bonn: International Food Policy Research Institute.

E3 | PEOPLE LIVING WITH HIV IN INDIA: THE STRUGGLE FOR ACCESS

The first case of HIV in India was reported in 1986. Three decades later, there are an estimated 2.1 million Indians living with HIV (NACO, 2015). AIDS-related deaths have decreased by 54 per cent since 2007 and according to the government, this decline has been accompanied by an expansion in access to anti-retrovirals (ARVs) in the country. It is estimated that between 2004 and 2014 around 450,000 lives have been saved in India as a consequence of enhanced access to ARVs[1].

A story of consistent struggles waged by People living with HIV (PLHIV) in India, supported by national and international solidarity, lies behind the successes achieved as regards HIV treatment in India. In many ways it mirrors the struggles of PLHIV in many countries across the world; by taking on legal battles to challenge patent monopolies on HIV treatment, networks of PLHIV in India have had a lasting impact not only nationally but globally. By the late 1990s triple combination therapy for HIV was approved, revolutionizing the lives and treatment of PLHIV. But treatment cost as much as US$ 15,000 per patient per year (MSF, 2005) – unaffordable to almost all patients in low- and middle-income countries (LMICs). In 2001 the situation changed dramatically when an Indian generic manufacturer (Cipla) offered treatment at less than a dollar a day (US$ 350 per year) – representing a 97 per cent drop in prices. (WHO, 2001). From a death sentence for millions in LMICs, almost overnight, HIV patients were offered a chance to live normal and fulfilling lives.

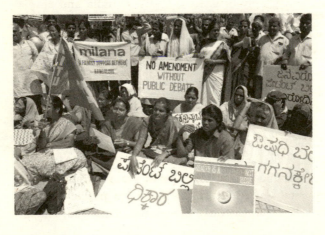

Image E3.1 Demonstration in 2005 against amendment of Indian Patent Act (Kajal Bhardwaj)

These dramatic events had little meaning for Indians living with HIV. While Indian companies started providing medicines to government-sponsored treatment programmes abroad, the Indian government continued to resist starting its own treatment programme. This forced Indian PLHIV networks to undertake a massive campaign for access to ARVs in India. After years of struggle and advocacy, the Indian government finally announced its plan to provide free anti-retroviral treatment on 1 December 2003[2]. Since then the role of PLHIV networks in treatment access in India has taken many shapes and forms; a key aspect of this work relates to trade, intellectual property and generic competition.

Changes in India's patent law

India's engagement with the issues of patents and access to medicines pre-dates the formation of the World Trade Organization (WTO) in 1995. India, after independence from British rule in 1947, retained the colonial patent system that allowed 14 years of patent protection on medicines. As a consequence India primarily depended on imported medicines and medicine prices in India were one of the highest in the world. In 1972 India introduced a new patent regime, and product patents on medicines were abolished, thus allowing domestic companies to manufacture and sell patented medicines at 1/10 to 1/5 of their price in the global market. This led to the establishment of a strong and vibrant generic pharmaceutical industry in India. By the late 1990s Indian generic medicines had become the lifeline for patients in most LMICs.

In 2005 India amended its patent law to fully comply with its obligations under the WTO Agreement on Trade Related Aspects of Intellectual Property Rights (TRIPS)[3]. TRIPS required India to start granting 20 year product patents on medicines that give patent holders exclusive rights over the manufacture, sale, use, offer for sale and import of the patented medicine. The exclusion of competition usually results in high prices and restricted availability. The impending change in India's patent regime and its impact on the continued production and supply of generic ARVs in India and abroad attracted significant national and international concern from public interest groups and the United Nations[4].

PLHIV networks in India, other health and public interest groups like the National Working Group on Patent Laws (NWGPL) and the Jan Swasthya Abhiyan (Peoples Health Movement, India) that had long been active on these issues, became critical sources of technical information and analysis. Multiple national and international letters of concern were written asking the Prime Minister, various ministries and members of Parliament to consider the serious implications of the amendments on public health (Health GAP, 2004) In February 2005, PLHIV marched along with health groups, trade unions, farmers' groups, environmental groups and many others in public rallies in Delhi, Mumbai, Bangalore, Kolkata, Chennai, Hyderabad, Dharwad, Panjim,

Pune and Thirupati[5] to protest the amendments. Working with the Affordable Medicines and Treatment Campaign (AMTC) of the Lawyers Collective, the networks demanded that the amendments to the patent law include[6]:

1. A clear definition of patentable criteria;
2. No patents for new usage and dosage of known medicines;
3. Provision for pre-grant opposition as before, to stop frivolous patents;
4. Simple procedures with a time limit for the granting of compulsory licences; and
5. (The) introduction of a ceiling on royalties to multinational corporations.

In reaching out to Members of Parliament, Indian PLHIV groups were joined by colleagues and representatives of international organisations who happened to be in India at the time. Wearing 'HIV-positive' t-shirts, the activists met several members of Parliament to explain the impact the amendments could have on the drugs they imported from India. In the parliamentary debates that took place over the amendments, access to HIV treatment featured repeatedly in the statements of various MPs. As one MP noted, "we all accept the fact that this Bill is perhaps one of the most important pieces of legislation that this Parliament is considering. I say this because it directly concerns the lives of billions of people and the livelihood of millions of people not only in India but in the lesser developed countries which are dependent on India for medical treatment from where medicines go. To give you an example, 70 per cent of the medicines used for AIDS treatment in the lesser developed countries are medicines made in India. They go from here only for the reason that they are available at prices which are affordable. Therefore, rushing through with a Bill of this importance is something that we should not do because we will be letting down our country and more importantly, or as importantly, we will be letting down countries that are dependent on us, that look up to India as a leader and look up to India as a country from where treatment is available to them at affordable costs."[7]

In their quest to balance public interest with India's WTO obligations, the Indian Parliament turned to the 2001 Doha Declaration on TRIPS and Public Health. Signed by all WTO members, the Doha Declaration states categorically that, TRIPS "can and should be interpreted and implemented in a manner supportive of WTO members' right to protect public health and, in particular, to promote access to medicines for all' (WTO, 2001). The Indian Parliament included multiple health safeguards in the patent law amendments including compulsory licences, the bolar and research exceptions, parallel imports, automatic licencing for medicines produced before 2005 and ensuring that the medicine registration system was separate from the patent regime. An additional key health safeguard was a provision restricting evergreening, i.e. the practice of pharmaceutical companies to extend their exclusive rights on a medicine by making minor or obvious changes to the medicine and applying for additional patents. Section 3(d) of India's patent law prohibits patents on new uses of known medicines. It also prohibits patents on new forms of existing medicines unless the patent applicant can show a significant increase in efficacy[8]. The law also allows challenges to patent applications (pre-grant) and to patents (post-grant) by a broad range of parties.

'Patent oppositions' by PHLIV groups

Two of the public health safeguards described above have been used extensively by PLHIV groups in India since 2005, i.e. Section 3(d) and the patent opposition mechanisms. The first pre-grant opposition filed against a patent application for an ARV concerned a fixed-dose combination of zidovudine/lamivudine (AZT/3TC) marketed by GlaxoSmithkline (GSK) as 'Combivir'. Indian PLHIV groups collaborated with Thai groups who were also opposing GSK's patent application for this medicine in their own country, sharing information and holding joint public actions. Before the patent office could take a decision in this matter, GSK withdrew its patent application.

The first victory at the patent office for PLHIV networks came in the case of the pediatric version of the ARV Nevirapine. In 2006, the Indian Network of People living with HIV/AIDS and the Positive Womens Network filed a joint opposition against Boehringer Ingelheim's application for Nevirapine Hemihydrate, a syrup form of Nevirapine often used for treating children. Nevirapine was not patentable in India as it was a pre-1995 medicine. Applying for an Indian patent on the syrup form of this medicine in 1998, the PLHIV networks argued, was an attempt at evergreening by Boehringer. The patent opposition argued that the medicine was not patentable under Indian law because the hemihydrate form of Nevirapine was "obvious to a person skilled in the art", that it was just a "new form" of an already known substance without any increased efficacy, and that the product was a "mere admixture" of ingredients that did not demonstrate any synergistic effects (Lawyers Collective, 2008). After a hearing, in June 2008 the Delhi Patent Office rejected Boehringer's application[9].

Explaining their involvement in the case, P Kousalya, president of Positive Women's Network (PWN) stated, "we have been involved in looking at the issues of women and children in the context of HIV. We opposed the patent application on nevirapine hemihydrate to ensure that it remains available for our children and to make sure that the government doesn't say it is too expensive to provide. This is important not just for us but for PLHIV across the world. Accessing appropriate pediatric formulations of AIDS drugs is a particular problem around the world, and we hope that this decision can be a first step in making them more available" (Mathew, 2008).

Several victories in courts for PLHIV groups has ensured that generic versions of most ARVs continue to be available in India, and importantly,

TABLE E3.1: Patent oppositions filed by PLHIV networks in India

MEDICINE	PATENT APPLICANT	PATENT OPPONENT	STATUS
Zidovudine/ lamivudine First-line ARV	GSK	Manipur Network of People living with HIV/AIDS, Indian Network for People living with HIV/AIDS	Patent Application Withdrawn
Nevaripine Hemihydrate (syrup) First-line ARV	Boehringer Ingelheim	Positive Womens Network and Indian Network for People living with HIV/AIDS	Patent Application Rejected
Tenofovir Fumarate or TDF (two applications) Preferred first -line ARV	Gilead Sciences	Delhi Network of Positive People and Indian Network for People living with HIV/AIDS; Brazilian Interdisciplinary AIDS Association (ABIA) and Sahara (Centre for Residential Care and Rehabilitation)	Patent Application Rejected
Amprenavir Second-line ARV	GSK	Uttar Pradesh Network of Positive People and Indian Network for People living with HIV/AIDS	Pending
Atazanavir Second-line ARV	Novartis	Karnataka Network for People Living with HIV and AIDS and Indian Network for People living with HIV/AIDS	ABANDONED; APPLICATION ON BISULPHATE REJECTED
Valgancyclovir OI medicine	F Hoffmann-La Roche	Tamil Nadu Network of Positive People and Indian Network for People living with HIV/AIDS	PATENT OVERTURNED
Abacavir Second-line arv	GSK	Indian Network for People living with HIV/AIDS	PATENT APPLICATION WITHDRAWN
Lopinavir Second-line arv	Abbott Laboratories	Delhi Network of Positive People, Network of Maharashtra by People living with HIV and AIDS and Indian Network for People living with HIV/AIDS	PATENT APPLICATION REJECTED
Lopinavir/Ritonavir (Soft Gel) Second-line ARV	Abbott Laboratories	Delhi Network of Positive People, and Indian Network for People living with HIV/AIDS	Patent Application Deemed Abandoned
Tenofovir or td First-line ARV	Gilead Sciences	Delhi Network of Positive People, and Indian Network for People living with HIV/AIDS	PATENT APPLICATION REJECTED
Ritonavir Second-line ARV	Abbott Laboratories	Delhi Network of Positive People, and Indian Network for People living with HIV/AIDS	PATENT APPLICATION REJECTED
Efavirenz (post-grant opposition) First-line ARV	Bristol Myers Squibb	Delhi Network of Positive People	Pending
Valgancyclovir (post-grant opposition) OI medicine	F Hoffmann-La Roche	Delhi Network of Positive People	PATENT OVERTURNED

Source: Adapted from Asia Pacific Network of People Living with HIV/AIDS (APN+) 2016

ensures that India continues to be a source of affordable ARVs for patients across the world. Table E3.1 summarizes cases where generic availability was ensured as a result of interventions by PLHIV groups. As can be seen, the threat of patent rejection often leads to companies withdrawing their applications. PLHIV networks have also been active in opposing patents on treatment for opportunistic infections and co-infections like TB and Hepatitis-C (Datta, 2015).

The Novartis Case

Between 2006 and 2013, the critical provision relied on by PLHIV groups in their patent oppositions was under a legal challenge in Indian courts, mounted by Novartis, the Swiss pharmaceutical company. The case related to the rejection of Novartis' patent application on *imatinib mesylate*, an important anti-cancer medicine used in the treatment of chronic myloid leukaemia (CML). Novartis sold its version, called Glivec (or Gleevec), at a global price of US$ 2,500 per person per month while generic companies marketed their versions at one-tenth this price. Novartis originally obtained the patent on imatinib in 1993. Unable to get a patent on the molecule which pre-dated the TRIPS Agreement, in 1998, Novartis filed a patent application on the 'beta-crystalline' form of imatinib mesylate at the Chennai Patent office. In 2006, the patent application was rejected for, among other things, failing the criteria set in Section 3(d) of India's Patent Act.

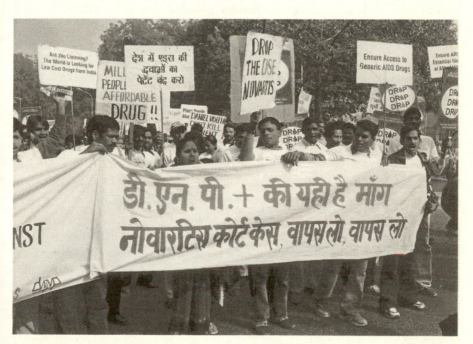

Image E3.2 Protest against Novartis for challenging Indian Law (Delhi Network of Positive People)

Over the next eight years, Novartis first challenged the provision (Section 3(d)) itself claiming it violated the Indian Constitution and India's TRIPS obligations and then the interpretation of the provision, arguing for a lower standard of interpreting 'efficacy.' If successful, Novartis's challenge to Section 3(d) would have impacted access to medicines across the board – not just the cancer medicine in question but also other medicines for HIV. As the case progressed in the Indian courts, PLHIV groups took on the task of challenging the public positions of Novartis which claimed that nothing in its case challenged or impacted access to medicines. Legal battles over intellectual property rights, particularly where they impinge on public interest or public health are fought as much in the court of public opinion as they are in the courts of law. Over the duration of the case, PLHIV and health groups undertook protests, press conferences and various other activities to maintain public focus on the case. They also kept an eye on how the Indian government was defending Section 3(d) and Indian Network for People Living with HIV/AIDS (INP+) wrote to the government, requesting that it deploy its best lawyers to argue the case[10].

On 1 April 2013, the case finally ended with the Supreme Court upholding the strict interpretation of Section 3(d). The importance of the decision for HIV treatment was underscored by Loon Gangte of Delhi Network for People: "We are extremely pleased and relieved that the Supreme Court has recognised the public health importance of section 3(d). We have been filing several oppositions to patent applications on ARV medicines on the basis of section 3(d). This is a crucial victory for people living with HIV and other diseases who can continue to rely on India for access to affordable treatment."

The free trade agreements

In 2007, a new challenge emerged as India started negotiating free trade agreements (FTAs) with Japan and the EU. FTAs negotiated with developed countries usually feature commitments far in excess of those made at the WTO, including on intellectual property. Known as 'TRIPS-plus' measures, the provisions demanded by developed countries in these negotiations typically require longer and newer exclusive rights on medicines. They also feature investment chapters that allow 'investors' to sue sovereign governments over health policies. (See Chapter D5 on Investment agreements.)

In the case of the India-Japan FTA, leaked versions of the IP chapter indicated that Japan's interests lay in streamlining administrative matters and IP enforcement. In detailed submissions to the Indian government on the impact of Japan's demands, DNP+ highlighted not only the TRIPS-plus measures but also the potential impact of the investment chapter, noting that, "we expect the Indian government to deal with high prices of patented medicines not only through compulsory licences but also price control and regulation. However, we fear that the government may have tied its hands in taking such measures by signing on to an investment chapter like those contained in other Japanese trade agreements" (Ahuja, 2010). In 2011, the India-Japan Comprehensive Economic Partnership Agreement was signed and in the final text, TRIPS-plus provisions appeared to have largely been rejected by the Indian government while the investment chapter included a specific exclusion for the use of TRIPS flexibilities.

Box E3.1: Campaign on the EU-India FTA

In 2009, a small group of protestors from networks of people living with HIV and other groups stood with banners outside the office of the European Union Delegation to India in New Delhi. As they chanted against the FTA and the demands being made of India by the EC, they were detained by the police. In 2010, people living with HIV continued to gather and protest outside the offices of the Indian Ministry of Commerce and Industry. In 2011, over 3,000 people from across India were joined by colleagues from South East Asia to march through New Delhi to voice their objection to the TRIPS-plus provisions of the EU-India FTA. A Press Conference held right after the rally, which included the former UN Health Rapporteur on the right to Health, a representative from a cancer group and representatives from other countries who came for the rally, was heavily reported in the media. The next day along with activists from Asia, the local networks met with various Indian official and the UN to raise community concerns on the harmful provisions in the EU-India FTA.

In 2012, as the EU-India Summit kicked off in Delhi in February with progress on the FTA identified as one its primary objectives, DNP+ delivered black coffins to the office of the Delegation of the EU in Delhi on one of the coldest mornings of the year. The motive was to highlight the deaths of people living with HIV/AIDS across regions who are reliant on production of Indian generic pharmaceutical that will be trammelled due to India-EU FTA. After that over 2000 people living with HIV marched through Delhi once more while protests against the EU-India FTA were also held in Asia, Africa, Latin America and the EU.

As a result of the persistent advocacy by PLHIV networks, the Commerce Ministry and Health Ministry started consulting them and other civil society groups on the text being proposed by the EU. In collaboration with legal experts an analysis of the EU text was submitted to the Indian government. Treatment literacy and outreach have been at the heart of this mobilization. The PLHIV networks spread information and awareness through community meetings. They have organized trainings on FTAs, Intellectual Property Rights for their members on an annual basis since 2010.

The EU-India talks have now gone on for a decade. Leaked negotiating texts of the IP Chapter and the Investment Chapter in 2009, 2010 and 2011 showed that the EU was demanding ambitious TRIPS-plus measures including longer patent terms and new exclusive rights on medicines in the form of data exclusivity and TRIPS-plus IP enforcement measures[11]. The alarm on these negotiations was raised by PLHIV groups who continue to make detailed submissions to the government of India, follow and report on each round of negotiations and hold regular rallies and public actions. (See Box E3.1.)

As global concern over this FTA increased over its potential impact on the manufacture, supply and distribution of generic medicines in and from India, even the European Parliament repeatedly issued resolutions directing the European Commission to ensure that access to medicines is not affected by the FTA. In May 2011, the European Parliament specifically asked the EC not to demand data exclusivity of the Indian government and recognized the importance of the use of TRIPS flexibilities by India. In April 2011, the Indian Prime Minister's Office issued a press release stating that nothing in the EU-India FTA would go beyond TRIPS or India's domestic law (PMO, 2011). Even as key TRIPS-plus demands like patent term extension were dropped by the EU negotiators, others remain on the table. As attempts to restart the negotiations on the EU-India FTA were made in 2017, PLHIV networks once more protested outside the EU offices in Delhi highlighting their ongoing concerns on the negotiations.

The Voluntary Licences

The introduction of product patents in India law has also had an impact on the business models and commercial considerations of Indian generic companies. Several top Indian companies have been acquired by MNCs or have tie-ups with them. But these buy-outs and tie-ups also mean that these companies are now unlikely to challenge patents, launch new medicines and take on MNCs in legal battles. MNCs have also altered their approach over time to offer voluntary licences to leading Indian generic exporters to counter the impact of the use of TRIPS flexibilities in India.

For instance, in 2006, patent oppositions were filed by PLHIV networks and generic companies against the patent applications filed by US MNC Gilead Sciences related to the ARV *tenofovir*. Within a week, Gilead offered voluntary licences to generic companies for the production and supply of *tenofovir* in a limited number of developing countries. Several generic companies took these licenses even though Gilead had no product patents on *tenofovir* and as a condition of taking those licenses withdrew their patent oppositions. As public interest groups and at least one generic company persisted with their oppositions, these product patent applications were later rejected by the patent office. Later in 2011, Gilead issued fresh licences to four generic companies and to the Medicines Patent Pool with a limited number of countries for these companies to supply to. Despite the health safeguards in the Indian law and the restrictions on their ability to manufacture and supply medicines in key developing countries, generic companies have continued to sign similar voluntary licenses on other medicines as well (Lawyers Collective, 2012).

The voluntary licences, particularly those issued through the Medicines Patent Pool have revealed interesting differences in approach within public-interest groups. Voluntary licences are among the few options for improving treatment access available to patient groups in countries where pharmaceutical companies have obtained patents. Accordingly, some international groups welcomed the issue of voluntary licences. However, in India where the patent system is quite different from other countries, it remains to be seen which medicines receive patents. Only then will the matter of considering voluntary licences arise. With the current licences there has been growing concern that these may be undermining the patent opposition process (I-MAK, 2011). As in the case of the Gilead licences, once licences are signed, generic companies have withdrawn their patent oppositions leaving only the PLHIV networks to oppose the applications. This occurred recently with the licenses for the new hepatitis C medicines (Babu, 2015).

Although India is included in each of these licences, PLHIV networks persist with their patent opposition work. As they commented: "Why are we still opposing the Tenofovir patents in India? Well, what guarantees are there with the voluntary licences? How long will they last? Mostly we are standing up for our Brazilian and Chinese colleagues who will suffer as a result of this game that Gilead is playing. In all respects, as long as one company and one company alone makes decisions about how and by whom medicines will be supplied, we will remain at their mercy. This is an unacceptable situation when it comes to protecting health and saving lives. In any case they don't even deserve a patent under Indian law, so where does the question of voluntary licences arise?[12]"

Future struggles

Since 2005, PLHIV networks have successfully raised the visibility of the debate around the very complicated issue of patents and health. The successful use of patent oppositions has inspired similar work in other countries while some developing countries have adopted or are considering adopting legal provisions similar to those in India's patent law. The Philippines introduced a provision similar to Section 3(d) in its own patents law in 2008 (Dalangin-Fernandez, 2008).

These successes have not come easily. PLHIV groups are under-resourced and over-stretched. The safeguards in the Indian law are facing a persistent onslaught from several MNCs; Novartis was just one of them. Bayer sued the Indian government in its attempt to enforce patent linkage (demanding that drug regulatory agencies enforce patent protection) in India; something

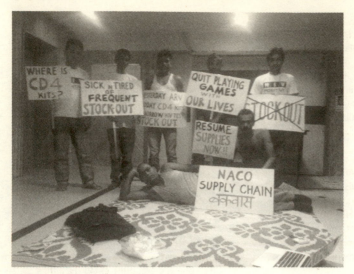

Image E3.3 HIV activists occupy office of the National Aids Control Organisation (NACO) to protest against stock-outs of medicines (Delhi Network of Positive People)

Bayer does not even enjoy under EU law[13]. Roche has used litigation in an attempt to enforce higher standards for the granting of temporary injunctions in patent infringement cases[14]. Developed countries are not only using FTA negotiations but are also using bilateral pressure such as though the US Special 301 law. This highlights the role and responsibility of the Indian government in safeguarding and using the public health safeguards in India's patent law. PHLIV groups face fresh challenges in a situation where the Indian Government has shifted its position on Intellectual Property Rights (IPRs) and there are fears it is beginning to align its positions with those of developed countries (Galhot and Krishnan, 2016). This comes at a particularly worrying time as pressure from Japan to adopt TRIPS-plus measures has re-emerged in the context of the ongoing negotiations on the Regional Comprehensive Economic Partnership (RCEP).

As difficult as the work on patents and health is, the Indian experience shows the benefits of using the legal system for making full use of the flexibilities under the TRIPS Agreement. But most importantly it shows that community groups like people living with HIV are at the heart of the successful use of these flexibilities.

Notes

1 See: http://naco.gov.in/sites/default/files/HIV%20Facts%20&%20Figures.pdf

2 World Health Organization, "Accelerating the scale-up of HIV/AIDS treatment and care," available at http://www.whoindia.org/en/Section3/Section125_1433.htm

3 Amendments to India's patent regime to comply with TRIPS started with the Patents (Amendment) Act, 1999, followed by the Patents (Amendment) Act 2002 which, among other things, extended the patent term to 20 years and the final set of amendments was made in 2005 in the Patents (Amendment) Act 2005 which introduced the product

patent regime in India as well as key health safeguards. See Patents (Amendment) Act, 1999, No. 17 of 1999 available at http://ipindia. nic.in/ipr/patent/patact_99.PDF, Patents (Amendment) Act, 2002, No. 38 of 2002 available at http://ipindia.nic.in/Ipr/patent/ patentg.pdf and Patents (Amendment) Act, 2005, No. 15 of 2005 available at http://ipindia. nic.in/ipr/patent/patent_2005.pdf.

4 See Letters from:

Nafis Sadik, M.D. Special Envoy of the UN Secretary-General HIV/AIDS in Asia and the Pacific and Stephen Lewis, Special Envoy of the UN Secretary-General HIV/AIDS in Africa U.N. Special Envoys for HIV/AIDS to the Prime Minister and President of India, 11 March 2005; http://www.pambazuka.org/global-south/ africaglobal-india-should-ensure-global-access-through-patent-law

Achmat Dangor, UNAIDS to Minister of Commerce and Industry, 23 February 2005; http://www.cptech.org/ip/health/c/india/ unaids02232005.html

Jim Yong Kim, HIV/AIDS Director of the World Health Organization to Minister of Health and Family Welfare, 17 December 2004 http://www.cptech.org/ip/health/c/india/ who12172004.html

5 See Global Events around Feb 26th 2005 at: http://www.apnplus. org/wp-content/uploads/2016/01/ Our-Health-Our-Right-The-roles-and-experiences-of-PLHIV-networks-in-securing-access-to-generic-ARV-medicines-in-Asia.pdf pp. 30-31

6 See: Affordable Medicines and Treatment Campaign, "Concerns Regarding Patents Bill 2005 Introduced in the Loksabha," 18 March 2005. See: http://www.cptech.org/ip/health/c/ india/amtco3182005.html

7 See: https://indiankanoon.org/ doc/1704755/

8 Section 3(d) of India's Patents Act, 1970 reads: "The following are not inventions within the meaning of this Act...the mere discovery of a new form of a known substance which does not result in the enhancement of the known efficacy of that substance or the mere discovery of any new property or new use for a known substance or of the mere use of a known process, machine or apparatus unless such known process results in a new product or employs at least one new reactant. *Explanation*:

For the purposes of this clause, salts, esters, ethers, polymorphs, metabolites, pure form, particle size, isomers, mixtures of isomers, comp-lexes, combinations and other derivatives of a known substance shall be considered to be the same substance, unless they differ significantly in properties with regard to efficacy."

9 The decision of the Patent Office in the Nevirapine syrup case is available at http:// www.lawyerscollective.org/content/patent-nevirapine-rejected

10 Letter from INP+ to the Prime Minister, 24 January 2007, see: http://www.tribuneindia. com/2007/20070131/nation.htm

11 See Text of Free Trade Agreements: EU, available at http://www.bilaterals.org/spip. php?rubrique52

12 Loon Gangte, DNP+ cf Our Health, Our Rights, APN+ http://www.apnplus. org/wp-content/uploads/2016/01/ Our-Health-Our-Right-The-roles-and-experiences-of-PLHIV-networks-in-securing-access-to-generic-ARV-medicines-in-Asia.pdf

13 See: https://www.escr-net.org/ caselaw/2013/bayer-corporation-and-anr-v-union-india-ors

14 See : https://indiankanoon.org/ doc/131401110/

References

Ahuja V 2010, Indian groups protest secret Japan-India CEPA, www.bilateral.org http://www.bilaterals.org/?indian-groups-protest-secret-japan

Asia Pacific Network of People Living with HIV/AIDS (APN+) 2016 'Our Health Our Right, The roles and experiences of PLHIV networks in securing access to generic ARV medicines in Asia, Asia Pacific Network of People Living with HIV/AIDS (APN+)', 2016. p 36 http://www.apnplus.org/wp-content/uploads/2016/01/Our-Health-Our-Right-The-roles-and-experiences-of-PLHIV-networks-in-securing-access-to-generic-ARV-medicines-in-Asia.pdf

Babu G 2015, 'IPA, Natco withdraw opposition to Gilead's drug' Business Standard, September 14, 2015 http://www.business-standard.com/article/companies/ipa-natco-withdraw-opposition-to-gilead-s-drug-115091300385_1.html

Dalangin-Fernandez L 2008, 'Philippine's Arroyo signs cheaper medicines law', Philippine Daily Inquirer, 6 June 2008.

Datta J 2015, 'More patent-opposition on Gilead's hepatitis C drug, sofosbuvir' The Hindu Business Line, Feb 2 2015 http://www.thehindubusinessline.com/companies/more-patentopposition-on-gileads-hepatitis-c-drug-sofosbuvir/article6847904.ece

Galhot M and Krishnan V 2016, Drug Deals: How big pharma and the Indian government are letting millions of patients down, The Caravan, 1 March 2016, http://www.caravanmagazine.in/reportage/drug-deals

Health GAP 2004, "International sign-on letter of concern to Prime Minister Manmohan Singh of India regarding the government's proposed amendments to the Patents Act and undermining medicines access for people in need—in India and around the world," 16 December 2004.

I-MAK 2011, Financial Impact of Medicines Patent Pool: I-MAK/ITPC Counter Analysis, September 2011, http://apps.who.int/medicinedocs/en/d/Js19792en/

Lawyers Collective 2012, 'Patent Pool: Legitimising Big Pharma's Practices?,' ACCESS (A newsletter from the Lawyers Collective HIV/AIDS Unit), Vol III, Issue No. 1, February 2012, available at http://www.lawyerscollective.org/files/Access%20-%20Vol%20III,%20No_%20I.pdf

Lawyers Collective 2013, 'Supreme Court Rejects Novartis Appeal; Upholds high standard for Section 3(d)', Lawyers Collecttive, April 1 2013 http://www.lawyerscollective.org/updates/supreme-court-rejects-novartis-appeal-upholds-high-standard-section-3d

Lawyers Collective HIV/AIDS Unit (2008), "Indian patent office rejects AIDS drug patent application," Press Release, 19 June 2008.

Mathew J C 2008, 'Govt turns down German pharma firm`s patent plea,' Business Standard, 20 June 2008

Medecins Sans Fronetieres (MSF), 2005 'The Future of Generic Medicines in India,' 21 April 2005 http://www.msf.org/msfinternational/invoke.cfm?objectid=63C0C1F1-E018-0C72-093AB3D906C4C469&component=toolkit.art"icle&method=full_html

National AIDS Control Organization (NACO) 2015, 'India HIV estimations-Technical Report' 2015 http://www.naco.gov.in/sites/default/files/India%20HIV%20Estimations%202015.pdf

Prime Minister's Office (PMO), 2011, Trade Negotiator's Given Guidelines, Press Information Bureau, Government of India, 30 April 2011 http://pib.nic.in/newsite/PrintRelease.aspx?relid=71881

Purailatpam S and Bhardwaj K 2017, 'RCEP and Health: This Kind of 'Progress' is Not What India and the World Need', The Wire, 27/02/2017 https://thewire.in/112260/rcep-this-kind-of-progress-is-not-what-india-and-the-world-need/

World Health Organization 2001, "New offers of low cost anti-retroviral medicines: A statement from the World Health Organization," Statement/WHO 04, 9 February 2001

World Trade Organization (WTO) 2001, Declaration on the TRIPS agreement and public health, WT/MIN(01)/DEC/2, 14 Doha, November 2001, available at http://www.wto.org/english/thewto_e/minist_e/min01_e/mindecl_trips_e.htm

The neoliberal order affects people' lives in myriad ways and it is thus contingent that the struggle for health be conceived and constructed as a very broad struggle. It incorporates different strands, different objectives of an immediate nature and diverse strategies, while upholding the vision of a globe that is free of the ills of neoliberal globalization. This chapter focuses on two struggles from Italy of communities, defending and reclaiming their rights, in the face of the neoliberal onslaught. The first relates the collective endeavor to defend land and food sovereignty; the second recounts the struggle for justice by families of victims who fell prey to the Asbestos industry.

Genuino Clandestino: struggle for food and land sovereignty

Genuino Clandestino (GC) is an Italian network of collectives, associations and individuals who advocate and practice the re-appropriation and collectivization of land for autonomous, self-managed small scale farming, as an anti-capitalist politics/way of life. It includes small-scale producers, urban and rural groups as well as individuals engaged in the struggle for food and land sovereignty. GC's actions are designed to re-build local communities and organize resistance against the expropriation of land.

The roots of this movement lie in the formation of many local networks of small-scale producers at the end of the 1990s, as part of the anti-globalization movement. GC itself was launched in 2009, as a response to new regulations, regarding 'direct-sale' markets and processed food, issued in the city of Bologna. The regulations sought to equate the processing of food produced by individual and small producers with that produced by the large-scale food industries[1]. This led to a campaign by small-scale producers and consumers for 'Genuine Clandestine Products'. The campaign promotes home-made processed food (which have long been part of rural traditions) and advocates that it is impossible for small producers to abide by the same norms that are applied on the organized food industry. The campaign soon spread across Italy and is currently loosely structured as a network of local groups, rooted in their own lands and communities.

In 2012, Genuino Clandestino launched a campaign called 'TerrABC' ('Terra Bene Comune' meaning land as a commons) in the attempt to bridge the separation between urban and rural resistances and to build a common global analysis on the process of expropriation of land. This campaign denounced the (mis)appropriation of land belonging to communities, by industrial agriculture, extractive industries and other corporations, where land was taken over for construction projects, for building road networks, factories, supermarkets, military bases, and for real estate speculation. TerrABC soon led to a wider movement for the re-appropriation of land. It focused on reclaiming access to land by local communities and also developed links with other movements, like the ones against imposed 'mega projects', movements for housing, and the movement for reclaiming of the 'commons' and for self-organized public spaces. Genuino Clandestino defines itself as a movement of communities that struggle for self-determination regarding practices related to food. The manifesto of GC declares that it is an anti-racist, anti-fascist, anti-sexist movement, based on the need to mobilize rural and urban resistances in the common struggle against expropriation and exploitation.

The practices of GC GC advocates that radical analysis regarding food sovereignty needs to be rooted in practice. This becomes necessary given the global debate on sustainability of local agricultural practices in the face of advocacy by agribusiness about the 'superiority' of industrial modes of food production. GC represents 'a movement of practices': one of the major planks of its activities relates to sharing experiences regarding different practices among different local networks. These practices are intrinsically linked to the specific needs of local communities.

The movement advocates for and promotes small-scale organic food markets, participatory certification of products, self-organized popular kitchens and access to land.

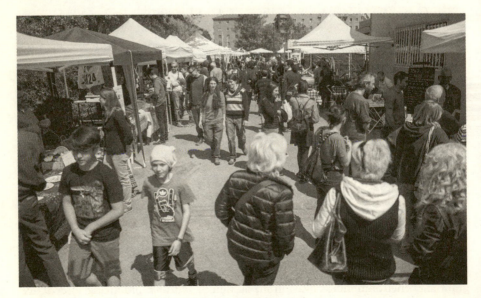

Image E4.1 Self organised farmers' market (Michele Lapini)

Self-organized small-scale organic markets are mainly located in urban social spaces. The farmers' markets promote rural organic agriculture, and also promote respect for biodiversity of the region, short food-production chain, and co-production – involving a direct relationship between the producer and the consumer. The markets are also public spaces for conducting public debates, concerts, drama, videos, meetings; and for agitating in support of food and land sovereignty and the re-appropriation land.

Participatory certification is an alternative practice of GC that seeks to replace official certification of products as 'organic'. In Italy, small farmers are particularly handicapped as official certification procedures are designed for large-scale food producers. Participatory certification involves quality control by a voluntary open group of people that follow practices of the producers by observing, participating and knowing their *modus operandi*. This practice offers an alternative method of certification based on the development of trust between producers and co-producers, and questions the legitimacy of the institutional apparatus as guarantor of the 'genuineness' of products.

Self-organized popular kitchen: Industrial modes of food production and large-scale distributions systems may lead to reduction in food prices, but they are predicated on a model of agricultural practices that promotes exploitation of workers employed in all sectors of the food production chain. On the other hand, rural organic agriculture can lead to higher cost of products, thus making them inaccessible to a majority of the people. Popular kitchen are designed to break free from the dichotomy where the rich can eat healthy food while the poor can only access low quality cheap food. Self-organized popular kitchens promote self-organization and collective forms of mutual support.

Access to land: In 2012 in Italy, as a response to the public debt crisis, reforms were approved that allowed public land to be sold to private entities. As a response to this, some initiatives were developed to safeguard and re-appropriate state-owned land that had fallen into disuse. In 2014 the TerrABC campaign initiated a struggle against the appropriation of land for mega projects and for real estate speculation. Since then, state-owned land has been utilized as common and open spaces, where local communities manage public land.

Significant aspects of GC Re-appropriation is the keyword and underlying principle of the movement. In Italy, as in many other parts of the world, food and land sovereignty movements represent a break with top-down governance structures and an experiment in 'direct democracy' involving grass-root communities. The act of claiming access to land is supplemented by actions on the right to housing, basic income, public health, education and self-determination in other aspects of life. Food-sovereignty movements show that the access to healthy food cannot be possible without fighting against exploitation, land grabbing, environmental devastation, as well as without practising alternative forms of governance, which are rooted in local and autonomous communities.

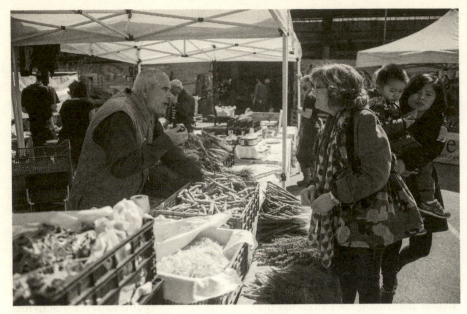

Image E4.2 Selling directly to consumers (Michele Lapini)

Rebuilding Legitimacy: Re-appropriation also requires defining again, what is fair, and what is not. It challenges the situation where a polluting factory is allowed and supported by governmental institutions, though it is harmful for health and the environment, while a hand-made bread is defined illegal because it has not been prepared in a laboratory compliant with legal standards. This is the focus of the claim of food and land sovereignty movements. On the other hand, current food and employment related laws do not address issues regarding the nutritional value of food, the working conditions of people employed in agriculture, and the use of pesticides, antibiotics and other substances in industrial modes of food production. The struggle for genuine and clandestine products seeks to affirm the legitimacy of rural traditions and to defend popular knowledge and habits that are now defined as illegal.

Self-organization and decentralization: In Genuino Clandestino self-organization is not a mere principle but also a practice that leads to the nurturing of a non-hierarchical organization. This is a novel and challenging aspect of a national movement that has the ambition to be large and inclusive, involving the participation of several struggles. In the network there are no representatives, no spokespersons, no delegates; the life of the movement is rooted in the autonomy of the local networks that adopt the practices and the organizational forms that are appropriate for their specific context. Their inclusion in the national movement is based on the respect of its principles and manifesto; on the daily struggle for food and territorial self-determination; and on the exchange of practices and knowledge between people and networks.

The movement organizes at least two national assemblies every year, in which people have the opportunity to share experiences, discuss common perspectives and take decisions that concern the entire movement.

Communities and relationships: The organizing principles described above can work only through the creation of relationships based on trust. The reconstruction of local communities is a crucial issue in the struggles today, as the defence of land is tightly linked to the aspirations of people living on it. Both at local and at national level, mutual support allows people to create communities based on solidarity, to practise alternatives that claim legitimacy, and to experiment practices that are explicitly against the dominant system which is based on expropriation and exploitation.

Supporting community struggle against effects of asbestos[2]

This is the story of citizens' resistance in Casale Monferrato (a town in the Piedmont region in Italy) against asbestos-related health and environmental hazards. The story originates in an action-research led by a group of psychologists named DUPP (Diritti Umani Psicologi Piemonte – Human Rights Psychologists Piedmon) that, in 2015–2016, organized several activities (focus group and meetings) in Casale involving citizens' organizations (such as AfeVA[3] – the association of asbestos victims and their families), local schools, representatives from local authorities and the regional psychology board.

There are no 'safe' levels of exposure for asbestos The effects of exposure to asbestos have been widely known for decades. 'Asbestosis' is a chronic disease that leads to shortness of breath (most prominent among workers who handle the material), and in some to pleural mesothelioma, an incurable and extremely aggressive form of cancer, with an average survival rate of 8–10 months. Exposure to asbestos also increases the risk of other forms of lung cancer. Unlike other carcinogens, there are no 'safe' levels of exposure to asbestos. The World Health Organization (WHO) estimates asbestos related annual deaths at more than 107,000 worldwide and has asked for a global ban on all forms of asbestos. Before 1970 there were very few regulations against the use of asbestos despite increasing scientific evidence about the carcinogenic effect of asbestos. Things have changed since, and now, primarily as a result of pressure from social movements around the world, asbestos has been banned in over 50 countries. Despite this, asbestos is still used in many low- and middle-income countries, often with few, if any, protective measures. At present an estimated 125 million people worldwide are exposed to asbestos. (WHO, 2014; Castelman, 2005)

While some countries have prohibited use of asbestos entirely, emerging economies such as India, China and Russia continue to allow the use and production of asbestos. In spite of evidence to the contrary it is claimed that protection against risks are possible through the use of protective measures.

In the 1980s and 90s, some directives against exposure to risk agents were adopted in the EU, and from 2005 the exchange and use of all asbestos fibres and products containing them, has been finally banned. (WHO, 2006).

Italy banned asbestos in 1992. Under Italian law, those whose properties are contaminated with asbestos, are required to notify the health authorities, so that they can determine the extent of asbestos contamination. In the event of an established risk from dispersion of asbestos fibres, the authorities can proceed for immediate remediation of the property (involving steps to remove asbestos).

The Center for Epidemiology and Cancer Prevention in Piedmont estimates that in the health district which includes Casale, pleural mesothelioma has an incidence of 59.4 per 100,000 among men and 24.7 per 100,000 among women. Incidence in the city of Casale is 101.9 and 43.4 for men and women respectively. People are also more likely to develop laryngeal and ovarian cancers (Maule, 2007).

The struggle against asbestos in Casale Monferrato The production facility of the Eternit company (Eternit is the trademark of a particular form of cement that includes 10 per cent of asbetsos) in Casale Monferrato extended over an area of about 94,000 square metres, of which about 50,000 were covered cement slabs that contain asbestos[4]. The plant was the biggest in Italy. Production started on 1907 and continued till 1986. At its peak the facility employed 3,500 workers. For years Eternit's workers believed that the plant was a boon for

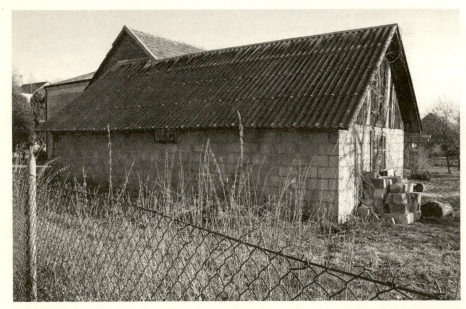

Image E4.3 A roof shed with Eternit (Di Karol Pilch (Karol91) - Opera propria, Pubblicodominio, https://commons.wikimedia.org/w/index.php?curid=1497806)

them as it provided secure employment. Eternit did not inform the workers of the extreme dangers posed by asbestos. Being totally unaware of the risks, workers returned home with their bodies and clothes covered and impregnated with asbestos fibres, embraced their wives and children and thus passed on to them the risks associated with asbestos.

In the 1970s, the news started emerged of the hazards associated with working in Eternit's factory. In the following years, complaints and lawsuits were initiated and the issue seized the entire community of Casale Monferrato. Some newspapers wrote about the Eternit factory as a producer of cancer and death. On 18 May, 1984, the national trade union CGIL held a national conference in Casale Monferrato to address the issue, exposing the fact that the asbestos-related diseases were affecting not only the workers, but also their families and the whole community.

Eternit shut down on 6 June, 1986. The first epidemiological survey of former Eternit workers was published in 1987, and in the same year, the local mayor issued an order prohibiting commercial production and use of materials containing asbestos, thus preventing the opening of new Eternit factories. At the conference titled, 'No To Asbestos' in 1989, the legal ban on asbestos was enforced. In the same year, the Association of Relatives of Deceased Eternit Workers (AFLED) was formed. On 27 March, 1992, a law was promulgated to ban asbestos in Italy, which provided for compensation to former workers. In 1998, AFLED changed its name to AFeVA (Association of Asbestos Victims and their Families), with the aim to represent all victims, not just victims who worked at the plant.

AFeVA's founding objectives were: 'justice, remediation and search'. The association supports the need to build a different culture, which respects the environment and the health of the population. To advocate for this the association has organized, from its inception, activities in schools and other public institutions, through which information is provided on health and environmental protection. This has led to engagement of students in campaigns and advocacy on environmental issues and in research work. AEeVA also played an important role in the legal and civil suit in the Torino court, in which the last owner of Eternit, was sentenced to 18 years in prison.

Law, memory and awareness The DUPP working group[5], together with AfeVA, worked with families of victims affected by asbestos. In the context of interpersonal relationships they explored the suffering and pain of affected families. The interaction was premised on an understanding that when an individual becomes isolated and loses connection with personal relationships, she ultimately loses hope and the strength to face major challenges. A community that gathers around a common struggle adds value to the accountability and participation of each individual. In spite of procedural delays in delivery of justice the social commitment to defend rights is maintained.

Three pillars were identifies, around which Casale's resilience is built: law, memory and awareness.

The knowledge of the law is useful to find possible legal weapons to defend those who are affected and to incriminate those who are responsible. It also helps and create precedents for others fighting against environmental pollution. Memory is necessary to pass on this story to future generations, and together with awareness regarding dangers that are still present, helps find solutions to problems.

When communities are pitted against the interests of multinational companies, the struggle is not easy. The three pillars of community resilience have consolidated on the work of health workers who have played an important role in supporting individuals and families. International support networks, which prevent local struggles from being isolated and place them in a larger context, reinforce the awareness of not being alone. The experience of Casale Monferrato, has become an example and an inspiration internationally, for the struggle against environmental pollution, and violence in many communities. This long process has allowed the city to find trust and hope.

Notes

1 See: http://autonomies.org/ru/2014/10/the-autonomous-self-management-of-landfood-genuino-clandestino/

2 We acknowledge help received, in putting together this case study, from: Afeva; Assunta Prato; Paolo Liedholm; Enza Gastaldi (Association Alt 76); Federica Grosso (ASL Casale Monferrato – MAIDASOLI); and Barry Castelman (Absestos Disease Awarness Organization)

3 See Afeva website: http://www.afeva.it/

4 See: http://www.comune.casale-monferrato.al.it/flex/cm/pages/ServeBLOB.php/L/IT/IDPagina/277

5 See: http://www.souqonline.it/home2_2_eng.asp?idpadre=2431&idtesto=2436#.WV3vzoSGOig

References

Maule M M, Magnani C, Dalmasso P,Mirabelli P, et al. 2007, 'Modeling Mesothelioma Risk Associated with Environmental Asbestos Exposure', Environ Health Perspect. 2007 Jul; 115(7): 1066–1071. doi: 10.1289/ehp.9900

World Health Organization (WHO) 2014, Asbestos-related diseases. World Health Organization, 2014. http://www.who.int/occupational_health/topics/asbestos_documents/en/

Castleman, B. I. (2005). *Asbestos: medical and legal aspects*. Aspen Publishers.

World Health Organization (WHO) 2006, 'Elimination of Asbestos-Related Diseases' World Health Organization, 2006. Geneva. http://apps.who.int/iris/bitstream/10665/69479/1/WHO_SDE_OEH_06.03_eng.pdf

LIST OF CONTRIBUTORS

Amit Sengupta, Associate Global Coordinator, People's Health Movement, India

Ananya Basu, independent researcher, Delhi, India

Andrea A. Cortinois, Lead, Masters Global Public Health Emphasis program, Dalla Lana School of Public Health, Toronto, Canada

Andrew Harmer, Lecturer Global Health Policy, Centre for Primary Care and Public Health, Blizard Institute, Queen Mary Institute of London, UK

Anna Engström, People's Health Movement, Scandinavia

Anna Kuehne, Berlin Health Collective, Berlin, Germany

Anne-Emanuelle Birn, Professor, Dalla Lana School of Public Health, University of Toronto, Canada

Asa Cristina Laurell, independent consultant and physician, Mexico

Barbara Adams, Global Policy Forum, New York, USA

Ben Brisbois, Postdoctoral Fellow, Centre for Urban Health Solutions, St. Michael's Hospital, Toronto, Canada

Cem Terzi, Surgeon in Izmir, Turkey, People's Health Movement, Turkey, and 'Bridging People' (*Halklarin Koprusu*)

Chiara Bodini, Centre for International Health, University of Bologna, Italy, and Co-Chair, People's Health Movement

David Legge, School of Public Health, La Trobe University, Victoria, Australia, and People's Health Movement

David McCoy, Queen Mary's University, London; Director, Medact, UK; and People's Health Movement, UK

David Ruben Barbaglia, Psychologist, Sportello Connessioni, Dupp (*Diritti Umani Psicologi Piemonte*), Italy

David Sanders, Emeritus Professor, School of Public Health, University of the Western Cape, Cape Town, South Africa, and Chair, People's Health Movement

Deepa Venkatachalam, Sama, Resource Group for Women and Health, and People's Health Movement, India

Fran Baum, Professor, Southgate Institute for Health, Society and Equity, Flinders University, Adelaide, Australia, and Chair, Advisory Council, People's Health Movement

Gabriela Alvarez Minte, Birkbeck, University of London, UK

Gargeya Telakapalli, Research Associate, People's Health Movement, India

Guido Leonti, Psychologist, Orientamente, Dupp (*Diritti Umani Psicologi Piemonte*), Italy

Jasmine Gideon, Senior Lecturer in Development Studies, Birkbeck, University of London, UK

Jens Martens, Executive Director, Global Policy Forum (New York/Bonn)

Jonathan Kennedy, Lecturer, Global Health Policy, Centre for Primary Care and Public Health, Blizard Institute, Queen Mary Institute of London, UK

José Félix Hoyo, President of Médicos del Mundo España

Julie Steendam, Policy Officer, G3W-M3M-Third World Health Aid (TWHA), Belgium

Kajal Bhardwaj, lawyer working on HIV, health and human rights, and independent researcher, India

Karolin Seitz, Global Policy Forum, Bonn, Germany

Liesbet Vangeel, Policy Officer, FOS - Socialistische Solidariteit, Belgium

Louis Reynolds, Pediatrician, People's Health Movement, South Africa

Maria Hamlin Zuniga, People's Health Movement, Nicaragua

Mariajosé Aguilera, Dalla Lana School of Public Health, University of Toronto, Canada

Marianna Parisotto, Centre for International Health (CSI) Bologna, Italy

Marine Buissonniere, independent researcher and consultant, humanitarian action, global health and human rights

Martin Drewry, Health Poverty Action, UK

Matteo Bessone, Psychologist, Sportello TiAscolto!, Dupp (*Diritti Umani Psicologi Piemonte*), Italy

Matthew Anderson, Associate Professor Department of Family and Social Medicine Montefiore Medical Center, New York, USA, and Editor, *Social Medicine*

Mia Appelbäck, People's Health Movement, Scandinavia

Muneer Mammi Kutty, Public Health Resource Network (PHRN), New Delhi, India

Natasha Horsfield, Health Poverty Action, UK

Oscar Feo, Latin American Association of Social Medicine (ALAMES), Venezuela

Pol De Vos, Public Health Department, Institute of Tropical Medicine, Antwerp, Belgium

Rafael Gonzales, Department of Public Health, School of Medicine, Universidad Nacional Autónoma de Mexico (UNAM), and Asociación Latinoamericana de Medicina Social (ALAMES)

Rene Loewenson, Training and Research Support Centre, Zimbabwe, and Regional Network on Equity in Health in East and Southern Africa (EQUINET)

Renee De Jong, Global Health Advocate, Wemos, The Netherlands

Robb Burlage, independent researcher and consultant, New York, USA

Ronald Labonte, Canada Research Chair, Globalization/Health Equity and Professor, Faculty of Medicine, Institute of Population Health, University of Ottawa, Canada

Samir Garg, State Health Resource Centre, Chhattisgarh, India

Sangeeta Shashikant, Legal and Policy Advisor, Third World Network

Sanya Reid Smith, Legal Adviser and Senior Researcher, Third World Network

Sarojini Nadimpally, Sama, Resource Group for Women and Health, and People's Health Movement, India

Shilpa Modi Pandav, independent researcher, India

Sneha Banerjee, Sama, Resource Group for Women and Health, and People's Health Movement, India

Stella Brancato, Psychologist, Dupp (*Diritti Umani Psicologi Piemonte*), Italy

Sulakshana Nandi, Public Health Resource Network (PHRN), New Delhi, and People's Health Movement, India

Susana Barria, Public Services International and People's Health Movement, India

Toby Freeman, Senior Research Fellow, Southgate Institute for Health, Society, and Equity Flinders University, Adelaide, Australia

Valeria Gentilini, Centre for International Health (CSI) Bologna, Italy

Vandana Prasad, National Convenor, Public Health Resource Network (PHRN), New Delhi, and People's Health Movement, India

We would also like to acknowledge the following for providing overall suggestions and inputs to the structure and contents of the book:

Claudio Schuftan (People's Health Movement), **David Woodward** (New Economics Foundation), **Dhananjay Kakakde** (Open Society Foundations), **Hani Serag** (People's Health Movement), **Indranil Mukhopadhyay** (People's Health Movement), **K. M. Gopakumar** (Third World Network), **Linda Mans** (Wemos), **Mirza Alas** (Third World Network), **Nicoletta Dentico** (Italian Observatory for Global Health), **Remco van de Pas** (Institute of Tropical Medicine, Antwerp), **Thomas Gebauer** (Medico International), Thomas Schwarz (MMI) and **Wim De Ceukelaire** (People's Health Movement).

We also acknowledge contributions from the **Asia-Pacific Network of People Living with HIV** (APN+) and **Delhi Network of Positive People** (DNP+).

INDEX